QUICK DRAW ANATOMY

ANATOMY

for Medical Students

QUICK DRAW ANATOMY

for Medical Students

Step-by-step instructions on how to draw, learn and interpret anatomy

Joanna Oram Fox

MBBCh, FRCA, FAcadMEd
Consultant Anaesthetist, Regional Anaesthesia Lead
Cardiff

Scion

© **Scion Publishing Ltd, 2024**

First published 2024

A CIP catalogue record for this book is available from the British Library.

ISBN 9781911510512

Scion Publishing Limited

The Old Hayloft, Vantage Business Park, Bloxham Road, Banbury OX16 9UX, UK

www.scionpublishing.com

Important Note from the Publisher

The information contained within this book was obtained by Scion Publishing Ltd from sources believed by us to be reliable. However, while every effort has been made to ensure its accuracy, no responsibility for loss or injury whatsoever occasioned to any person acting or refraining from action as a result of information contained herein can be accepted by the authors or publishers.

Readers are reminded that medicine is a constantly evolving science and while the authors and publishers have ensured that all dosages, applications and practices are based on current indications, there may be specific practices which differ between communities. You should always follow the guidelines laid down by the manufacturers of specific products and the relevant authorities in the country in which you are practising.

Although every effort has been made to ensure that all owners of copyright material have been acknowledged in this publication, we would be pleased to acknowledge in subsequent reprints or editions any omissions brought to our attention.

Registered names, trademarks, etc. used in this book, even when not marked as such, are not to be considered unprotected by law.

Cover and text design by AM Graphic Design Ltd, Oxford, UK
Illustrations by Hilary Strickland, Bath, UK
Typeset by Medlar Publishing Solutions Pvt Ltd, India
Printed in the UK by Ashford Colour Press Ltd

Last digit is the print number: 10 9 8 7 6 5 4 3 2

Contents

Detailed contents

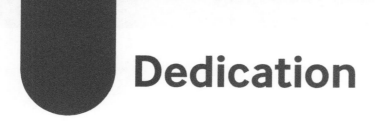

Dedication

For my wonderful grandparents, Flora and Edmund.

My grandparents met at the bus stop to their shared medical school in Glasgow. My Grannie was from Rothesay, a small island off the west coast of Scotland. It was very unusual for women to become doctors back then. She passed her medical degree and did her registration years before having three children. This is when her journey as a doctor ended. At that time it wasn't easy for women in medicine to have a family and continue to work. I believe my Grannie would have made an excellent doctor. She returned to work in the medical field as a phlebotomist when my mother and her siblings were older.

My grandparents and family are my biggest supporters, I think they were rather surprised when I wrote my first book, let alone the three I have now completed! Sadly, my Grandad didn't get to see this, and my Grannie passed away in January 2023 so didn't see the final copy of *Quick Draw Anatomy for Medical Students*. My other books took pride of place in their house. I know they would have been super proud at how much work I have put into this book to try and improve medical student learning of anatomy.

I would like to recognise all the women in medicine who couldn't or can't work due to circumstance, but who now, against the odds, can have both a family and a career. I wish you all the greatest success in both.

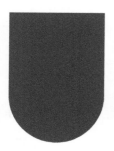

Acknowledgements

This book would not have happened if it weren't for my 'study buddy' (for anaesthetic exams), Dr Kiran Singh Kandola. He helped me understand so many things, and developing early versions of some of these diagrams was part of our revision.

I would also like to thank my editor, Alison Whitehouse, for her meticulous work. She spent a lot of time looking at my drawings and words, making sure they were accurate and made sense.

The artist and team at Scion Publishing who turned my Sharpie pen drawings on graph paper into the electronic versions you now see in the book have done a brilliant job. I am so pleased with how they turned out. I appreciate your skill and also your patience working through my comments and altering the text and illustrations over and over to ensure they were right.

I am so grateful to those staff at Cardiff University Anatomy Department (Jittima Muensoongnoen, Shiby Stephens, Kirsty Richardson, Helen McCarthy, Isaac Myers and Hannah Shaw) who checked through the proofs, making sure that the book was consistent and accurate. It was a pleasure to work with you.

And lastly, I send my love and gratitude to my family and friends who have offered me unwavering support throughout my life. It is so lovely that you are all so proud of me. These books are something I would never have thought I could do, were it not for your encouragement. If my daughter Hope studies medicine/anatomy I look forward to her thoughts and comments!

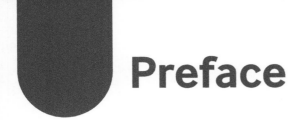

Preface

Anatomy was always a subject I found difficult. I've always been someone who does better with remembering things through understanding. When studying for my first anaesthetic exams I followed the norm and left anatomy as one of the last things to learn. I crammed just before and forgot most of what I had learnt fairly quickly afterwards.

For my final FRCA I developed some line diagrams, like Tube maps, so that I could easily apply them to actual anatomical specimens or images. I found this helped me to remember. The diagrams were all different shapes as an additional memory aid; for example, the popliteal fossa was 'the diamond'. Although the diagrams took time for me to develop, I found them really helpful for learning anatomy properly. During my training I developed the diagrams I had and published them all in my first book, *Quick Draw Anatomy for Anaesthetists* (winning first prize in the BMA Book Awards for Anaesthesia along the way). Ironically, I now teach anatomy more than any other subject in anaesthetics.

I knew these anatomy diagrams would have helped me at medical school. I also knew that it would be a lot of work to develop diagrams for all the areas of anatomy not covered in the anaesthetic syllabus, but well worthwhile. The writing of *Quick Draw Anatomy for Medical Students* has been a long, hard job. The first draft was completed in 2018 during a post-fellowship CCT in Australia. I have since revised the material at least five times, working with the editor, publisher, artist and also Cardiff University Anatomy Department staff. I apologise for any errors that remain, but we have all worked extremely hard to minimise these.

I hope this book can help medical and non-medical professionals who want to improve their anatomical knowledge. Good luck with your studying.

Joanna Oram Fox

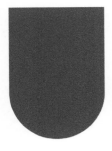

How to use the book

For the anatomical sections that have step-by-step drawings, the idea is to learn how to draw each diagram quickly and efficiently.

At each stage the diagram follows conventional labelling:

- Green for nerves
- Blue for veins
- Red for arteries
- Black for structures

For subsequent steps the colours are shown as tints to allow you to easily see the new lines drawn in the next step.

Once you can draw diagrams without thinking (e.g. using the shape memos like 'diamond' for the popliteal fossa), then you should learn to label them.

Finally, you should learn to explain what you are drawing. For example, the brachial plexus can be drawn in less than 15 seconds. Then you explain it whilst drawing, which should take around a minute. This will give an excellent impression in viva or OSCE examinations.

Happy drawing!

Chapter 1
Head, neck and neuro-anatomy

01

1.1 Skull and brain

1.1.1 Skull

Here you will find simplified images of the skull from different views to try to make it easy to understand and remember. The skull is composed of many bones that join at sutures. Neonates have fontanelles, incompletely fused suture lines, leaving membranous gaps between the bones; this allows growth of the brain and skull during childhood and adolescence. Intramembranous ossification of the bones of the calvaria takes place and the bones fuse by approximately 20 years of age.

The skull encloses and protects the brain, meninges and cerebral vasculature. It is divided into a roof (calvarium) and base:

- **calvarium:** frontal, 2 parietal and occipital bones
- **base:** frontal, sphenoid, ethmoid, occipital, parietal and temporal bones.

E   ethmoid bone
L   lacrimal bone
S   sphenoid bone
Z   zygomatic bone

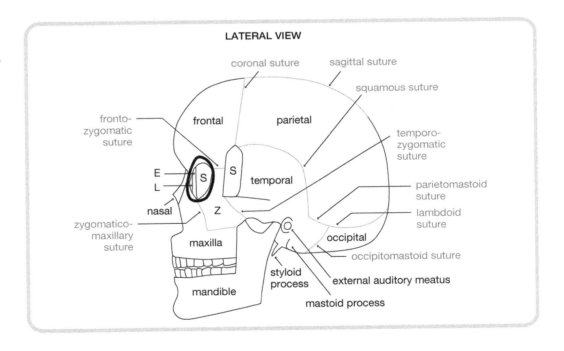

LATERAL VIEW

coronal suture · sagittal suture · squamous suture · fronto-zygomatic suture · frontal · parietal · temporo-zygomatic suture · E · L · S · S · temporal · parietomastoid suture · nasal · Z · lambdoid suture · zygomatico-maxillary suture · maxilla · occipital · occipitomastoid suture · styloid process · external auditory meatus · mandible · mastoid process

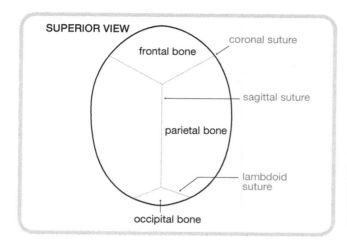

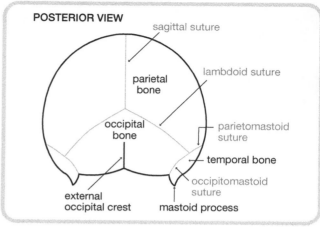

NATURAL POINT OF WEAKNESS IN THE SKULL

Pterion: junction between the temporal, parietal, frontal and sphenoid bone. Thinnest part of the skull. Very near middle meningeal artery. Injury here can lead to extradural haemorrhage.

FRACTURE TYPES

- **Depression:** bone pushed inwards. Result of direct blow. Skull indentation and possible underlying brain injury.
- **Linear:** simple break traversing full thickness. Radiating lines from point of impact (most common).
- **Base of skull:** can present with Battle's sign (bruising behind the ears) and raccoon eyes (bruising around orbits). Note history of trauma for likelihood of fracture.
- **Diastatic:** along suture lines leading to a wide suture, more common in children.

FACIAL BONES

Most are in pairs, 6 pairs plus 2 other bones.

- 2 zygomatic
- 2 lacrimal
- 2 nasal
- 2 inferior nasal conchae (not shown)
- 2 palatine (forming roof of palate, not shown)
- 2 maxillary (joined centrally by the intermaxillary suture, not shown)
- 1 vomer (posterior aspect of nasal septum, not shown)
- 1 mandible

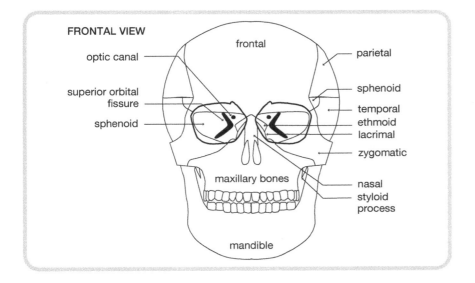

FRONTAL VIEW

- optic canal
- superior orbital fissure
- sphenoid
- frontal
- maxillary bones
- mandible
- parietal
- sphenoid
- temporal
- ethmoid
- lacrimal
- zygomatic
- nasal
- styloid process

BASE OF THE SKULL

List of cranial nerves

I	olfactory nerve
II	optic nerve
III	oculomotor nerve
IV	trochlear nerve
V	trigeminal nerve –
	1 ophthalmic division
	2 maxillary division
	3 mandibular division
VI	abducens nerve
VII	facial nerve
VIII	vestibular nerve
IX	glossopharyngeal nerve
X	vagus nerve
XI	accessory nerve
XII	hypoglossal nerve

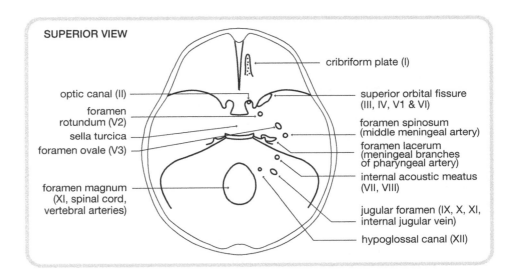

SUPERIOR VIEW

- optic canal (II)
- foramen rotundum (V2)
- sella turcica
- foramen ovale (V3)
- foramen magnum (XI, spinal cord, vertebral arteries)
- cribriform plate (I)
- superior orbital fissure (III, IV, V1 & VI)
- foramen spinosum (middle meningeal artery)
- foramen lacerum (meningeal branches of pharyngeal artery)
- internal acoustic meatus (VII, VIII)
- jugular foramen (IX, X, XI, internal jugular vein)
- hypoglossal canal (XII)

Learning how to draw the base of skull in sections will help you remember the foramina more easily.

 How to draw

STEP 1

- Draw the bone structure as shown here. The bones are labelled as shown: the frontal bone anteriorly, the temporal bone in the middle and the parietal and occipital bones posteriorly. Between the two frontal bones is the ethmoid bone. The sphenoid bone is central between the frontal bone and the temporal bone, in a butterfly shape. The sella turcica is central to this.
- Draw a big hole in the lower third of the skull. This is the foramen magnum (the biggest hole). This allows the spinal cord, vertebral arteries and the spinal root of the accessory nerve (CN XI) to pass through the skull.

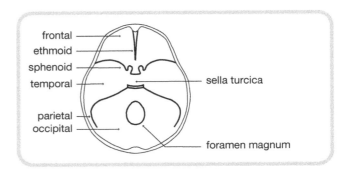

- frontal
- ethmoid
- sphenoid
- temporal
- parietal
- occipital
- sella turcica
- foramen magnum

STEP 2

- Draw a dotted area lateral to the middle of the ethmoid bone which represents the cribriform plate (this is part of the ethmoid bone). This is where the olfactory nerve (CN I) passes through the base of skull.
- Draw the optic canal, a small circle anterolateral to the sella turcica. This is where the optic nerve (CN II) passes through the skull.
- The superior orbital fissure is an elliptical shape just along the sphenoid ridge. This is where the oculomotor (CN III), trochlear (CN IV), abducens (CN VI) and the ophthalmic division (V1) of the trigeminal nerve (CN V) pass through the skull.

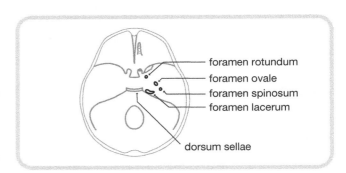

STEP 3

- Draw 1 circle, 1 oval-shaped hole and another small circle lateral to the centre of the sphenoid bone, each one slightly lower and further to the right than the last.
- The upper hole is the foramen rotundum (see the section on the trigeminal nerve in *Section 1.3.1: Cranial nerves*) where the maxillary branch (V2) of the trigeminal nerve passes.
- The next hole is the foramen ovale, where the mandibular branch (V3) of the trigeminal nerve passes through the skull.
- The third hole is small and is called the foramen spinosum; this is a hole for the middle meningeal artery to pass through.
- The next hole to add is an elliptical shape just lateral to the dorsum sellae. This is the foramen lacerum; it allows the meningeal branches of the ascending pharyngeal artery to pass through the skull.

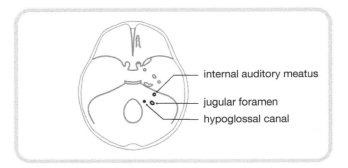

STEP 4

- Next you need to draw in 2 small circles and an oval hole laterally (see image for exact positions).
- The hole on the parietal bone ridge is the internal auditory meatus. As suggested in the name, the vestibulocochlear nerve (CN VIII) passes through here, as does the facial nerve (CN VII).
- The larger oval hole is the jugular foramen; 3 cranial nerves pass through here, the glossopharyngeal nerve (CN IX), the vagus nerve (CN X) and the accessory nerve (CN XI).
- The final small hole is the hypoglossal canal and, unsurprisingly, the hypoglossal nerve (CN XII) passes through here.

1.1.2   Brain and scalp

The brain controls most functions of the body. Approximate adult brain weight is:

- **males:** 1340 g
- **females:** 1200 g.

The central nervous system (CNS) is made up of the brain and the spinal cord, cranial nerves I and II are often included here too. The peripheral nervous system (PNS) consists of the nerves and ganglia outside of the brain and the spinal cord. This includes cranial nerves III to XII and spinal nerves. The PNS can be divided into the somatic and the autonomic nervous systems.

The nervous system is made of 2 types of cells, glial cells which provide support and nutrition, and neurones which send and receive nerve impulses. There are about 50 times more glial cells than neurones.

LOBES AND VENTRICLES OF THE BRAIN

Lobes

- Draw the cerebrum in lateral view. The frontal lobe is at the front, the parietal lobe posteriorly, the occipital lobe below the parietal lobe and the temporal lobe beneath the posterior half of the frontal lobe and the anterior half of the parietal lobe.
- Draw the cerebellum below the occipital lobe.
- Draw the brainstem. The midbrain is out of view but is situated above the pons and the medulla oblongata. It is visible in the sagittal section (see below). The spinal cord is a continuation of the brainstem.

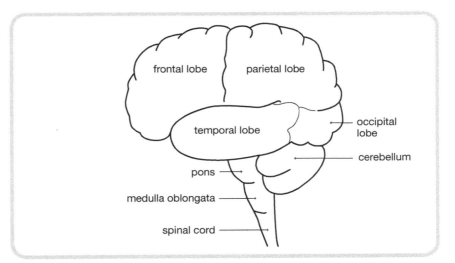

Ventricles and other structures

- The sagittal section of the brain is not that simple to learn. Here I have made it as simple as possible without losing too much detail. I have drawn the image slightly off centre so you can see the ventricles too.
- The structure labelled as the limbic lobe is the cingulate gyrus which is part of the limbic lobe. It can be seen beneath the frontal and parietal lobes. This lies just above the corpus callosum, fornix and thalamus. The fourth ventricle is continuous inferiorly with the central canal. This allows some CSF to flow inferiorly through the central canal to the spinal cord.

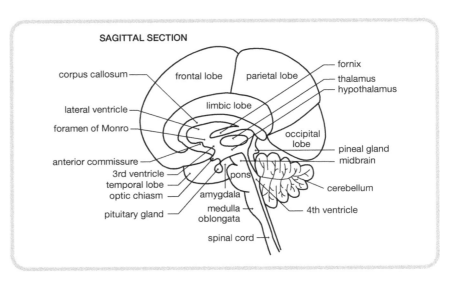

GYRI OF THE BRAIN

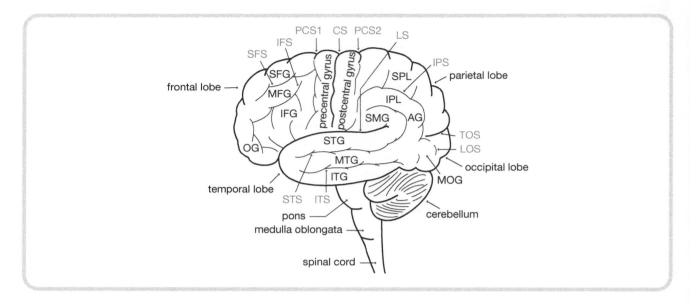

AG	angular gyrus	LOS	lateral occipital sulcus	SFG	superior frontal gyrus
CS	central sulcus	LS	lateral sulcus (Sylvian fissure)	SFS	superior frontal sulcus
IFG	inferior frontal gyrus	MFG	middle frontal gyrus	SMG	supramarginal gyrus
IFS	inferior frontal sulcus	MOG	middle occipital gyrus	SPL	superior parietal lobule
IPL	inferior parietal lobule	MTG	middle temporal gyrus	STG	superior temporal gyrus
IPS	intraparietal sulcus	OG	orbital gyrus	STS	superior temporal sulcus
ITG	inferior temporal gyrus	PCS1	precentral sulcus	TOS	transverse occipital sulcus
ITS	inferior temporal sulcus	PCS2	postcentral sulcus		

 How to draw

STEP ①

- Copy the outline of the lobes (see earlier), redrawing the line that divides the frontal lobe from the parietal lobe in more detail. This is the central sulcus (CS).
- Label the horizontal line that comprises the superior edge of the temporal lobe: it is the lateral sulcus (also called Sylvian fissure).

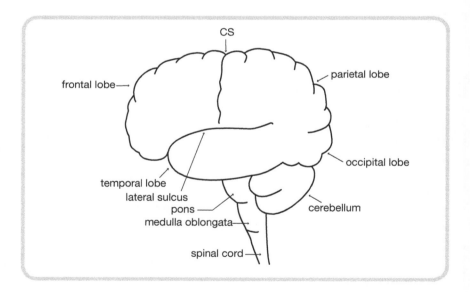

STEP **2**

- Starting with the frontal lobe, draw a line down in front of the central sulcus. The area between these two sulci is the precentral gyrus.
- Then divide the frontal area further with 2 horizontal lines, the superior frontal sulcus and the inferior frontal sulcus. Easy when you know! These lines split the frontal area into 3: the superior frontal gyrus, the middle frontal gyrus and the inferior frontal gyrus (IFG).
- Draw curves down from the anterior end of the IFG to separate the orbital gyrus anteriorly.

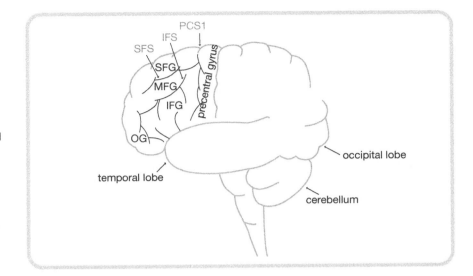

STEP **3**

- Draw a line behind the central sulcus. This is the postcentral sulcus; the postcentral gyrus is anterior to it.
- Posterior to this draw 1 horizontal line that curves posteriorly. This separates the superior parietal lobule and the inferior parietal lobule (IPL). The IPL consists of the supramarginal gyrus that caps the terminal part of the posterior ramus of the lateral sulcus and the angular gyrus (AG) that caps the posterior termination of the superior temporal sulcus.
- Below the AG, there are 3 main gyri in the occipital lobe, the superior occipital gyrus (not shown), the middle occipital gyrus and the inferior

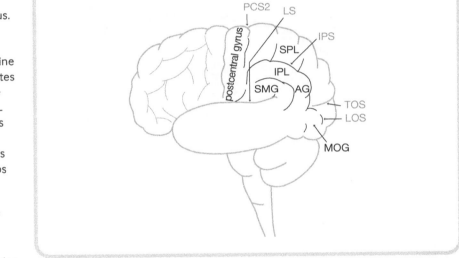

occipital gyrus (not shown). These are separated by the superior and inferior occipital sulci.
- The lateral occipital sulcus divides the middle (or lateral) occipital gyrus into a superior and inferior part which are continuous with the parietal and temporal lobes.

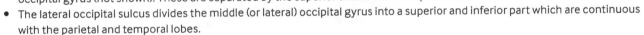

STEP **4**

- Divide the temporal lobe into 3 gyri: the superior, middle and inferior (like the frontal lobe). They are separated by the superior temporal sulcus and inferior temporal sulcus.
- Draw surface detail onto the cerebellum.
- Label the pons, medulla oblongata and spinal cord.

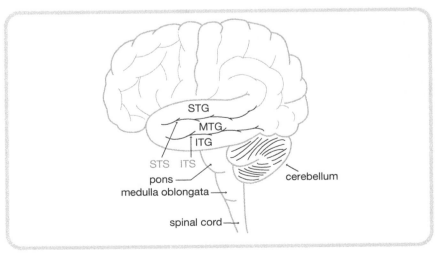

SCALP AND MENINGES

The meninges are the connective tissues that cover the brain.

- **Dura mater:** outer layer. Lines entire skull. 2 important dural folds to hold brain in position: (1) the falx cerebri (separates right and left cerebral hemispheres), and (2) the tentorium (separates the occipital lobes from the cerebrum).
- **Arachnoid mater:** intermediate layer. Thin and delicate, covers entire brain. Made of delicate elastic tissue and contains blood vessels. The space between the dura mater and the arachnoid mater is known as the subdural space.
- **Pia mater:** tightly adheres to the brain and follows the gyri and sulci of the brain. The space between the arachnoid mater and the pia mater is known as the subarachnoid space (this is where cerebrospinal fluid flows).

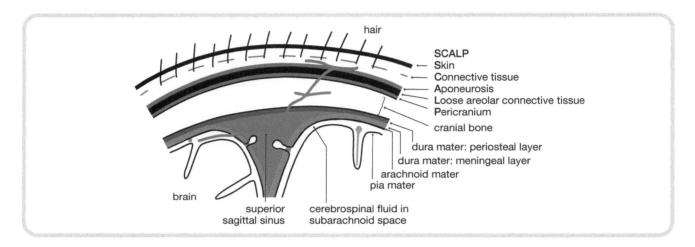

How to draw

STEP 1

Draw 5 layers of the SCALP. From exterior to interior these are:

- **S**kin
- **C**onnective tissue
- **A**poneurosis
- **L**oose areolar connective tissue
- **P**ericranium.

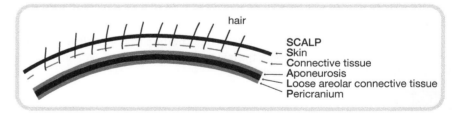

STEP 2

Draw the cranial bone as 2 lines, its inner and outer surfaces in sagittal section.

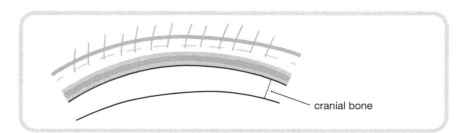

STEP 3

The dura mater is directly beneath the cranium. It has a periosteal layer and a meningeal layer; these meet and project downwards between the cerebral hemispheres as the falx cerebri, as shown.

- Draw the 2 layers of the dura mater; use a lighter colour or pencil for the meningeal layer (other structures will pass through it in step 4).

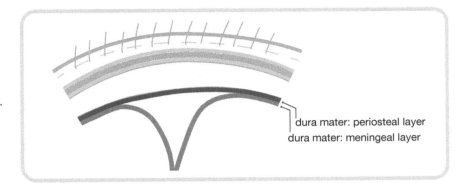

dura mater: periosteal layer
dura mater: meningeal layer

STEP 4

- Draw the arachnoid mater, with the arachnoid villi projecting through the meningeal layer of the cranial dura mater into the superior sagittal sinus.
- The subdural space is a potential space between the dura and the arachnoid.

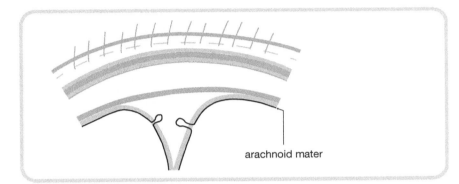

arachnoid mater

STEP 5

- Draw the pia mater (directly on the brain's outer surface, with the same outline).
- The subarachnoid space is between the arachnoid and the pia, and is filled with cerebrospinal fluid.

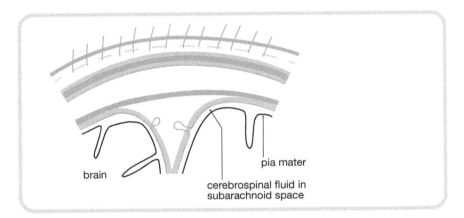

brain

pia mater

cerebrospinal fluid in subarachnoid space

STEP 6

- Add the superior sagittal sinus and veins in blue as shown.
- Draw in cerebral arteries in red as shown.

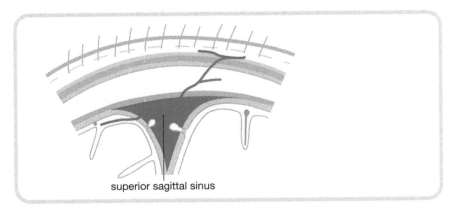

superior sagittal sinus

1.1.3   Endocrine organs of the head and neck

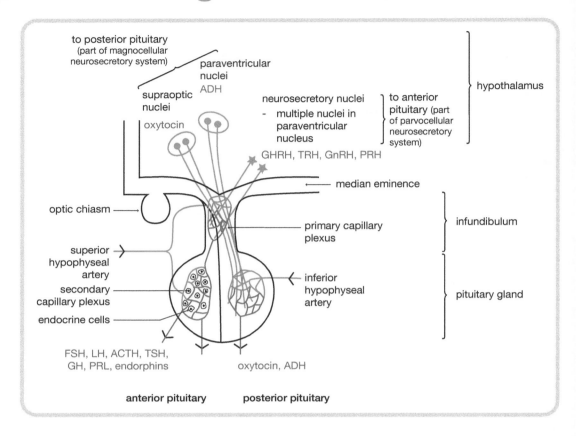

Abbrev.	Full term	Abbrev.	Full term
ACTH	adrenocorticotropic hormone	LH	luteinising hormone
ADH	antidiuretic hormone	PRH	prolactin-releasing hormone
FSH	follicle-stimulating hormone	PRL	prolactin
GH	growth hormone	TRH	thyrotropin-releasing hormone
GHRH	growth-hormone-releasing hormone	TSH	thyroid-stimulating hormone
GnRH	gonadotropin-releasing hormone		

HYPOTHALAMUS AND PITUITARY GLAND

In this drawing, hormones of the hypothalamus and pituitary gland are labelled in colour (see also Tables 1.1 and 1.2).

Table 1.1. Different hypothalamic nuclei release different hormones

Hypothalamic nucleus	Hormone
Supraoptic nuclei	Oxytocin
Paraventricular nuclei	Antidiuretic hormone (ADH)
Neurosecretory nuclei	Growth-hormone-releasing hormone (GHRH) Thyrotropin-releasing hormone (TRH) Gonadotropin-releasing hormone (GnRH) Prolactin-releasing hormone (PRH)

Table 1.2. Different hormones are released from each part of the pituitary gland

Pituitary	Hormones
Anterior	Follicle-stimulating hormone (FSH)
	Luteinising hormone (LH)
	Adrenocorticotropic hormone (ACTH)
	Thyroid-stimulating hormone (TSH)
	Growth hormone (GH)
	Prolactin (PRL)
	Endorphins
Posterior	Oxytocin
	Antidiuretic hormone (ADH)

Superior hypophyseal artery

The SHA often only supplies the infundibular part of the pituitary gland. In some individuals it will be as shown to both the infundibulum and the pituitary. Most people have two SHAs, one from each internal carotid artery; if blood supply is interrupted then the endocrine function isn't necessarily lost because there is blood supply from the other side.

 How to draw

STEP 1

- Draw the framework: a large 'hanging grape' (the pituitary gland or hypophysis) with a small 'bud' (the optic chiasm) in front of it.
- Label 3 regions: hypothalamus, infundibulum and pituitary gland.
- The hypothalamus is located above the pituitary gland and below the thalamus. It links the nervous system with the endocrine system in the pituitary and is involved in the actions of the limbic system.
- The pituitary gland lies in the sella turcica of the sphenoid bone below the hypothalamus.
- The infundibulum connects the hypothalamus and pituitary gland.

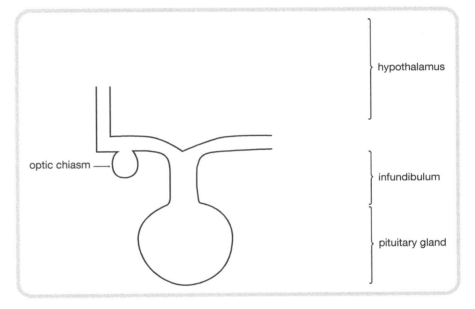

STEP 2

- Draw a line from the anterior part of the infundibulum down to approximately the middle of the inferior edge of the grape-shaped pituitary gland. This divides the anterior pituitary (adenohypophysis) and the posterior pituitary (neurohypophysis).
- Label the median eminence, an area superior to the infundibulum. Hormones collect here before being released into the portal system and then the general circulation.

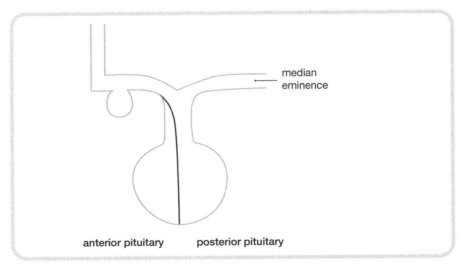

STEP 3

- Draw blue and red ovals in the infundibulum, the anterior pituitary and the posterior pituitary; these represent the 3 capillary plexuses.
- Add a vein to join the upper plexus to the lower one in the anterior pituitary; this is the portal hypophyseal vein. Draw 2 arrows exiting inferiorly to represent venous drainage. Draw one arrow exiting inferiorly from the posterior circle. Venous drainage is into the cavernous sinus.
- Draw a red line to represent each artery. The superior hypophyseal artery supplies the infundibulum and the anterior pituitary gland. The inferior hypophyseal artery supplies the posterior pituitary gland. They are both branches of the internal carotid artery.

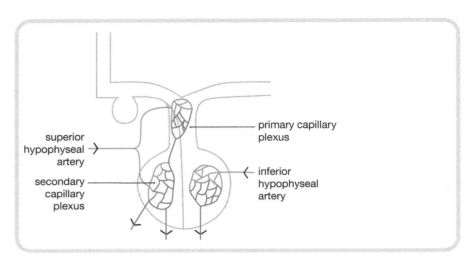

STEP 4

- Draw 2 green circles in the hypothalamus to represent the supraoptic nuclei anteriorly and the paraventricular nuclei posteriorly.
- Then draw 2 green dots in each circle, with 2 lines passing down the infundibulum to the posterior pituitary. These represent the secretory neurones that release hormones near the capillary networks in the posterior pituitary gland — the hypothalamo-hypophyseal tract.

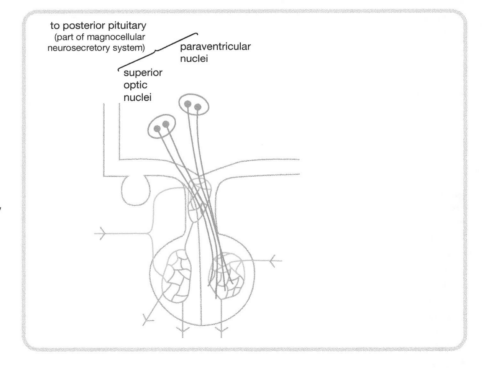

STEP 5

- Draw 2 star shapes in green posterior to the 2 circles. These represent the parvocellular neurosecretory cells which are part of the paraventricular nucleus. They project to the median eminence and release hormones here as listed in Step 6 below.
- Draw a line from each nucleus to the primary capillary plexus. The neurosecretory nuclei release inhibiting and releasing hormones, which are then transported via the hypothalamic–hypophyseal portal veins to the anterior pituitary to inhibit or stimulate hormone release.

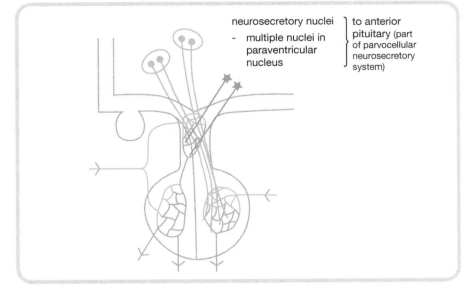

STEP 6

- Add the hormones released by the hypothalamic nuclei (see Table 1.1).
- Add hormones released by the anterior and posterior pituitary (see Table 1.2).
- Add endocrine cells between vessels of the anterior pituitary plexus.

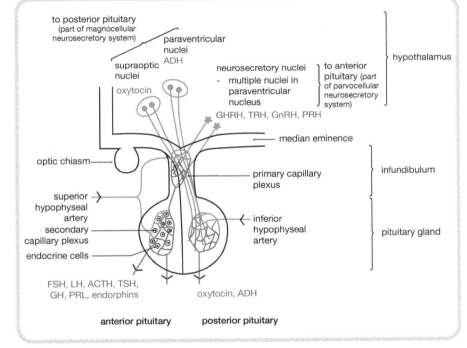

THYROID AND PARATHYROID GLANDS

The thyroid gland is an endocrine gland found in the front of the neck. It secretes two thyroid hormones, thyroxine (T4) and triiodothyronine (T3), and calcitonin. Hormone release is regulated by thyroid-stimulating hormone (TSH), which is secreted from the anterior pituitary gland. This itself is controlled by thyrotropin-releasing hormone (TRH) produced by the hypothalamus.

The thyroid hormones are produced by the combination of iodine and tyrosine. T3 has 3 atoms of iodine and T4 has 4. These two hormones play roles in metabolism, growth and development and the catecholamine effect (fight or flight response).

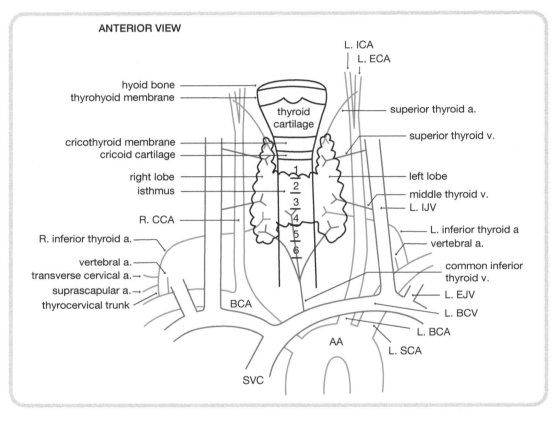

AA	aortic arch	**ECA**	external carotid artery	**SCA**	subclavian artery
BCA	brachiocephalic artery	**EJV**	external jugular vein	**SVC**	superior vena cava
BCV	brachiocephalic vein	**ICA**	internal carotid artery		
CCA	common carotid artery	**IJV**	internal jugular vein		

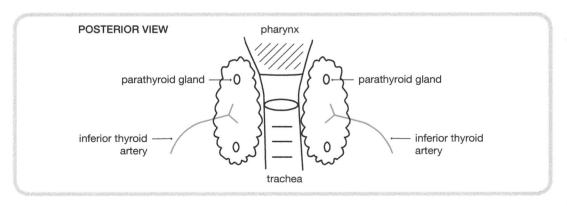

How to draw

Thyroid gland

STEP 1

- Draw 2 vertical lines to represent the trachea, and mark the boundaries of tracheal rings 1 to 6.
- Then draw the outline of the hyoid, thyrohyoid membrane, thyroid cartilage, cricoid cartilage and cricothyroid membrane.

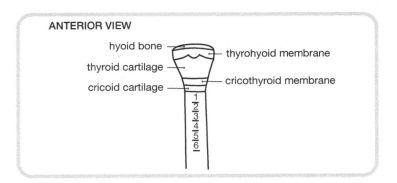

STEP 2

- Draw a 'cloud', H in shape and passing anteriorly across tracheal rings 2 to 4 from one side to the other.
- Label the left lobe, right lobe and the isthmus that joins them. This is the thyroid gland.

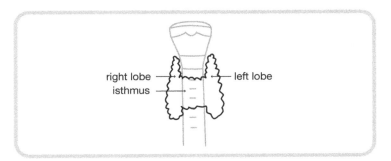

STEP 3

The next 2 steps are to add the venous drainage, starting with the major veins.

- Draw the superior vena cava and left and right brachiocephalic veins (an 'm' shape).
- On the left draw 2 vessels superiorly: the medial branch is the left internal jugular vein (IJV) and the lateral branch is the external jugular vein. Do the same on the right.

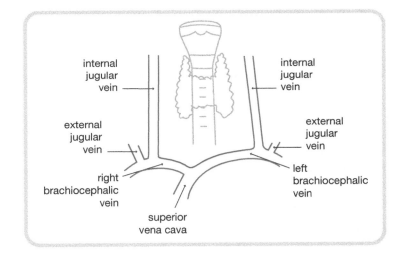

STEP 4

- Draw 2 pairs of veins, 1 on each side draining to each IJV at approximately the height of tracheal ring 1 and 3. The superior pair are the left and right superior thyroid veins. The inferior pair are the left and right middle thyroid veins.
- Draw a vein draining from each lobe and the isthmus (in the 6 o'clock position) into the left brachiocephalic vein. This is the common inferior thyroid vein.

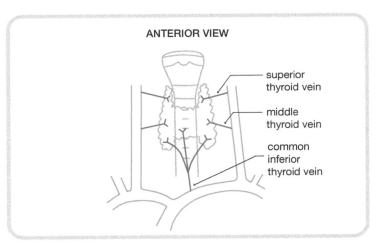

STEP 5

Next add the arterial supply, again starting with the major vessels.

- Draw the arch of the aorta, with 3 branches. On the right side is a single branch, the brachiocephalic artery. This divides into the right subclavian artery (heads towards the arm) and the right common carotid artery. On the left side there are 2 branches: the left common carotid, which branches off the arch of the aorta directly, and the left subclavian artery.
- Draw the common carotid arteries coursing upwards and show the bifurcation into internal and external carotid arteries.

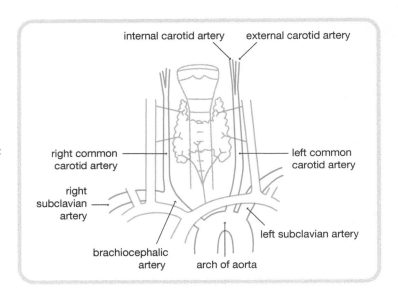

STEP 6

- On each side, draw a red line from the external carotid artery, arising just below the level of the hyoid bone and supplying the thyroid gland. This is the superior thyroid artery, the first branch of the external carotid artery, and it divides into many branches to supply the gland. Sometimes the ascending pharyngeal artery arises as the first branch.
- Then draw a line from the right subclavian artery to the inferior right lobe. The first portion is the thyrocervical trunk. Its main branch is the right inferior thyroid artery. Draw 2 other branches: the transverse cervical and suprascapular arteries.

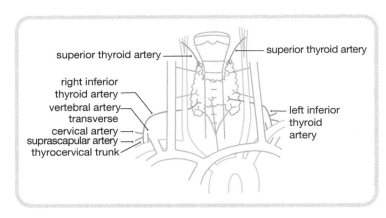

- Draw the corresponding arteries branching from the left subclavian artery.
- On each side add a branch from the subclavian artery, just medial to the thyrocervical trunk; this represents the vertebral artery.

Parathyroid glands

STEP 7

- In black pen draw the same outline as in Step 1 of the thyroid (see earlier). It is going to be a posterior view of the same region of the neck.

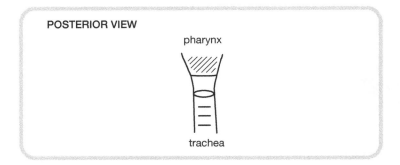

STEP 8

- Draw a 'cloud' shape on each side to represent the lobes of the thyroid. Add 4 circles, 2 superiorly and 2 inferiorly; these are the 4 parathyroid glands.
- Draw the inferior thyroid arteries entering the lobes.

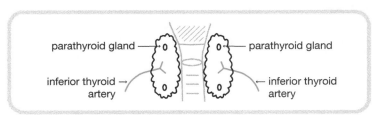

1.2 Blood supply and venous drainage of the head and neck

1.2.1 Arteries of the head and neck

The arteries of the head and neck can be thought of as an external system, supplying most of the head outside the brain, and an internal system, the circle of Willis (see *Section 1.2.2: Circle of Willis*). The network of arteries making up the circle of Willis is supplied by the internal carotid arteries anteriorly, shown here, and the basilar artery posteriorly.

AA   aortic arch
BCA   brachiocephalic artery
CCA   common carotid artery
ECA   external carotid artery
ICA   internal carotid artery
SCA   subclavian artery
VA   vertebral artery

ICA usually lies posterolateral to ECA. Drawn in this position to allow the image to show where the circle of Willis lies.

The facial artery and lingual artery usually arise from the ECA in the upper neck region, but they are shown slightly higher in this image.

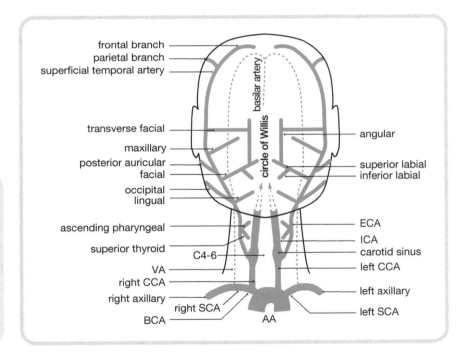

✏️ How to draw

STEP 1

- Draw the outline of the head and neck as shown.
- Draw the arch of the aorta with 3 main branches coming off it: the brachiocephalic on the right side and the left common carotid and left subclavian on the left side.
- Divide the brachiocephalic into the right subclavian and the right common carotid artery.

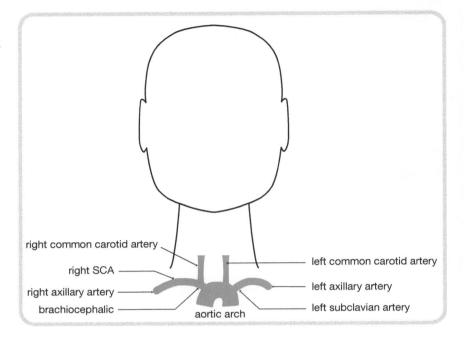

STEP 2

- From this step onwards, draw each side symmetrically. The steps describe the right side but draw the other side too.
- Divide the common carotid into the internal and external carotid branches (at level C4 to C6). Arrows show the internal branches feeding the circle of Willis.
- ICA usually lies posterolateral to ECA. It is drawn in this position to allow the image to show where the circle of Willis lies. The facial artery and lingual artery usually arise from the ECA in the upper neck region, but they are shown slightly higher in this image.

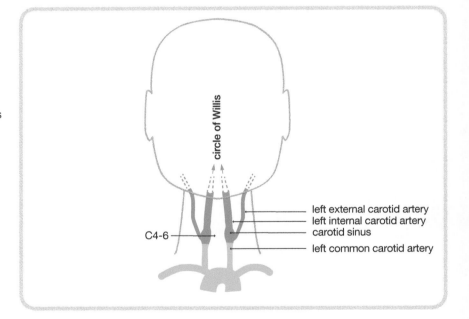

STEP 3

- Draw the external carotid coursing upwards; the ECA terminates by dividing into the maxillary and superficial temporal arteries.
- The superficial temporal artery splits into the frontal branch and the parietal branch.

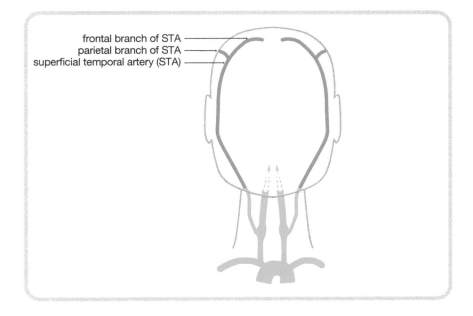

STEP 4

- Draw a sideways V from the external carotid in the neck. The arms represent the superior thyroid artery and the ascending pharyngeal artery as shown.
- Moving further up the face, draw lines as shown to represent in order: the lingual, occipital, facial (draw a snake's tongue shape for this one), posterior auricular and maxillary arteries.
- The snake's tongue shape represents the facial artery's division into the inferior and superior labial arteries to supply the lips and some of the nose.
- Draw a line from the upper part of the snake's tongue, the superior labial artery, joining to the transverse facial artery. This represents the angular artery, which is the terminal part of the facial artery.

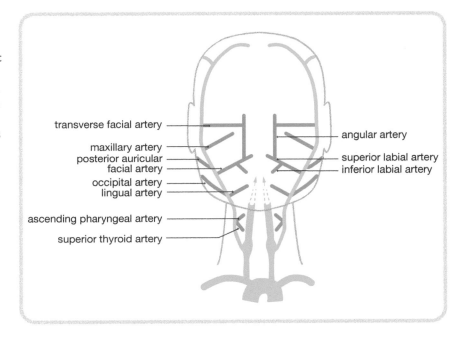

- In dotted lines draw the vertebral arteries from the subclavian arteries.
- The vertebral arteries join to become the basilar artery. This supplies the circle of Willis.

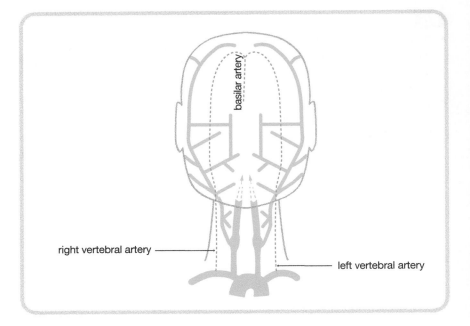

basilar artery

right vertebral artery

left vertebral artery

1.2.2 Circle of Willis

The circle of Willis is a difficult part of anatomy to learn. I hope this will help! It is the most simple diagram I could come up with that includes relevant and necessary branches. I like to think of it as an '**insect with a tail**'.

ICA internal carotid artery
MCA middle cerebral artery
PICA posterior inferior cerebellar artery

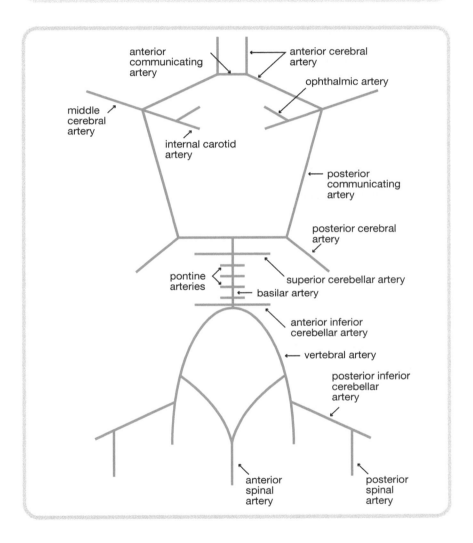

anterior communicating artery

anterior cerebral artery

ophthalmic artery

middle cerebral artery

internal carotid artery

posterior communicating artery

posterior cerebral artery

pontine arteries

superior cerebellar artery

basilar artery

anterior inferior cerebellar artery

vertebral artery

posterior inferior cerebellar artery

anterior spinal artery

posterior spinal artery

How to draw

STEP 1

- Draw an irregular hexagon with a small top horizontal line and a long bottom horizontal line (as shown). Draw two lines (antennae) up from the top two corners. These are the anterior cerebral arteries. The line joining them is the anterior communicating artery.
- The line going from the anterior cerebral artery to the posterior cerebral artery (see Step 3) represents the posterior communicating artery.

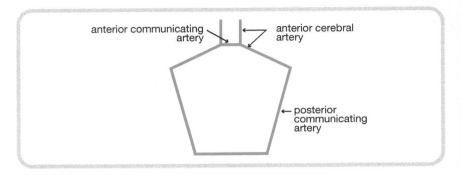

STEP 2

- Draw 2 lines (front legs) through the second and fifth angles on the hexagon. These represent the middle cerebral artery (MCA) laterally and the internal carotid artery (ICA) medially. The ophthalmic artery branches anteriorly from the ICA.

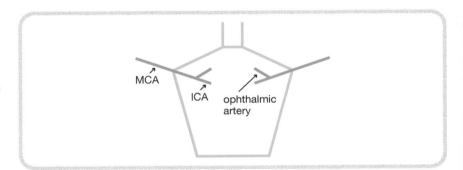

STEP 3

- Draw 2 lines (back legs) from the lower angles of the hexagon. These represent the posterior cerebral arteries.
- Draw 1 line from the centre of the lower, longer horizontal line on the hexagon. This represents the basilar artery.

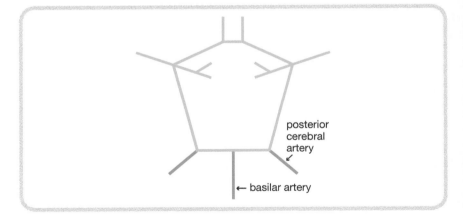

STEP 4

Drawing 'the tail':

- Draw 6 lines horizontally through the basilar artery; the top and bottom ones should be longer than the middle ones. The top one is the superior cerebellar artery (often implicated in trigeminal neuralgia), and the bottom one is the anterior inferior cerebellar artery. The small ones represent the pontine arteries.
- Draw a downward U shape from the base of the basilar artery. This represents the vertebral arteries.

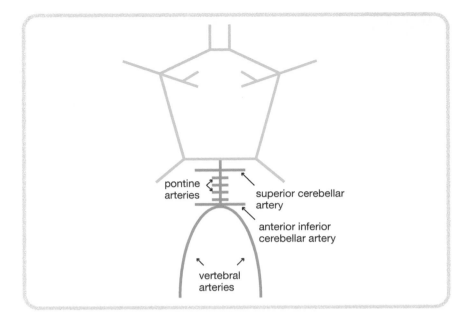

STEP 5

- Draw horizontal lines outwards from midway along each vertebral artery. These represent the posterior inferior cerebellar arteries (PICA).
- Draw a small line from each of these to represent the posterior spinal arteries.
- Draw two curved lines, one from the inside of each vertebral artery, that join in the middle to form the anterior spinal artery.

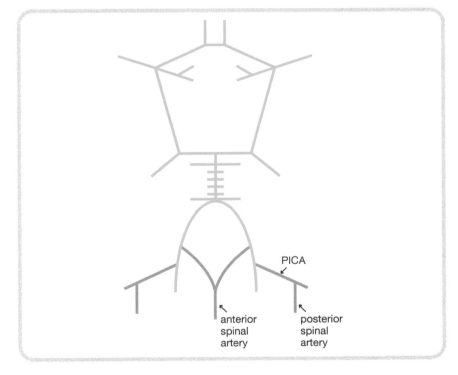

1.2.3 Venous drainage of the head

The venous drainage of the brain is often overlooked in revision. I have designed a simplified version which includes most of the important veins and sinuses you should learn.

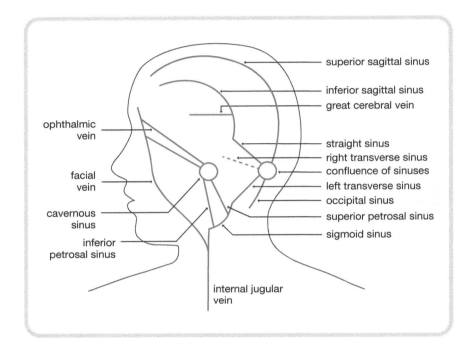

✏ How to draw

STEP ①

- Draw a head facing left. Draw the semicircle just inside the upper skull; this is the superior sagittal sinus.
- Draw a circle at the lower end of the semicircle. The circle represents the confluence of sinuses.

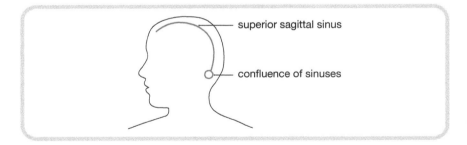

STEP ②

- From the confluence of sinuses draw a straight line heading towards just above the eye. This is the straight sinus.
- Then draw an arc curving around the eye and a line branching from this. The main arc is the inferior sagittal sinus. The branch is the great cerebral vein.

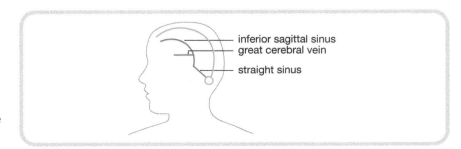

STEP 3

- Draw a line downwards from the confluence of sinuses; this is the occipital sinus.

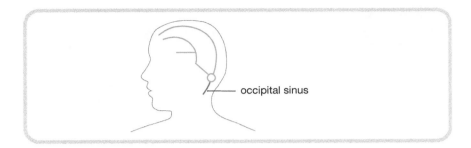

STEP 4

- Draw a line anterior to the occipital sinus as shown. This represents the left transverse sinus; it drains into the sigmoid sinus which in turn drains into the internal jugular vein (IJV).

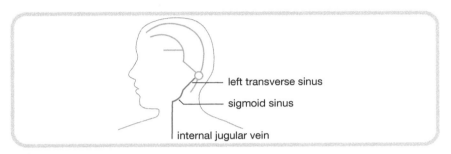

STEP 5

- Draw the facial vein draining into the IJV (it does so via the common facial vein).

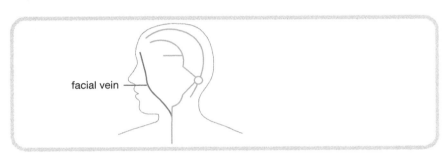

STEP 6

- Draw 2 lines (the inferior and superior petrosal sinuses) upwards from the sigmoid sinus that form a blue circle (the cavernous sinus). Draw 2 lines from the facial vein to the cavernous sinus; these are the ophthalmic veins.

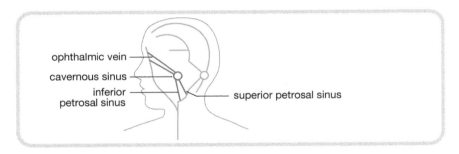

STEP 7

- Draw in a dotted line behind the left transverse sinus (to show that the line is further back). This is the right transverse sinus. Drawing all the veins on both sides would be much more complicated, but they would look similar to the left side.

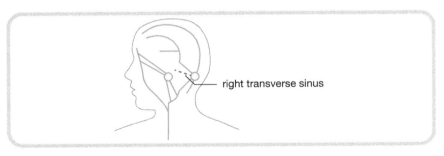

1.2.4   Venous drainage in the neck

The venous drainage of the neck is shown as a continuation downwards from the previous drawing. Deep vessels are shown in dotted lines.

EJV	external jugular vein
IJV	internal jugular vein
SCM	sternocleidomastoid muscle
SVC	superior vena cava

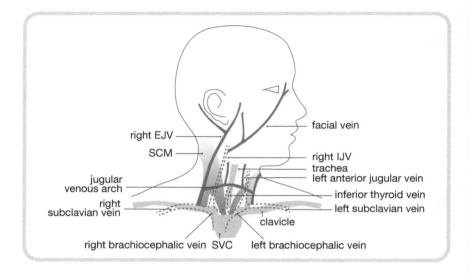

 How to draw

STEP 1

- Draw the head (facing right), neck, clavicles, sternum, sternocleidomastoid and trachea.
- With blue dotted lines to represent deep structures, draw the right and left internal jugular veins (IJV) draining into the brachiocephalic veins. These then meet on the right side of the body to form the superior vena cava (SVC).
- Between the 2 IJVs draw a line in front of the trachea to represent the inferior thyroid vein.

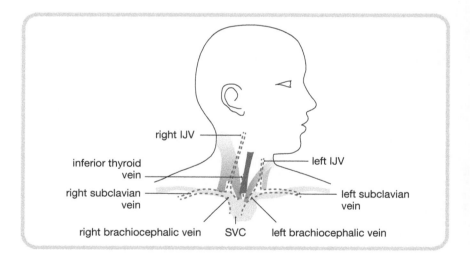

STEP 2

- With a full blue line draw the left and right external jugular veins. These drain the external cranium and the deep parts of the face.

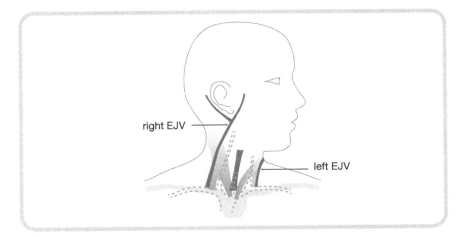

STEP 3

- Draw an arch that joins the 2 external jugular veins. This is the jugular venous arch. From here, draw the anterior jugular veins. There are normally two but sometimes there is only one.

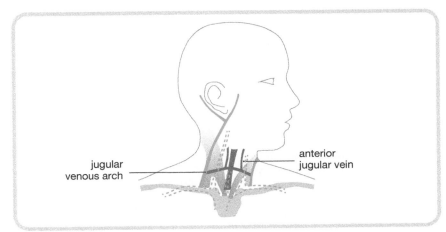

STEP 4

- Draw the facial vein draining into the common facial vein which drains into the IJV.

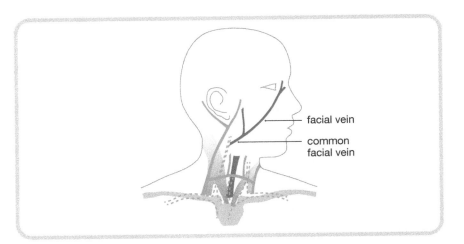

1.3 Nerves of the head and neck

1.3.1 Cranial nerves

There are 12 pairs of cranial nerves. They emerge directly from the brain and brainstem, in contrast to spinal nerves, which emerge from the spinal cord (it's in the name!).

At medical school you study how to examine the cranial nerves but their anatomy is notoriously difficult to learn and remember. The drawings in this chapter are designed to help you do this for each one. You will draw each one from the brainstem or brain to its effectors or sensors. Also, you will draw a 'map' of the brainstem to help learn where the nuclei lie in relation to each other.

These images are here to help you consolidate the anatomy, not to replace anatomical drawings and text. Good luck!

CRANIAL NERVE NUCLEI

This drawing is a summary or map of how to distinguish different cranial nerve nuclei in the brainstem. It will help you understand any image given to you.

Motor nuclei are labelled in purple and sensory nuclei are labelled in black. Draw nuclei and nerves in green, matching the book's colour scheme.

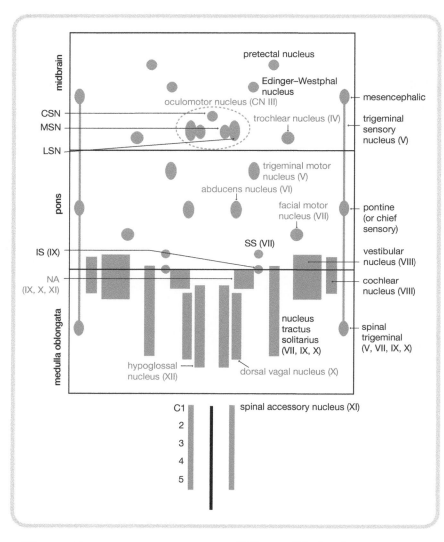

CN	cranial nerve	**MSN**	medial subnucleus
CSN	central subnucleus	**NA**	nucleus ambiguus (IX, X, XI)
IS	inferior salivatory nucleus (IX)	**SS**	superior salivatory nucleus (VII)
LSN	lateral subnucleus		

NOTE: the cranial nerve associated with each nucleus is mentioned in brackets throughout the chapter.

How to draw

STEP 1

- Draw a rectangle consisting of 3 sections filling the whole page: the midbrain, pons and medulla oblongata. Most cranial nerve drawings will start in this way.

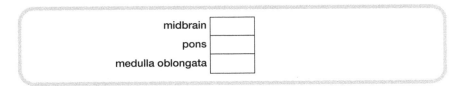

STEP 2

- Starting with the midbrain, draw the oculomotor nucleus (CN III), shown by the dotted outline, in the midline just above the junction with the pons.
- Show how the oculomotor nucleus consists of the central subnucleus (aka central caudal nucleus) superiorly and bilateral medial and lateral subnuclei inferiorly (LSN supplies ipsilateral inferior rectus, inferior oblique and medial rectus muscles; MSN supplies contralateral superior rectus muscle; CSN supplies both levator palpebrae superioris muscles).

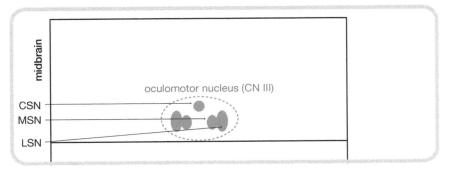

STEP 3

- Draw the pretectal nucleus, the Edinger–Westphal nucleus and trochlear (CN IV) nucleus on both sides as circles, in that order from superior to inferior.

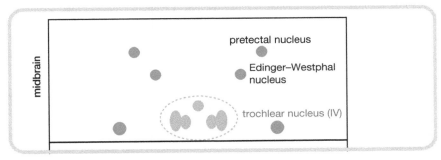

STEP 4

- At each side draw a circle at the midpoint of each rectangle, connected by a line which represents that these 3 nuclei are all part of the same trigeminal sensory nucleus (CN V). It is present in all 3 areas of the brainstem.
- Label nuclei as shown.

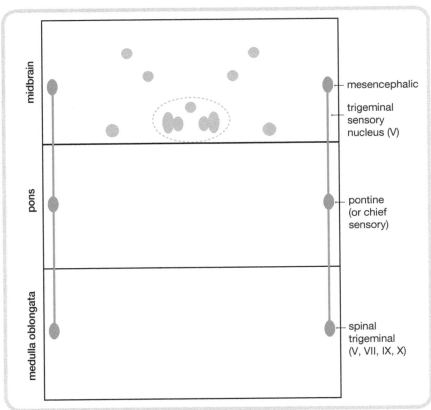

31

STEP 5

- In the pons, the middle rectangle, draw 3 circles to represent the trigeminal motor nucleus (CN V), abducens nucleus (CN VI) and facial motor nucleus (CN VII), from superior to inferior.

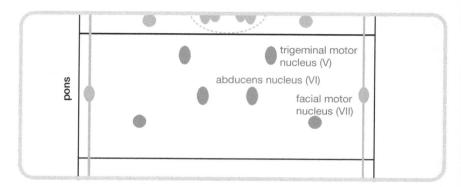

STEP 6

On the junction between the pons and medulla oblongata start drawing from the left side towards the middle and then the mirror image as you continue.

- First, next to the line representing the trigeminal sensory nucleus, draw a small vertical rectangle; this is the cochlear nucleus (CN VIII).
- Next to this draw a larger vertical rectangle; this is the vestibular nucleus (also CN VIII).
- Further in draw a long thin rectangle. This is the nucleus tractus solitarius, it contributes to the formation of cranial nerves VII, IX and X.

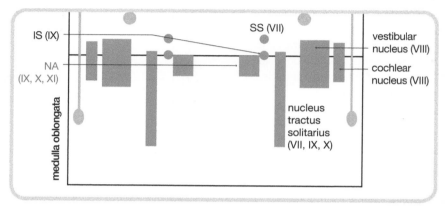

- Just inside of this draw 2 small circles, 1 above the other, and then a square in the medulla oblongata just below the line. These are the superior salivatory nucleus (CN VII), the inferior salivatory nucleus (CN IX) and the nucleus ambiguus (CN IX, X, XI).

STEP 7

- In the middle of the medulla oblongata, on each side draw 2 fairly midline vertical rectangles. These are the hypoglossal nuclei (CN XII) medially and the dorsal vagal nuclei (CN X) laterally.

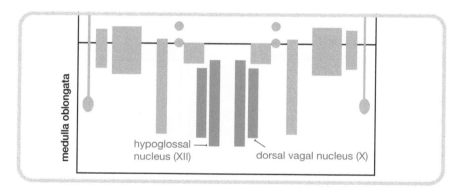

STEP 8

- Below the brainstem draw a black line to represent the spinal cord. The spinal accessory nucleus (CN XI) lies here.

Now you can draw ALL the nuclei of the brainstem!

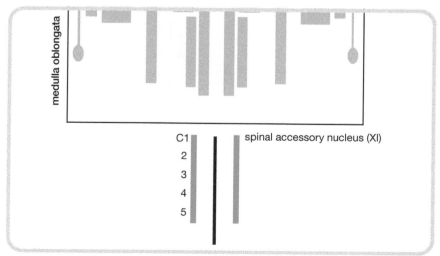

OLFACTORY NERVE (CN I)

This is the shortest cranial nerve and contains the sensory nerve fibres needed to detect smell (olfaction).

The axons of the olfactory nerve pass from the nasal cavity through the cribriform plate into the anterior cranial fossa. Here they enter the olfactory bulb, which lies in the olfactory groove. In the bulb they synapse with mitral cells (specialised neurones), and second-order nerves then pass back as the olfactory tract. The tract divides into 2:

- **The lateral olfactory stria** carries signals to the primary olfactory cortex in the temporal lobe. From here signals are sent to the piriform cortex, the amygdala and the entorhinal cortex. These areas are involved in memory of smells.
- **The medial olfactory stria** transmits signals to the hypothalamus and brainstem.

Destruction of the olfactory tract leads to ipsilateral loss of smell (anosmia).

Blood supply to the olfactory nerve is from the olfactory artery, which is a branch of the anterior cerebral artery. The nerve is also supplied by the anterior and posterior ethmoidal arteries (branches from the ophthalmic artery).

Venous drainage from the olfactory nerve is poorly understood and not well explained in textbooks.

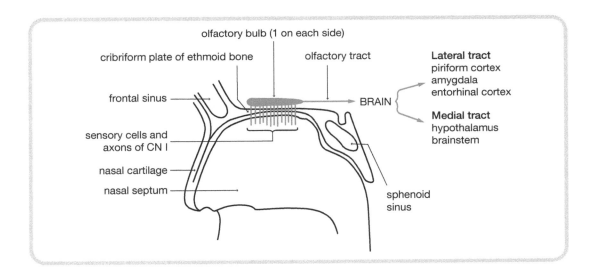

OPTIC NERVE (CN II)

The optic nerve (CN II) transmits visual information from the eye (retina) to the brain. It transmits all visual information including brightness, contrast and colour.

It is responsible for the afferent limb of the light reflex (constriction of both pupils when light is shone in either eye) and the accommodation reflex (lens adjustment for near vision).

- **Arterial supply:** from the posterior ciliary artery (main supply) and retinal circulation. Also branches from the pial arteries, which arises from the internal carotid artery, ophthalmic artery, anterior cerebral artery and anterior communicating artery.
- **Venous drainage:** the central retinal vein, ophthalmic vein and pial veins drain into the cavernous sinus.

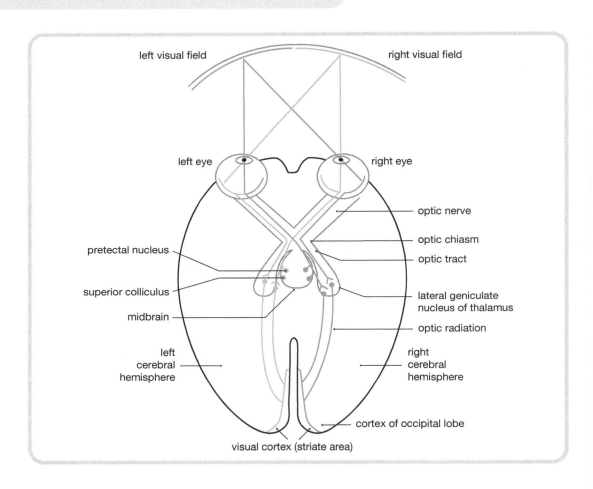

How to draw

- With a black pen draw the cross-section of a brain, and add 2 eyeballs in grey.
- Inside each grey eyeball draw a smaller oval anteriorly, with a black dot in the middle to represent the pupil.

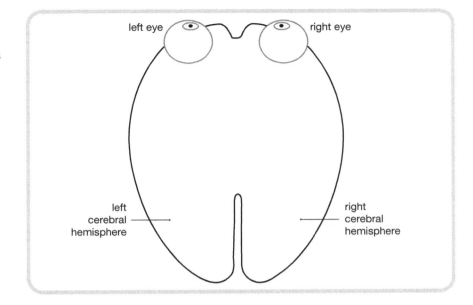

STEP 2

- From the back of the eye, with the grey pen draw an X shape which represents the optic nerve, optic chiasm and optic tract.
- Draw an oval between the base of the X to represent the midbrain.
- In front of the eyes draw a semicircle to represent the visual field.

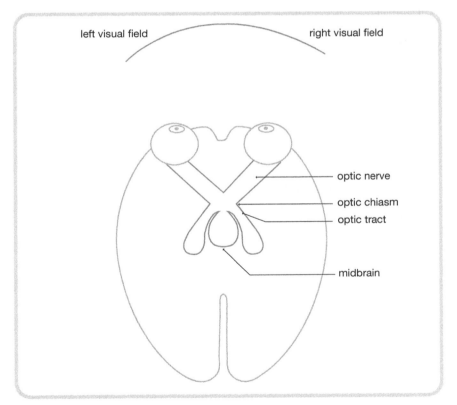

STEP 3

- Draw a curve to represent the right side of the visual field. From the middle of this draw 1 line straight to the back of the right eye and 1 to the back of the left; these represent light from this part of the field.
- Draw a green half semicircle in each eye to show which part of the retina 'sees' the right visual field.
- From the back of each eye draw nerve fibres that run to the left side of the optic chiasm. Show how they synapse with the lateral geniculate nucleus of the thalamus and pass back to the visual cortex. Draw the visual cortex as a line at the back of the brain in the cortex of the occipital lobe.
- In the midbrain draw 2 branches with dots representing the pretectal nucleus (pupillary light reflex) and the superior colliculus (part of the tectum, a complicated area that is involved in eye and head movements).

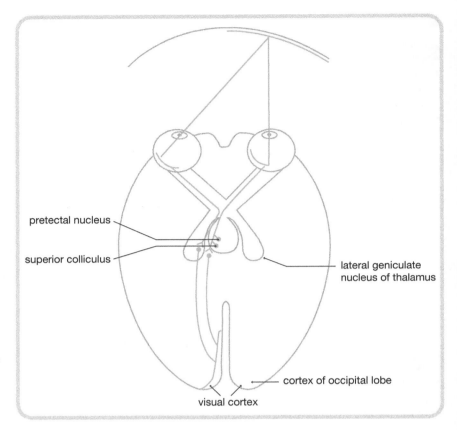

STEP 4

- Draw a mirror image of the pathways for the left visual field.
- The important thing to note is that the nerve crosses the centre on each side so that the right visual field is 'seen' in the left cerebral cortex and the left visual field is 'seen' on the right.

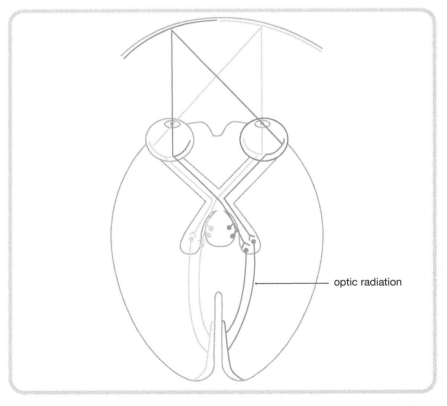

OCULOMOTOR, TROCHLEAR AND ABDUCENS NERVES (CN III, IV AND VI)

These 3 cranial nerves supply the extrinsic muscles of the eye (see *Box 1.1*). The oculomotor nerve controls eyelid movement and all 3 control movement of the eyeball. The oculomotor nerve also supplies some of the intrinsic muscles that control pupillary constriction and accommodation (see *Box 1.2*). Each nerve is drawn from the muscle(s) it innervates to the position of its nucleus within the brainstem. I have drawn the nuclei and nerves only on one side to make the image and hence the anatomy easier to draw.

I remember which nerve supplies which muscle by the memory aid **SO4LR6**: the **S**uperior **O**blique is supplied by trochlear nerve, CN **IV**, and the **L**ateral **R**ectus muscle is supplied by abducens nerve, CN **VI**. All other muscles are supplied by the oculomotor nerve, CN III.

All these nerves pass through the superior orbital fissure as shown.

In the lighter shade of green you can see the nerve supply to the pupil, also shown only on one side.

Nuclei positions are described in *Section 1.3.1: Brainstem nuclei*, above.

AN	abducens nucleus (VI)
CSN	central caudate subnucleus
EWN	Edinger–Westphal nucleus
LSN	lateral subnucleus
MSN	medial subnucleus
ON	oculomotor nucleus (III)
PTN	pretectal nucleus
TN	trochlear nucleus (IV)

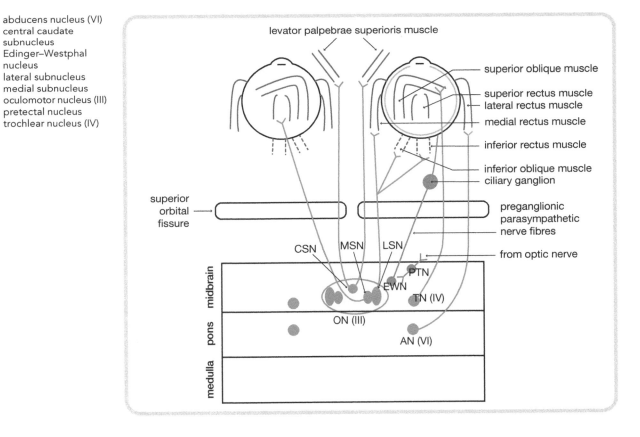

✎ How to draw

STEP ①

- At the top of a page, draw the eyeballs from above and add the muscles of movement.
- Further down (posterior to) each eye draw a lozenge to represent the superior orbital fissure.
- Below the fissures, draw 3 rectangles to represent the regions of the brainstem.

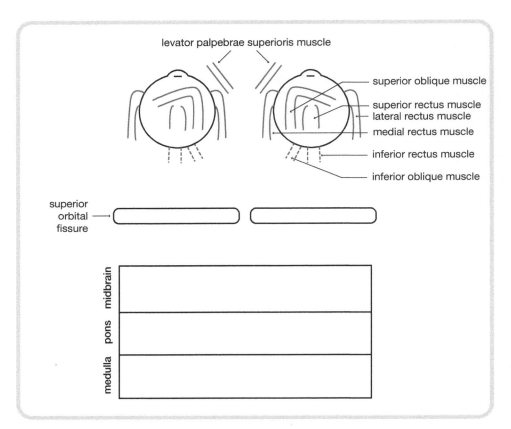

STEP ②

Now add the nuclei on both sides of the brainstem but show the nerves and labels just on one side to keep the drawing simple.

- In the midbrain, draw the trochlear nucleus and its nerve (CN IV) supplying the superior oblique.
- In the pons, draw the abducens nucleus and its nerve (CN VI) supplying the lateral rectus.
- Then draw the medial, central caudate and lateral nuclei of the oculomotor nucleus, with branches of CN III to the other muscles at the end (as shown).

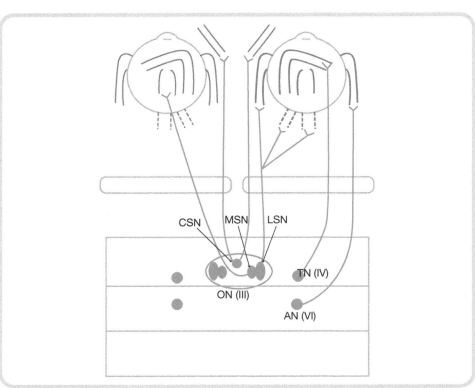

STEP ❸

Finally, draw the parasympathetic innervation to the sphincter pupillae and ciliary muscle, showing it only on one side to keep things simple:

- The optic nerve (CN II) sends a signal to the Edinger–Westphal nucleus (EWN) via the pretectal nucleus (PTN).
- Each pretectal nucleus sends bilateral projections to both the left and right EWN.
- Postganglionic fibres continue to the ciliary muscle (controls movement of the lens and pupil) and sphincter pupillae.

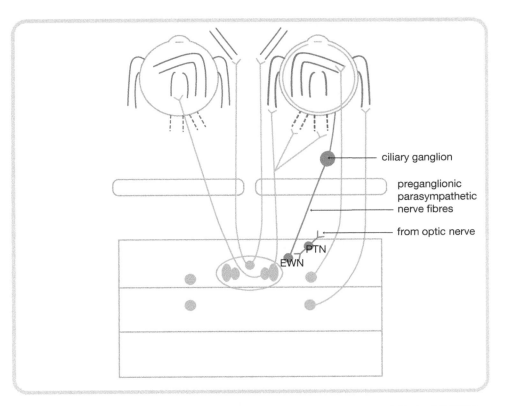

ciliary ganglion

preganglionic parasympathetic nerve fibres

from optic nerve

PTN

EWN

Box 1.1: Lesions of CN III, IV and VI

Oculomotor nerve (CN III)

Muscles supplied: levator palpebrae superioris, superior rectus, inferior rectus, medial rectus and inferior oblique.

Lesion: causes the eye to have a lateral deviation due to the lateral rectus muscle and an inferior deviation due to the superior oblique. The position is known as 'down and out'. You may also notice eyelid droop (ptosis).

Trochlear nerve (CN IV)

Muscle supplied: superior oblique.

Lesion: leads to paralysis of superior oblique, no obvious eyeball abnormality but the patient complains of diplopia (double vision) and may develop a head tilt away from the side of the lesion.

Abducens nerve (CN VI)

Muscle supplied: lateral rectus.

Lesion: leads to paralysis of lateral rectus, eye appears adducted.

Box 1.2: Consensual light reflex

When you see bright light a signal is sent via the optic nerve to the PTN and then the EWN, which in turn sends an excitatory response to the parasympathetic innervation of the smooth muscle of the iris. This leads to constriction (miosis) of the pupil, which reduces the amount of light entering the eye. Constriction occurs in both eyes even if light is shone in one eye; this is because fibres cross the midline as described above. This is the consensual light reflex. The direct light reflex refers to the reaction of the pupil in the eye that receives the light.

TRIGEMINAL NERVE (CN V)

A simple guide to drawing the complicated 5th cranial nerve. By the end of this section you will be able to draw up to 18 branches (there are a few more which I didn't include for simplification). This will put you miles ahead of anyone else who is asked about the anatomy of the trigeminal nerve.

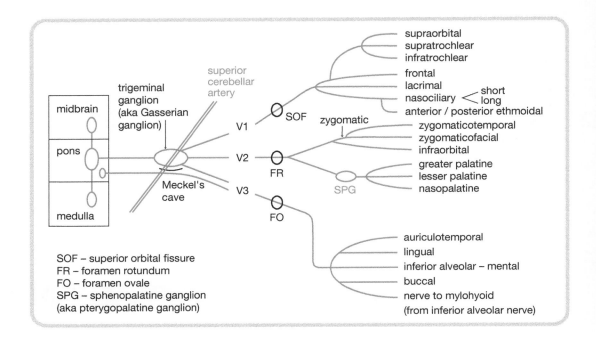

SOF – superior orbital fissure
FR – foramen rotundum
FO – foramen ovale
SPG – sphenopalatine ganglion
(aka pterygopalatine ganglion)

✏️ How to draw

STEP ①

Start by drawing the brainstem, where the trigeminal nerve starts.

- Draw a rectangle split into 3 squares. This represents the brainstem – the midbrain, pons and medulla oblongata.
- Draw an arc to represent Meckel's cave.

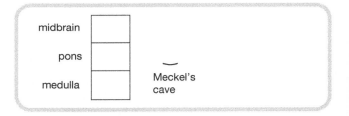

STEP ②

- Draw 3 sensory nuclei: mesencephalic (midbrain), chief sensory nucleus (pons), and the spinal trigeminal nucleus (medulla). Join the 3 nuclei with straight lines meeting in the middle nucleus.
- Draw the trigeminal ganglion in Meckel's cave.
- Draw one line horizontally to the trigeminal ganglion.
- Draw 3 lines laterally originating at the ganglion; these are the divisions V1, V2 and V3.

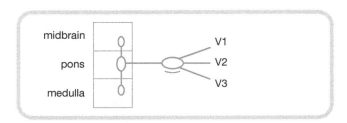

STEP 3

- Draw an artery across Meckel's cave, to represent that the artery runs near to the trigeminal nerve/ganglion and can cause compression. Compression of the ganglion leading to trigeminal neuralgia is most commonly caused by the superior cerebellar artery (60–90% of the time).
- Draw the motor nucleus in the pons and draw a line that bypasses the ganglion and Meckel's cave. It should run alongside V3.

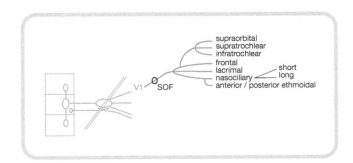

STEP 4

- From V1 draw one line going through the SOF. This then divides into 3 nerves: the frontal, lacrimal and nasociliary. The frontal nerve gives branches of the supraorbital and supratrochlear. The supratrochlear gives the branch of infratrochlear as shown.
- From the nasociliary nerve draw branches to the anterior and posterior ethmoidal nerves and the branches to the short and long ciliary nerves.

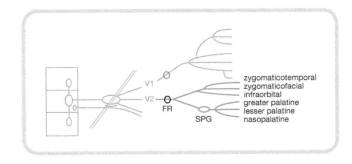

STEP 5

- Draw a line from V2 that passes through the foramen rotundum and then divides into 2.
- In this simplified version, the upper branch divides into 3: the infraorbital, the zygomaticotemporal and zygomaticofacial nerves.
- The lower branch forms the sphenopalatine ganglion and then divides into 3; the greater palatine, lesser palatine and nasopalatine nerves.

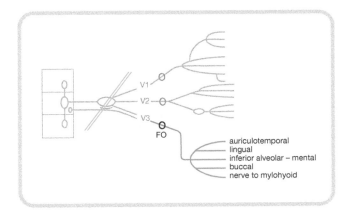

STEP 6

- Draw a line from V3 that passes through the foramen ovale. It then divides into 5 branches.
- I remember their names by the mnemonic ALIEN (the E is a back to front B in my head!). The branches are the **A**uriculotemporal, **L**ingual, **I**nferior alveolar (mental), **B**uccal and **N**erve to mylohyoid.

FACIAL NERVE (CN VII)

The facial nerve has motor, sensory and parasympathetic components:

- **Motor function:** control of the muscles of facial expression
- **Sensory function:** taste in the anterior 2/3 of the tongue
- **Parasympathetic activity:** control of the submandibular gland, sublingual gland and lacrimal glands.

It has 4 nuclei. Its motor nucleus is known as the facial motor nucleus. This controls most muscles of facial expression. There are 3 sensory nuclei:

- **Nucleus tractus solitarius:** fibres from the facial nerve (taste on anterior 2/3 of tongue), glossopharyngeal nerve (taste on posterior 1/3 of tongue) and vagus nerve (epiglottis) terminate in this nucleus.
- **Superior salivatory nucleus:** provides parasympathetic innervation to the submandibular and sublingual salivary glands. The lacrimal nucleus lies alongside the superior salivatory nucleus. It gives off the greater petrosal nerve which sends signals to the lacrimal gland.
- **Spinal trigeminal nucleus:** sends branches via the posterior auricular nerve to feed back sensation from the external ear.

The facial nerve is very complicated so I have tried to simplify it without losing the important anatomical points you need to learn.

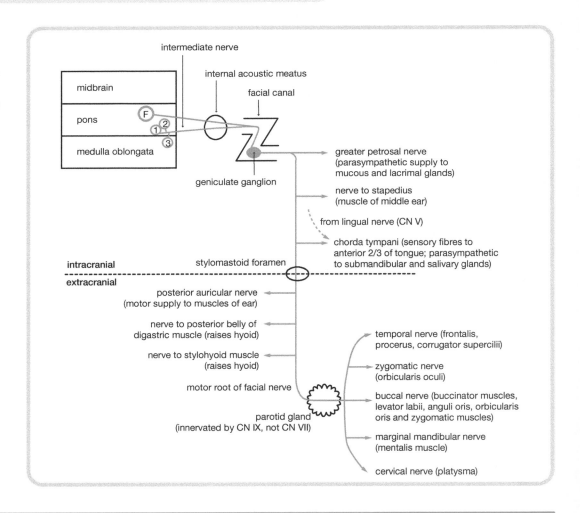

F   Facial motor nucleus

Sensory nuclei:
1   superior salivary nucleus
2   solitary nucleus
3   spinal nucleus of trigeminal nerve

intermediate nerve

internal acoustic meatus

facial canal

midbrain

pons

medulla oblongata

geniculate ganglion

greater petrosal nerve (parasympathetic supply to mucous and lacrimal glands)

nerve to stapedius (muscle of middle ear)

from lingual nerve (CN V)

chorda tympani (sensory fibres to anterior 2/3 of tongue; parasympathetic to submandibular and salivary glands)

intracranial

stylomastoid foramen

extracranial

posterior auricular nerve (motor supply to muscles of ear)

nerve to posterior belly of digastric muscle (raises hyoid)

nerve to stylohyoid muscle (raises hyoid)

motor root of facial nerve

parotid gland (innervated by CN IX, not CN VII)

temporal nerve (frontalis, procerus, corrugator supercilii)

zygomatic nerve (orbicularis oculi)

buccal nerve (buccinator muscles, levator labii, anguli oris, orbicularis oris and zygomatic muscles)

marginal mandibular nerve (mentalis muscle)

cervical nerve (platysma)

How to draw

STEP 1

- Draw a rectangle at the top left of the page; split this into 3 areas to depict the brainstem. Label midbrain, pons and medulla oblongata from top to bottom.
- Draw a dotted line across the middle of the page to show the intracranial and extracranial portion of the facial nerve.

| midbrain |
| pons |
| medulla oblongata |

intracranial
- -
extracranial

STEP 2

- Draw 1 large green circle and 3 small green circles in the pons and medulla oblongata as shown. These represent the nuclei, 1 motor and 3 sensory (lacrimatory nucleus not shown).

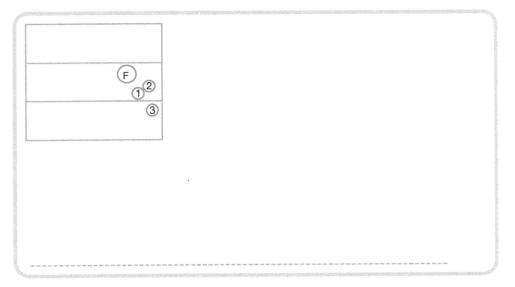

STEP 3

- Draw a black circle to represent the internal acoustic meatus (IAM). Draw 2 Z-shaped black lines to show the facial canal.
- Draw the intermediate nerve from the 3 sensory nuclei and another from the facial motor nucleus, to both pass through the IAM and join at the start of the facial canal.
- Continue the nerve through the facial canal. Add a green circle in the middle of it. This represents the geniculate ganglion.

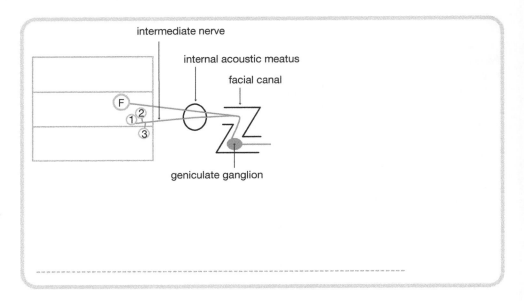

STEP 4

- From the exit of the facial canal draw the line of the nerve directly down through the dotted black line to 3/4 of the way down the page.
- In the intracranial part draw 3 branches horizontally from the facial nerve. These are the greater petrosal nerve, the nerve to stapedius muscle and the chorda tympani.
- Just above chorda tympani draw a dashed green line to join it; this represents a part of the trigeminal nerve (the lingual nerve) that conveys general sensation to the anterior 2/3 of the tongue.

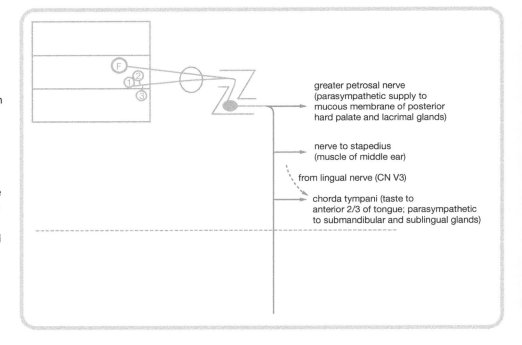

STEP 5

- Draw a black circle around the facial nerve, on the dashed line, to represent the stylomastoid foramen.
- Draw 3 branches from the facial nerve on the left side of the page. From the top down these are the posterior auricular nerve, the nerve to the digastric muscle and the nerve to the stylohyoid.

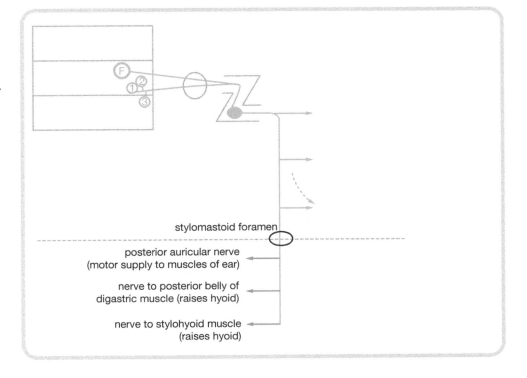

stylomastoid foramen

posterior auricular nerve
(motor supply to muscles of ear)

nerve to posterior belly of
digastric muscle (raises hyoid)

nerve to stylohyoid muscle
(raises hyoid)

STEP 6

- Continue the motor root of the facial nerve; it passes through the parotid gland (draw a black circular 'cloud' shape) but does not innervate it.
- Beyond the parotid gland draw 5 branches, from the top down: **T**emporal, **Z**ygomatic, **B**uccal nerve, **M**andibular and **C**ervical nerve. You can remember these branches using a mnemonic, for example '**T**wo **Z**ulus **B**efriended **M**y **C**at'.

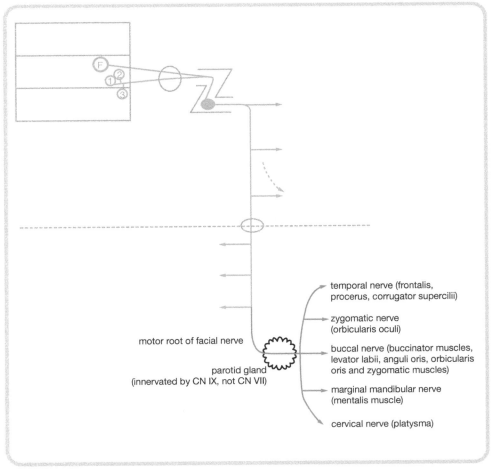

temporal nerve (frontalis,
procerus, corrugator supercilii)

zygomatic nerve
(orbicularis oculi)

motor root of facial nerve

buccal nerve (buccinator muscles,
levator labii, anguli oris, orbicularis
oris and zygomatic muscles)

parotid gland
(innervated by CN IX, not CN VII)

marginal mandibular nerve
(mentalis muscle)

cervical nerve (platysma)

SENSORY SUPPLY TO THE FACE AND MOTOR SUPPLY FOR MUSCLES OF FACIAL EXPRESSION (CN V AND VII)

Sensation

For your diagram the face can be split into 3 zones: V1, V2 and V3. Each zone has 3–5 branches. Use this image along with the trigeminal nerve diagram to learn the distribution of these nerves.

Motor supply

The motor supply to the muscles of facial expression is from the facial nerve (it's in the name!).

The branches can be remembered using various mnemonics; the one I use is 'Two Zulus Befriended My Cat'. Yes, it is a little odd, but it works for me!

- Temporal nerve: supplies frontalis, procerus, corrugator supercilii muscles.
- Zygomatic: supplies orbicularis oculi.
- Buccal: supplies buccinator muscles, levator labii, anguli oris, orbicularis oris and zygomatic muscles.
- Marginal mandibular: supplies mentalis muscle.
- Cervical: supplies platysma.

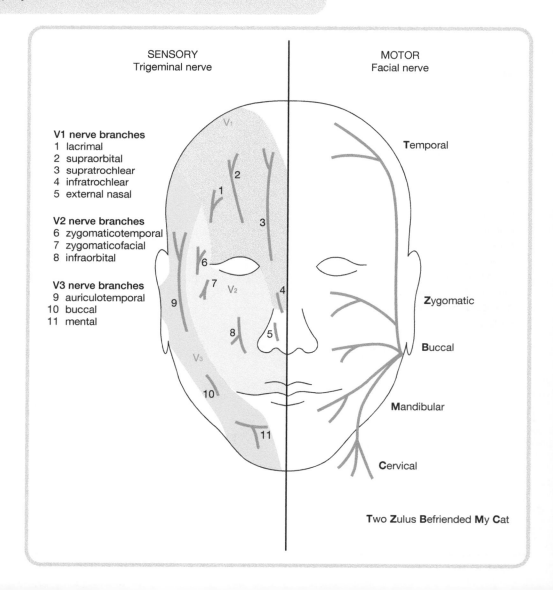

VESTIBULOCOCHLEAR NERVE (CN VIII)

This nerve transmits sound (cochlear part) and equilibrium/balance (vestibular part) from the inner ear to the brain. It is one of the most complicated cranial nerves to study so I have divided it into the vestibular and cochlear parts to make it easier to learn.

Vestibular part – balance

We will start by drawing a representation of the structures within the brain and spinal cord, and then will draw the nerve pathways.

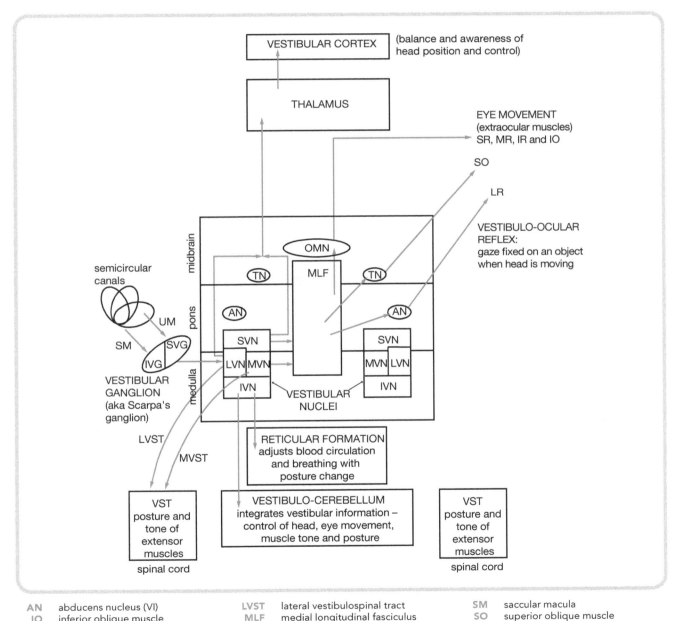

AN	abducens nucleus (VI)	LVST	lateral vestibulospinal tract	SM	saccular macula
IO	inferior oblique muscle	MLF	medial longitudinal fasciculus	SO	superior oblique muscle
IR	inferior rectus muscle	MR	medial rectus muscle	SR	superior rectus muscle
IVG	inferior vestibular ganglion	MVN	medial vestibular nucleus	SVG	superior vestibular ganglion
IVN	inferior vestibular nucleus	MVST	medial vestibulospinal tract	SVN	superior vestibular nucleus
LR	lateral rectus muscle	OMN	oculomotor nucleus (III)	TN	trochlear nucleus (IV)
LVN	lateral vestibular nucleus	RST	reticulospinal tract	UM	macula of utricle

47

✏️ How to draw

STEP 1

- Start by drawing a square in the middle of the page to represent the brainstem.
- Draw a vertical rectangle in its centre. This is the medial longitudinal fasciculus (MLF).
- Draw 2 horizontal lines dividing the square into 3; label the areas as the midbrain, pons and medulla oblongata (MO).

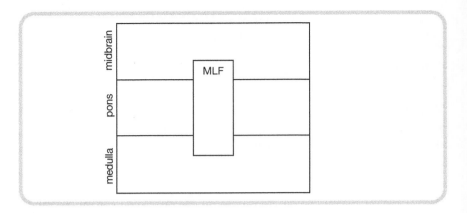

STEP 2

- At the top of the page draw 2 horizontal rectangles, 1 above the other. These represent the vestibular cortex above and the thalamus below.
- Above the MLF draw a horizontal oval; this is the oculomotor nucleus, CN III (OMN).
- Lateral to the MLF draw a circle on each side just above the pons. These are the trochlear nuclei (CN IV).

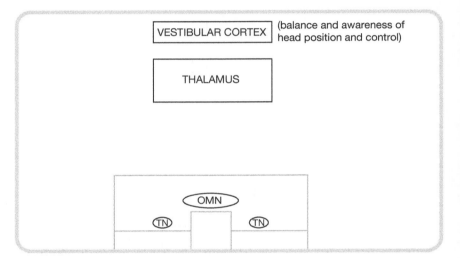

STEP 3

- In the pons draw 2 circles, 1 on each side centrally; these are the abducens nuclei (CN VI).
- Draw a vertical rectangle divided into 3, with the SVN and part of the LVN above the MO in the pons, and the MVN and IVN in the MO. This is the vestibular nucleus and the 4 nuclei are usually known together as the vestibular nuclear complex.

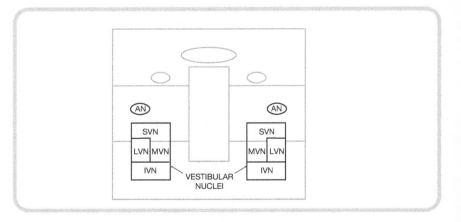

STEP 4

- Draw 2 horizontal rectangles below the brainstem; these are the reticular formation above and the vestibulo-cerebellum below.
- On each side of the vestibulo-cerebellum draw a vertical rectangle; these represent the vestibulospinal and reticulospinal tracts within the spinal cord. They are components of the balance posture reflex.

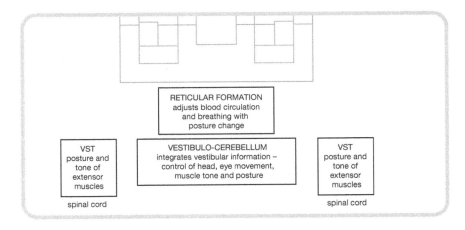

STEP 5

- Draw 3 loops together. These are the semicircular canals in the inner ear.
- Between the semicircular canals and the MO, draw an oval divided into 2. This represents the vestibular ganglion.

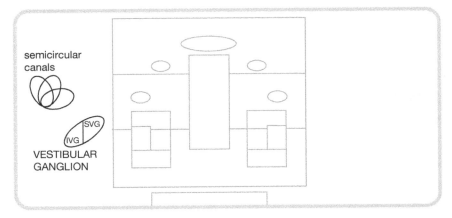

STEP 6

Now start drawing the nerves as green arrows, depicting the pathways in the brain:

- Draw 2 arrows from the semicircular canals to the vestibular nuclei – the saccular macula and the utricular macula. From here draw 1 arrow to the LVN.
- From the vestibular nucleus draw 4 arrows: the lateral vestibulospinal tract going from the LVN to the VST; the medial vestibulospinal tract going from the MVN to the VST; an arrow from the LVN towards the thalamus; and a final arrow going from the SVN towards the thalamus.

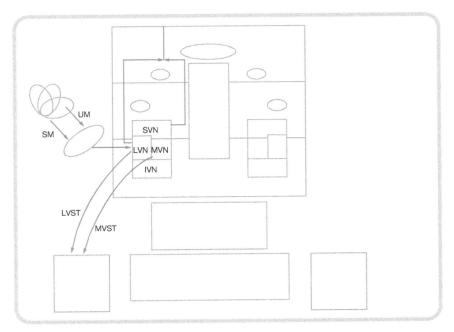

STEP 7

- Draw 2 arrows from the IVN: 1 to the reticular formation and 1 to the vestibulo-cerebellum.
- Draw 1 arrow from the SVN to MLF and 1 from MVN to MLF.

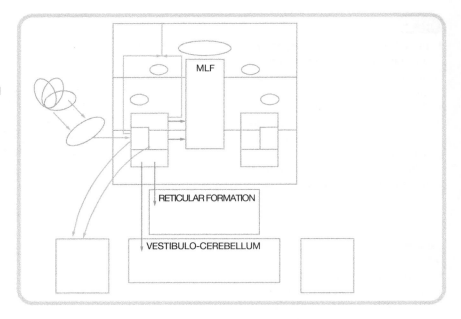

STEP 8

- From the MLF draw 3 arrows: 1 to oculomotor nucleus, 1 to trochlear nucleus and 1 to abducens nucleus.
- From each of the nuclei draw an arrow to the corresponding muscle of the eye and label muscles as shown. This is the pathway for the vestibulo-ocular reflex: your vision is fixed on a distant object whilst walking.

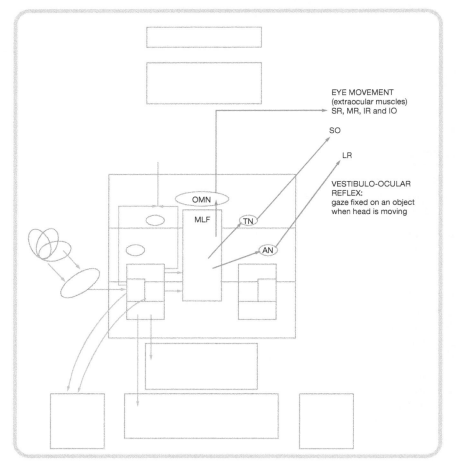

STEP 9

- Draw 1 arrow from the thalamus to the vestibular cortex. Extend the arrow into the thalamus from the midbrain.

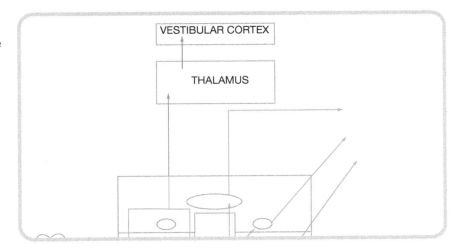

Cochlear part – sound

This is slightly more simple than the vestibular part of CN VIII.

Note each ear has bilateral representation in the primary auditory cortex – a unilateral lesion would not fully disrupt hearing.

DCN   dorsal cochlear nucleus
IC   inferior colliculus
MGN   medial geniculate nucleus (or body)
SON   superior olivary nucleus
VCN   ventral cochlear nucleus

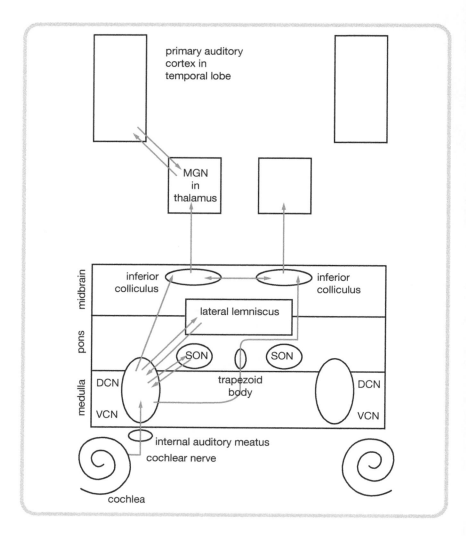

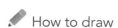 How to draw

STEP 1

- Draw 2 rectangles at the top of the page, 1 on each side to represent the primary auditory cortices in the temporal lobes.
- Draw 2 squares below to represent the medial geniculate nucleus (MGN) of thalamus.

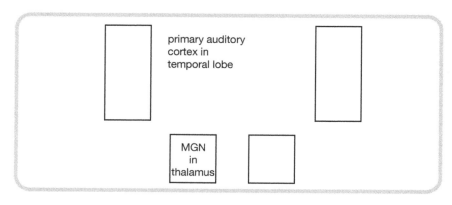

STEP 2

- Draw the brainstem as 1 large rectangle, divided into 3 in pencil.
- Add 1 small rectangle along the line between midbrain and pons. This is the lateral lemniscus.
- Above this draw 2 ovals, 1 on each side; these are the inferior colliculi.
- Draw 2 circles below the lateral lemniscus, the superior olivary nuclei (SON), and a smaller circle between them to represent the trapezoid body.

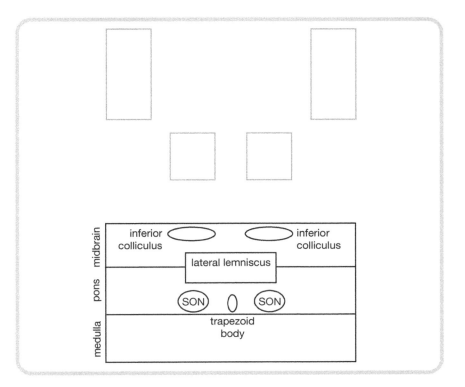

STEP 3

- Draw 2 large ovals interrupting the line between MO and pons; these are the cochlear nuclei (now the MO–pons boundary can be inked in). In each one, label the dorsal cochlear nucleus and the ventral cochlear nucleus.
- Below the brainstem draw 2 'snail shells', one for each cochlea.
- On one side draw an oval next to the cochlea to represent the internal auditory (or acoustic) meatus.

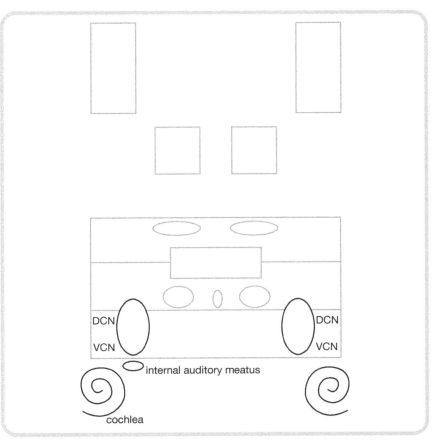

STEP 4

We will draw green arrows representing the nerves on just one side in Steps 4 and 5, for simplicity.

- From the left cochlea draw an arrow to represent the cochlear nerve passing through the internal auditory meatus to the cochlear nucleus.
- From the cochlear nucleus draw 2 pairs of arrows representing paths to and from the SON and the lateral lemniscus.

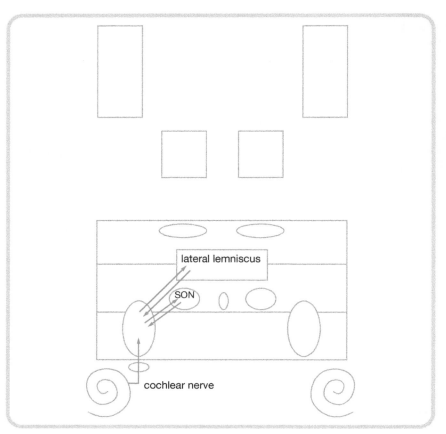

STEP 5

- Draw an arrow from the cochlear nucleus to the inferior colliculus on each side.
- Draw a 2-way arrow between each inferior colliculus.
- From each inferior colliculus draw an arrow directly upwards to the MGN.
- Draw 2 arrows, 1 each way from MGN to the primary auditory cortex.

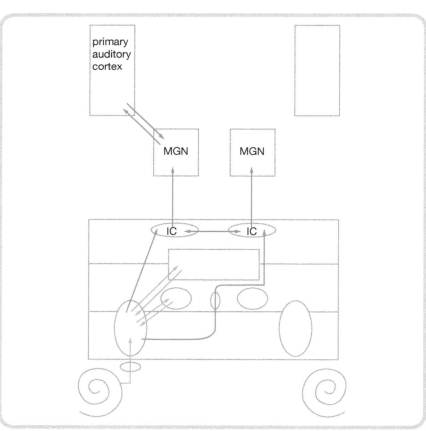

GLOSSOPHARYNGEAL NERVE (CN IX)

The glossopharyngeal nerve is a mixed motor and sensory nerve. It has 5 distinct general functions:

1. Branchial motor (special visceral efferent): supplies the stylopharyngeus muscle.
2. Visceral motor (general visceral efferent): parasympathetic innervation of the parotid gland
3. Visceral sensory (general visceral afferent): carries information from the carotid sinus and carotid body.
4. General sensory (general somatic afferent): carries information from inner surface of the tympanic membrane, upper pharynx, and posterior 1/3 of the tongue.
5. Visceral afferent (special visceral afferent): taste sensation from posterior 1/3 of tongue

TN   tympanic nerve

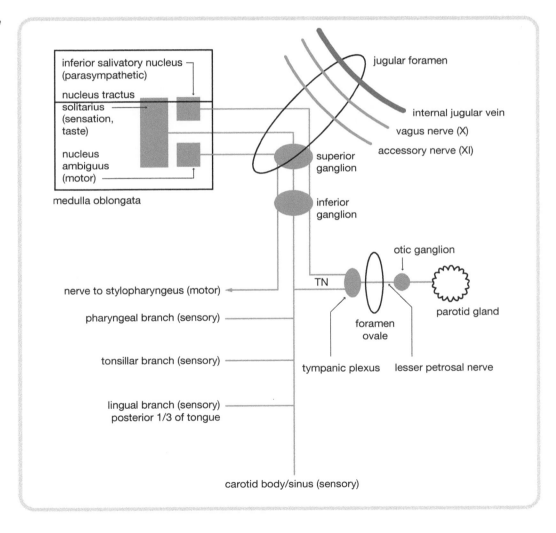

✏ How to draw

STEP ①

- Draw a black square divided into 2; the top represents the pons and the bottom the medulla oblongata.
- Draw an elliptical shape at 45° next to this, to represent the jugular foramen.

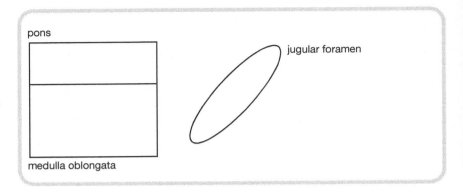

STEP ②

- Draw 3 nuclei, 1 vertical rectangle and 2 squares as shown.
- The rectangle represents nucleus tractus solitarius (fibres conveying taste and visceral sensation terminate here).
- The upper square is the inferior salivatory nucleus (parasympathetic) and the lower is the nucleus ambiguus (motor).

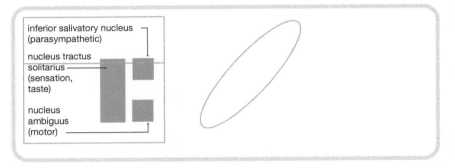

STEP ③

- From each of these draw a line towards the jugular foramen and then turn 90° downward to continue the lines to join the superior ganglion.
- Draw all 3 continuing to the inferior ganglion.

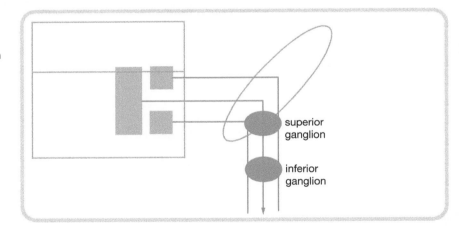

STEP 4

- From the inferior ganglion draw 2 lines downwards, 1 straight down representing the sensory nerve for the carotid body/sinus and another on the left, going down and turning 90° as an arrow to represent the motor nerve to stylopharyngeus.
- Draw 3 lines from the right line to show 3 sensory nerves: the pharyngeal branch, the tonsillar branch and the lingual branch.
- Do not confuse the lingual branch of the glossopharyngeal nerve with the lingual nerve from the trigeminal nerve (CN V3 division).

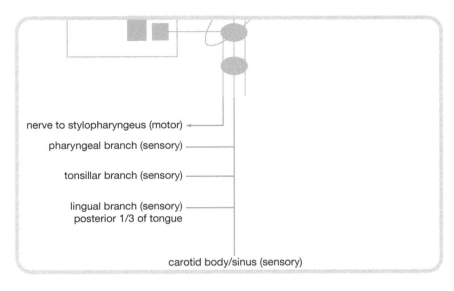

STEP 5

- Draw an oval shape representing the tympanic plexus, to one side of and below the inferior ganglion.
- Draw a short 3rd line down from the inferior ganglion and a branch off the nerve to the carotid body/sinus, both joining the tympanic plexus.
- From the plexus draw a line through a black oval (the foramen ovale) to a circle representing the otic ganglion. This is the lesser petrosal nerve. Finally continue this as a nerve (parasympathetic) to the parotid gland.

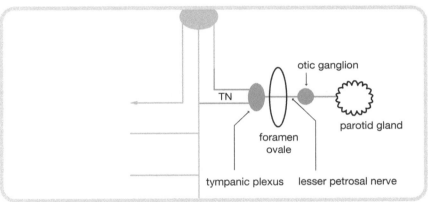

STEP 6

Draw a blue line representing the internal jugular vein, and 2 green lines representing CN X and XI, through the jugular foramen.

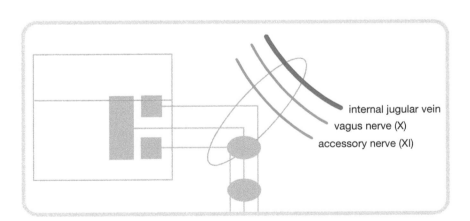

VAGUS NERVE (CN X)

The vagus nerve is a parasympathetic nerve that supplies many organs in the body. It is a complicated nerve and it runs a different course on each side. The important points are covered in the diagram but I would advise looking in available atlases/textbooks or on the internet at all the different anatomical images to get a comprehensive and clear idea of where it runs and what it looks like.

There are 4 nuclei in the medulla:

- the dorsal vagal nucleus is the parasympathetic supply to the viscera
- the nucleus ambiguus is for motor supply of pharynx, larynx and upper oesophagus
- the nucleus tractus solitarius is for afferent taste and visceral sensation
- the spinal trigeminal nucleus is for crude touch and pain and temperature.

It exits the skull through the jugular foramen.

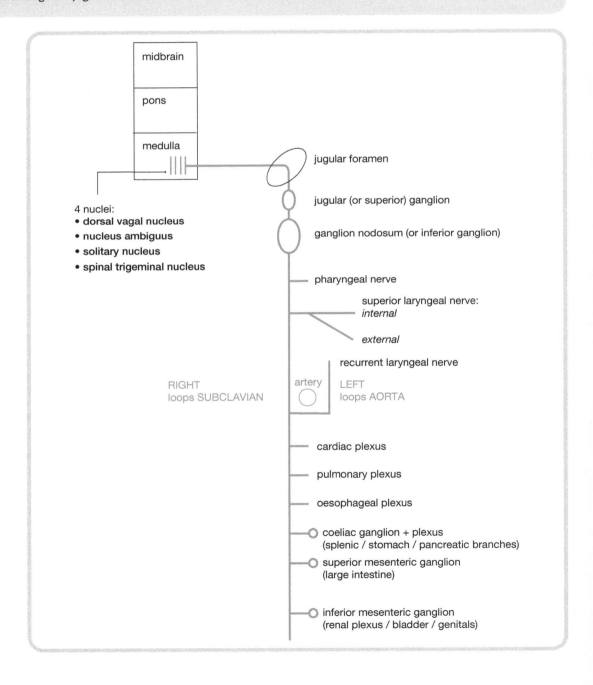

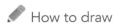 How to draw

STEP 1

- Draw the midbrain, pons and medulla as a box.

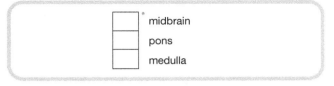

STEP 2

- Draw the 4 nuclei (see text above). Draw a line to the right that goes through the jugular foramen and ends in the jugular ganglion. Draw a further line to the ganglion nodosum.

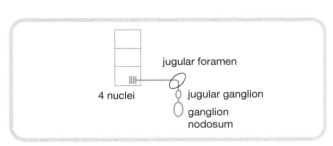

STEP 3

Draw a long line down from the ganglion nodosum. Draw 3 branches:

- The superior one is the pharyngeal nerve.
- The next one is the superior laryngeal nerve – this divides into the internal and external branches.
- The third branch represents the recurrent laryngeal nerve – this descends on the left and the right differently. On the right it descends and loops the subclavian artery before ascending into the neck between the trachea and the oesophagus to supply as well as innervate all of the intrinsic muscles of the larynx except the cricothyroid. On the left it descends into the thorax and then loops around the arch of the aorta before ascending.
- Draw the artery, labelled as above.

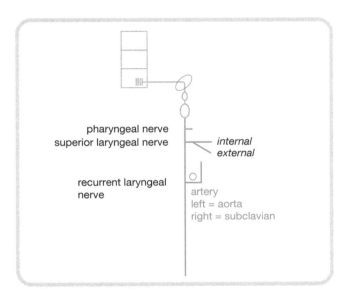

STEP 4

- Draw 4 more branches: these represent the cardiac plexus, pulmonary plexus, oesophageal plexus and the coeliac ganglion and plexus (a circle represents the ganglion).
- Draw 2 further branches – each branch has a circle to represent a ganglion. These are the superior mesenteric ganglion and the inferior mesenteric ganglion.
- The superior mesenteric ganglion has branches to spleen, stomach, pancreas and large intestine.
- The inferior mesenteric ganglion has branches to the renal plexus, bladder and genitals.

1	cardiac plexus
2	pulmonary plexus
3	oesophageal plexus
4	coeliac ganglion + plexus
5	superior mesenteric ganglion
6	inferior mesenteric ganglion

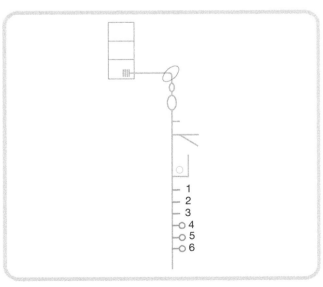

ACCESSORY NERVE (CN XI)

The accessory nerve (CN XI) has a cranial part and a spinal part. The cranial part joins the vagus nerve fairly 'early' and so people are normally referring to the spinal part and the motor supply of sternocleidomastoid and trapezius muscle when they talk about the accessory nerve.

The spinal accessory nerve supplies sternocleidomastoid muscle (SCM) and trapezius muscle.

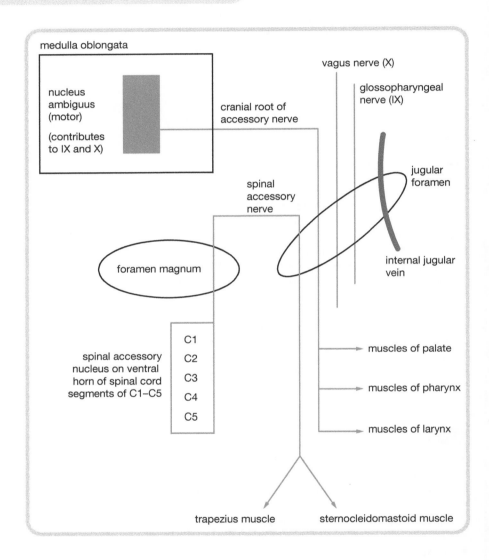

How to draw

STEP 1

- Draw a black square and label as the medulla oblongata (MO). Then draw an elliptical black ring, the jugular foramen (as you did in CN IX).
- Draw a 2nd black ellipse just below the MO to represent the foramen magnum.

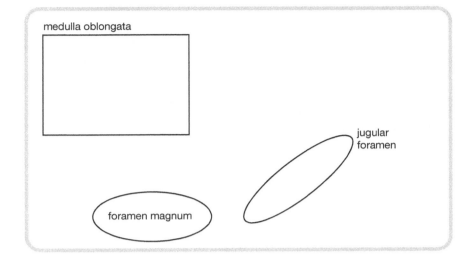

STEP 2

- Below the foramen magnum draw a green rectangle and label from C1 to C5; this represents the spinal accessory nucleus, located on the ventral horn of segments C1 to C5.
- From the upper right corner draw a vertical nerve up through the foramen magnum and then turn 90° twice to continue through the jugular foramen and downwards, splitting into 2 to innervate the sternocleidomastoid and trapezius muscles. This is the spinal accessory nerve.

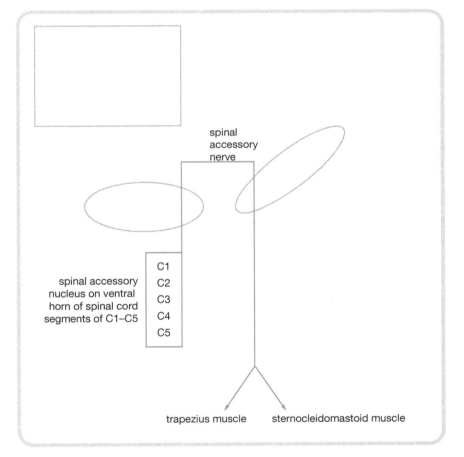

STEP 3

- Draw a green rectangle in the medulla oblongata; this is the nucleus ambiguus, also a nucleus for IX and X.
- From here draw a line to exit the medulla and pass down through the jugular foramen; this represents the cranial root of the accessory nerve.
- Add 3 branches to supply the muscles of the palate, pharynx and larynx.

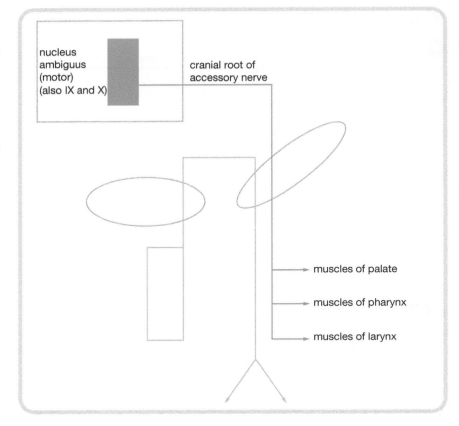

STEP 4

- Draw 2 vertical green lines through the jugular foramen to represent CN X and IX.
- Draw a blue line through the jugular foramen to represent the internal jugular vein.

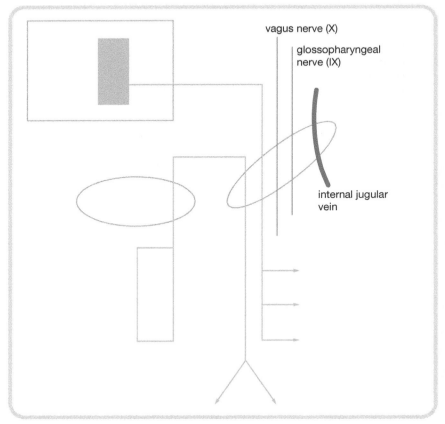

HYPOGLOSSAL NERVE (CN XII)

CN XII is a motor nerve. It innervates all intrinsic and extrinsic muscles of the tongue except palatoglossus (innervated by CN X).

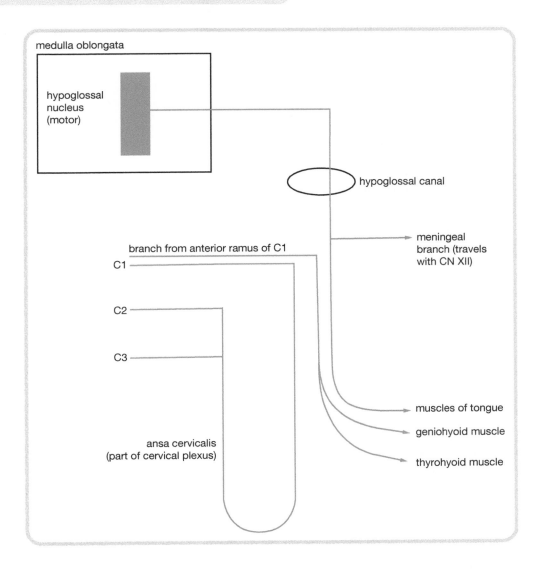

How to draw

STEP 1

- Draw a black square representing the medulla oblongata.
- Draw a black oval to represent the hypoglossal canal.

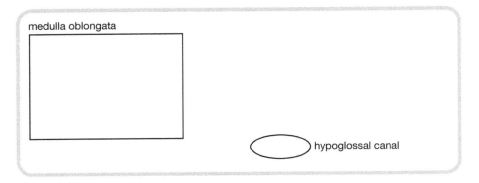

STEP 2

- Draw a green rectangle in the medulla to represent the hypoglossal nucleus.
- From here draw the hypoglossal nerve moving horizontally until above the hypoglossal canal. Here draw the nerve passing downwards to a branch in the lower part of the page supplying the muscles of the tongue.
- The extrinsic muscles of the tongue supplied by the hypoglossal nerve include the styloglossus, genioglossus and hyoglossus. The hypoglossal nerve also innervates intrinsic muscles (superior longitudinal, transverse and vertical, inferior longitudinal).
- Add a branch after the hypoglossal canal, the meningeal branch, which travels with CN XII.

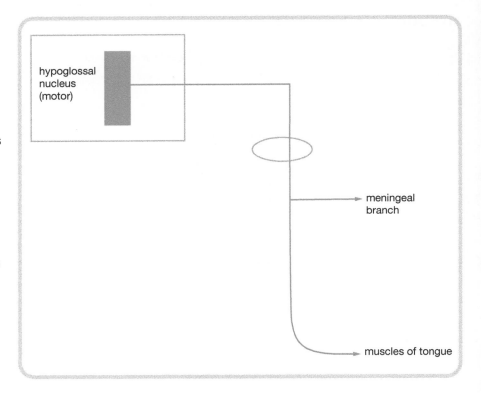

STEP 3

This final step shows the relationship of the hypoglossal nerve to the ansa cervicalis and major vessels.

- Draw and label C1, C2 and C3. Draw a loop that starts at C1 and loops round to C2 and C3 (as in the cervical plexus diagram – see *Section 1.3.2*); this is the ansa cervicalis. It is a motor loop that supplies omohyoid, sternohyoid and sternothyroid muscles. Thyrohyoid and geniohyoid muscles are supplied by C1 via CN XII.
- Draw a line alongside the branch from C1 and label as branch from the anterior ramus of C1. This line then descends alongside the hypoglossal nerve and supplies the geniohyoid and thyrohyoid.

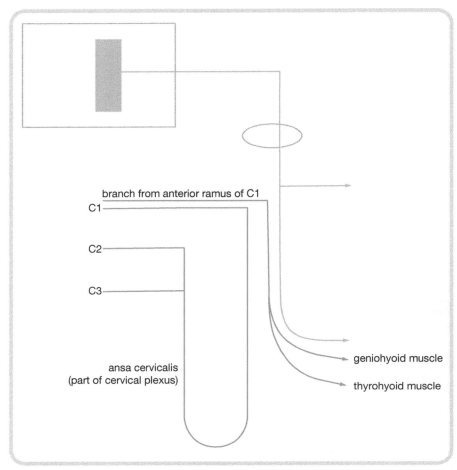

1.3.2 Cervical plexus

AC   ansa cervicalis
GA   greater auricular
LO   lesser occipital
SC   supraclavicular
TC   transverse cervicalis

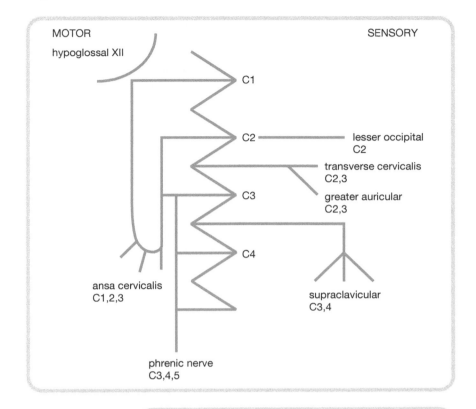

MOTOR

hypoglossal XII

C1

C2

C3

C4

ansa cervicalis
C1,2,3

phrenic nerve
C3,4,5

SENSORY

lesser occipital
C2

transverse cervicalis
C2,3

greater auricular
C2,3

supraclavicular
C3,4

 How to draw

STEP ①

- Draw 4.5 unfinished arrowheads facing to the right. Label them as C1, 2, 3 and 4.
- C5 is not labelled as it is not 'officially' part of the cervical plexus.

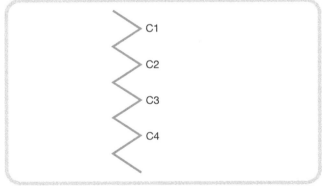

C1

C2

C3

C4

STEP ②

Add in the motor component.

- The ansa cervicalis (AC) has roots from C1, 2 and 3 and forms a loop. Three muscles are supplied by the ansa cervicalis (see Hypoglossal nerve (CN XII)) and this can be represented by drawing 3 lines from the bottom of the loop.
- Also, draw the phrenic nerve by taking roots from C3, 4 and 5 and joining them together as shown.

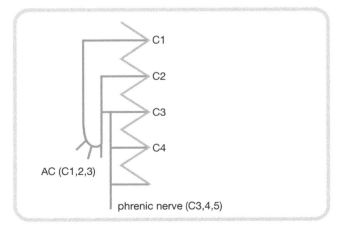

C1

C2

C3

C4

AC (C1,2,3)

phrenic nerve (C3,4,5)

STEP 3

Add the sensory nerves to the right side.

- One line from C2 to represent the lesser occipital nerve.
- One line between C2 and C3 splits into 2. This represents the transverse cervicalis and greater auricular nerves.
- Add a third line from between C3 and C4. This will split into 3; the medial, intermediate and lateral supraclavicular nerves.

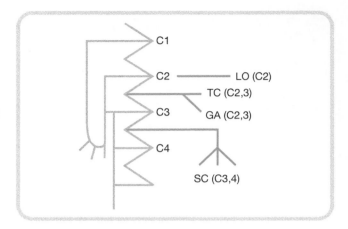

STEP 4

- Add in the hypoglossal nerve (CN XII). This carries some motor component of the cervical plexus.

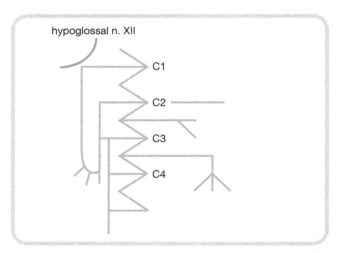

1.4 Sensory organs

1.4.1 Eye

NERVE SUPPLY TO THE EYE AND SURROUNDING STRUCTURES

Motor

- CN III – oculomotor nerve – levator palpebrae superioris muscle, superior rectus muscle, medial rectus muscle and inferior oblique muscle
- CN IV – trochlear nerve – superior oblique muscle
- CN VI – abducens nerve – lateral rectus muscle
- CN VII – facial nerve – orbicularis oculi muscle.

Sensory

- Trigeminal nerve (CN V, see *Section 1.3.1*)
- CN V1 (ophthalmic division) – skin/conjunctiva/upper eyelid/cornea/inner eyelid/inner canthus/outer eyelid
- CN V2 (maxillary division) – lower eyelid and its conjunctiva/lacrimal duct/lateral wall of nose.

Autonomic

- Sympathetic supply – long and short ciliary nerves from the superior cervical ganglion → these cause pupil dilation through contraction of dilator pupilae (mydriasis) and causes contraction of ciliaris which causes the lens to become rounded for far sight.
- Parasympathetic supply – fibres from the oculomotor nerve (CN III) → pupil constriction from contraction of constrictor pupilae (miosis) and causes relaxation of ciliaris which leads to the lens becoming flattened for near sight (accommodation).

ARTERIAL SUPPLY

Globe of the eye and orbital contents – ophthalmic artery (a branch of the internal carotid artery). The ophthalmic artery passes through the optic canal.

Intraocular pressure

Normal intraocular pressure (IOP) is 10–20 mmHg. This increases with age and there is a diurnal variation of 2–3 mmHg.

Aqueous humour

Clear fluid which fills posterior chamber of the eye. There is approximately 250 µl.

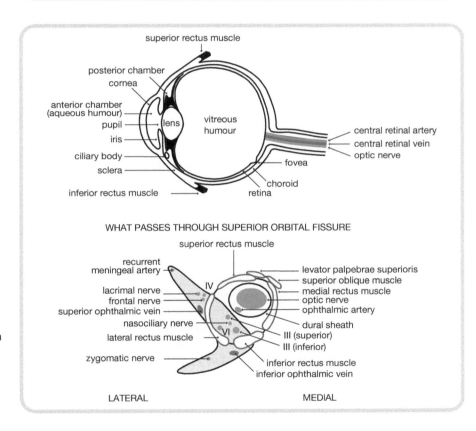

WHAT PASSES THROUGH SUPERIOR ORBITAL FISSURE

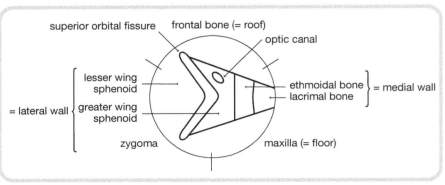

1.4.2 Nose

> First, we will look at cartilages of the nose and then the internal anatomy and blood supply. For nerve supply, see *Section 4.1: Airway sensation.*

NASAL CARTILAGES

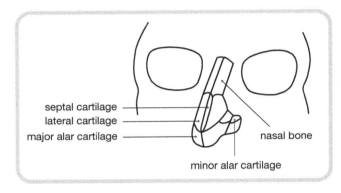

septal cartilage
lateral cartilage
major alar cartilage
nasal bone
minor alar cartilage

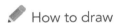 How to draw

STEP 1

- Draw the eye and nose area of a skull.
- Draw a line down left of centre to form a nose, and draw its tip and a left nostril so it is pointing to its right slightly.
- Draw 2 almost rectangular shapes in the upper part of the nose; these are the nasal bones.

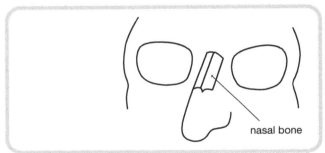

nasal bone

STEP 2

- Divide the area below the nasal bones with a downward arrow 2/3 of the way down; this is the inferior border of the nasal septal cartilages.
- Divide this area so that it has a slim segment in the middle and 2 sides. The slim part represents the septal cartilage. The lateral parts are the lateral cartilages (actually lateral processes of the septal cartilage).

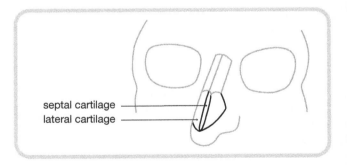

septal cartilage
lateral cartilage

STEP 3

- Below the downward arrow draw a line down the centre of the nose to the tip; this is the junction of the 2 major alar cartilages.
- Divide the posterior 1/3 of the left alar area of the nose into 3 as shown. The small area in the middle is the minor alar cartilage; there is a small area between the lateral and major cartilage called the accessory cartilage (not shown). The areas above and below the minor alar cartilage are the fibrofatty tissue.

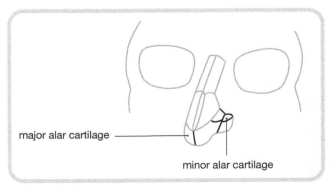

major alar cartilage

minor alar cartilage

NASAL SEPTUM, NASAL BONES AND PARANASAL SINUSES

To understand the nasal septum, nasal bones and paranasal sinuses we will draw a sagittal section. Paranasal sinuses are a group of 4 paired air-filled spaces around the nasal cavity (2 are shown here). The ethmoid sinuses are hollow spaces in the bones around the nose, (not shown). The maxillary sinuses are the largest and located laterally and inferiorly to the nose.

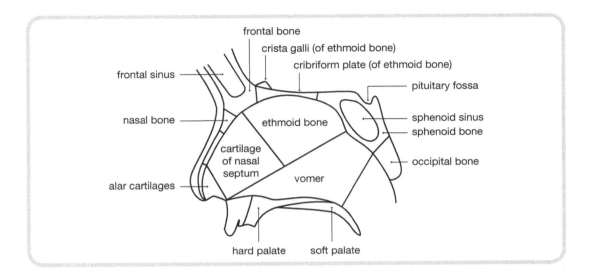

How to draw

STEP 1

- On the left side of the page starting approximately between the eyes, draw the profile of a face down to the upper lip. As you turn in from the upper lip flatten out the line for the gum and then make an arch to represent the palate.
- Draw a 2nd line in parallel with the facial profile, just behind it and ending at the tip of the nose.

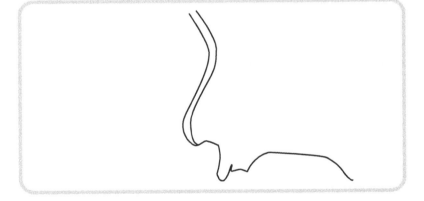

STEP 2

- From the tip of the nose draw a semicircle towards the right side of the page, with an indentation as shown.
- From the corner of the bottom of the nose draw a straight-ish line towards the right side of the page, joining the back of the palate.
- Draw a vertical line down from just behind the lip to the edge of the palate, separating the lip from the palate; then divide the palate area into 2 with a straight line running directly back from part way along the bottom of this area. The front part is the hard palate and the back is the soft palate.

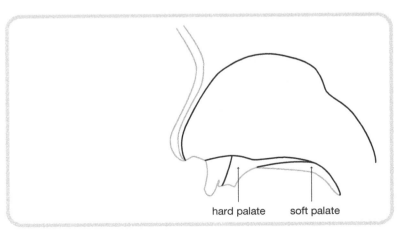

STEP 3

- Draw a 'U' shape just between the eye area; this is the frontal sinus.
- Draw 3 lines between the 2nd and 3rd lines in the 'profile' of the face. These divide the area into nasal bone, septal cartilage and major alar cartilage.

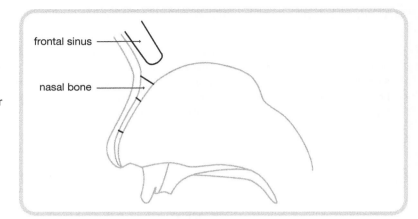

STEP 4

Divide the inside of the nasal passage into 4 areas: the small triangle at the front is the alar cartilage, the main area behind this is the cartilage of the nasal septum; behind this is the ethmoid bone and below this the vomer.

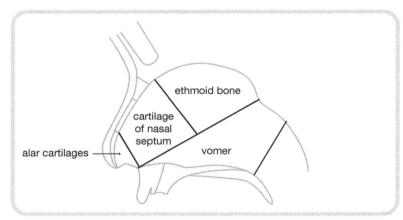

STEP 5

- Behind the ethmoid and vomer bones draw an oval shape; this is the sphenoid sinus.
- Draw a line starting just to the right of the frontal sinus heading down, almost parallel to the upper edge of the ethmoid bone and beyond it around the sphenoid sinus, including a small dip to represent the pituitary fossa; then continue the line down to join the boundary of the nasal cavity posterior to the vomer bone.
- Draw 2 vertical lines from this to the ethmoid bone, one anteriorly and one posteriorly; the cribriform plate of the ethmoid is between these and the frontal bone is anterior to that. Just above at the front of this draw a 'bump'; this is the crista galli of the ethmoid.
- Draw a straight line as shown behind the sphenoid sinus; this divides the sphenoid and occipital bones.

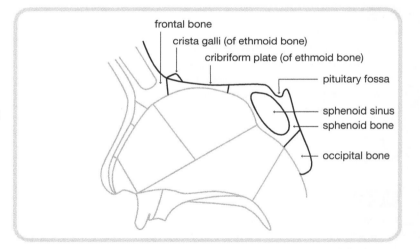

INTERNAL NASAL ANATOMY AND SINUS DRAINAGE

We will now look at the internal nasal anatomy and sinus drainage in more detail, drawing a section that shows the lateral wall of the nasal cavity.

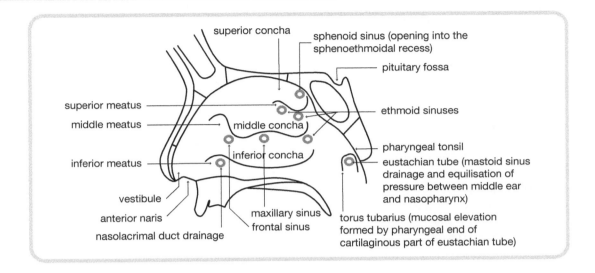

superior concha

sphenoid sinus (opening into the sphenoethmoidal recess)

pituitary fossa

superior meatus

middle meatus

middle concha

ethmoid sinuses

inferior concha

pharyngeal tonsil

inferior meatus

eustachian tube (mastoid sinus drainage and equilisation of pressure between middle ear and nasopharynx)

vestibule

anterior naris

maxillary sinus

frontal sinus

nasolacrimal duct drainage

torus tubarius (mucosal elevation formed by pharyngeal end of cartilaginous part of eustachian tube)

 How to draw

STEP ①

- Use the image you just learned to draw: copy the main outlines but leave out the lines within the nasal cavity.
- Label the anterior naris (nostril) and vestibule anteriorly and the pituitary fossa and the location of the pharyngeal tonsil posteriorly.
- Add in an upside-down U shape anterior to the location of the pharyngeal tonsil. This is the torus tubarius, a mucosal elevation formed by the pharyngeal end of the cartilaginous part of the eustachian tube.

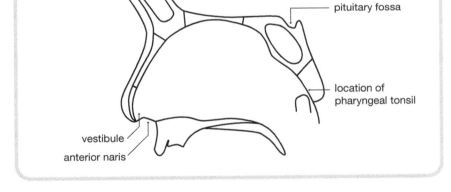

pituitary fossa

location of pharyngeal tonsil

vestibule

anterior naris

STEP ②

Draw 3 curved lines within the nasal cavity:

- Draw a curved line in the upper posterior part of the nasal cavity as shown.
- A line about 2/3 down and longer, with a Z-shaped curve at the front so you can imagine it 'protruding like a shelf'; this is the middle concha.
- A final line in a similar but more flattened curve; this is the inferior concha.

Label the middle meatus, the gap between the hanging middle concha and the nasal wall; add labels for the superior meatus and inferior meatus as shown. The meati are located beneath the conchae.

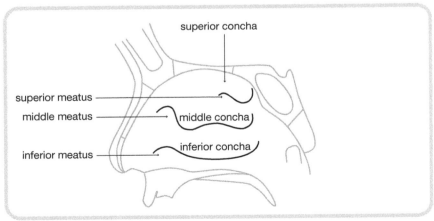

superior concha

superior meatus

middle meatus

middle concha

inferior concha

inferior meatus

STEP 3

For the sinus drainage we will draw small grey circles to represent their opening into the nasal cavity.

- Start with one above and posterior to the superior concha. This is where the sphenoid sinus drains in the sphenoethmoidal recess.
- Just below the superior concha draw 2 more circles; these represent ethmoid sinus drainage.
- Draw 1 circle below and posterior to the middle concha; the ethmoid sinus also drains here. The circles represent the approximate location of the sinuses.
- Anterior sinus opens onto the hiatus semilunaris (middle meatus).
- Middle sinus opens onto the lateral wall of the middle meatus.
- Posterior sinus opens onto the lateral wall of the superior meatus.

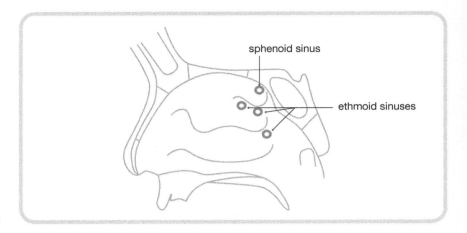

STEP 4

- Just below the centre of the middle concha draw a circle to represent the maxillary sinus drainage site (commonly in the middle of the hiatus semilunaris).
- Anterior to this but still below the middle concha, add the frontal sinus drainage area, in the anterior aspect of the hiatus semilunaris.
- Draw a grey circle below the anterior 1/3 of the inferior concha; this is where the nasolacrimal duct drains. This is the reason your nose drips when you cry!
- Draw a final circle in the posterior nasopharynx; this is where the eustachian tube connects the middle ear to the nasopharynx. It also allows some mastoid sinus drainage and equalisation of pressure between the middle ear and the nasopharynx.

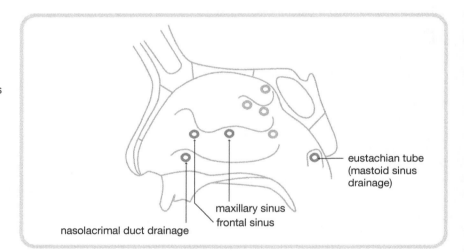

NASAL BLOOD SUPPLY

We will now look at the blood supply to the nose. This is particularly important when you are learning about epistaxis. The most common area in which nasal bleeds occur is Little's area, because it has blood supply from 5 main arteries.

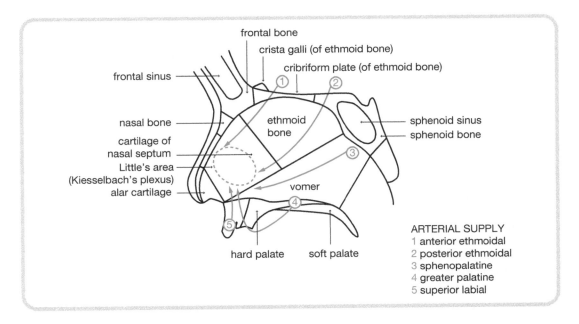

ARTERIAL SUPPLY
1 anterior ethmoidal
2 posterior ethmoidal
3 sphenopalatine
4 greater palatine
5 superior labial

How to draw

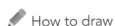

STEP 1

Once again draw the outlines for a sagittal section of the nose; this time include the septal cartilage and bones.

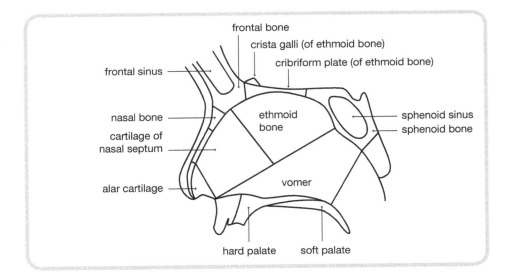

STEP 2

- Draw a dotted circle in the middle of the nasal septal cartilage. This is Little's area.
- Draw a red arrow from just above the cribriform plate to the top of Little's area. This represents the anterior ethmoid artery.
- Draw a 2nd arrow from just posterior to the cribriform plate to the 3 o'clock position on Little's area. This is the posterior ethmoid artery.

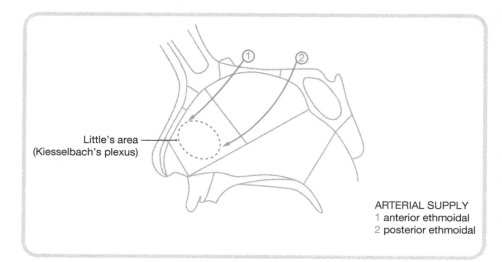

Little's area (Kiesselbach's plexus)

ARTERIAL SUPPLY
1 anterior ethmoidal
2 posterior ethmoidal

STEP 3

- Draw a red arrow from the posterior of the vestibule to approximately a 5 o'clock position on Little's area. This represents the sphenopalatine artery.
- Draw a 4th arrow from the soft palate to the 6 o'clock position, the greater palatine artery.
- Draw a final 5th arrow from the upper lip to the 7 o'clock position; this is the superior labial artery (septal branch).

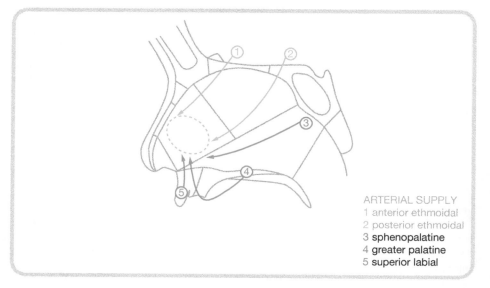

ARTERIAL SUPPLY
1 anterior ethmoidal
2 posterior ethmoidal
3 sphenopalatine
4 greater palatine
5 superior labial

1.4.3 Ear

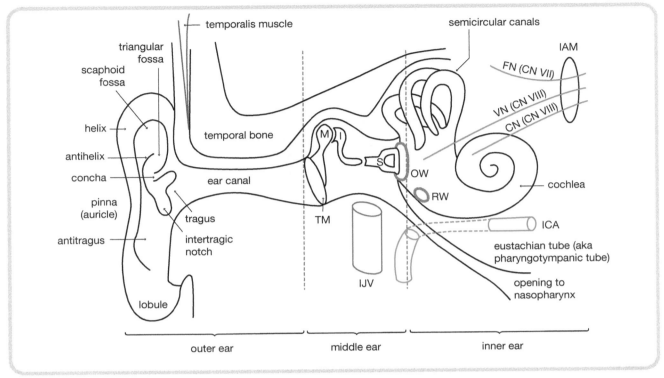

CN	cochlear nerve	**ICA**	internal carotid artery	**RW**	round window
FN	facial nerve	**IJV**	internal jugular vein	**S**	stapes (stirrup)
I	incus (anvil)	**M**	malleus (hammer)	**TM**	tympanic membrane (eardrum)
IAM	internal acoustic meatus	**OW**	oval window	**VN**	vestibular nerve

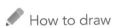 How to draw

STEP 1

- Draw the outer ear and label its features.
- Draw the temporal bone and temporalis muscle above.

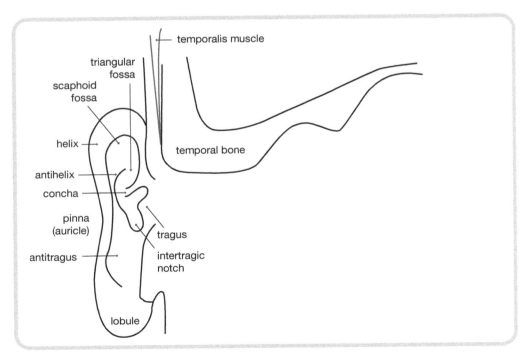

STEP 2

- Draw a 'channel' from the outer ear to the tympanic membrane (TM, eardrum).
- Add a vertical dashed grey line in line with the TM. This divides the outer ear and middle ear.

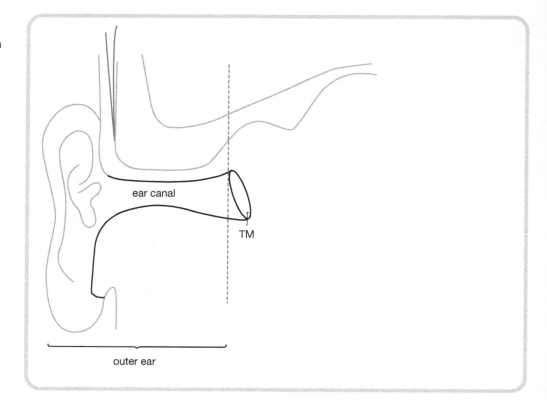

ear canal

TM

outer ear

STEP 3

- Draw a chamber as shown behind the TM, leaving an aperture where the oval window will be (see Step 4).
- Draw the eustachian tube leaving inferiorly and heading medially.
- Add a dashed grey line in line with where the oval window will be. This separates the middle and inner ear.
- Starting at the TM, draw the 3 ossicles: the malleus, incus and stapes.

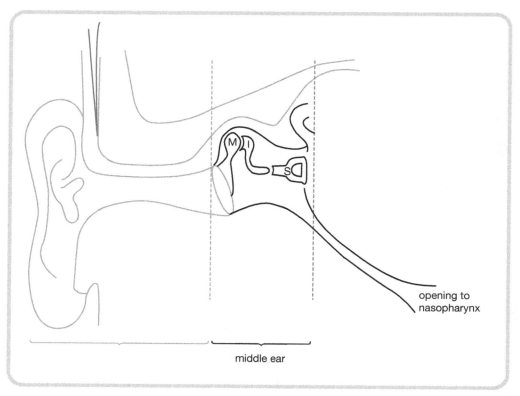

opening to nasopharynx

middle ear

STEP 4

- Draw the oval window, which sits at the edge of the inner ear.
- Draw 3 semicircular canals above and the cochlea (snail shape) below.
- Add the round window on the cochlea.
- Add the ICA and IJV: they run inferiorly to this.
- Label the inner ear.

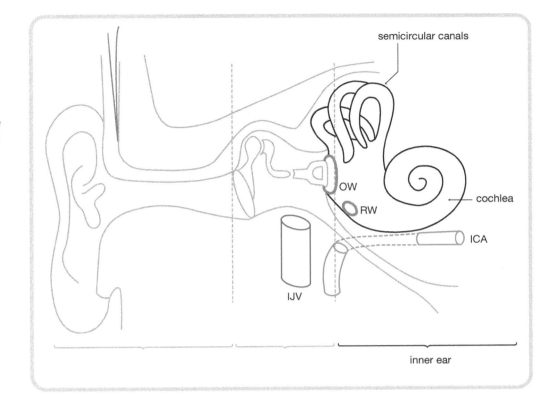

STEP 5

- Draw the internal acoustic meatus.
- Draw the cochlear nerve and vestibular nerve from the cochlear and semicircular canals, respectively; they pass through the internal acoustic meatus with the facial nerve. The chorda tympani (CN VII) is also closely related to the middle ear. This is why surgeons often require facial nerve monitoring with certain types of ear surgery.

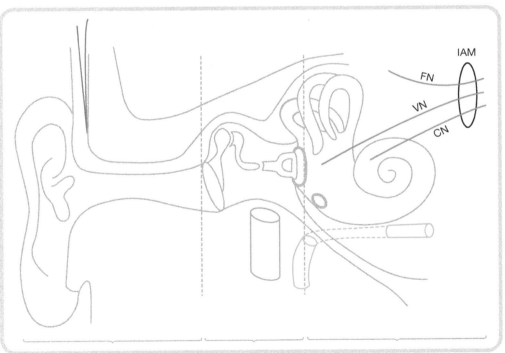

HEARING AND THE EAR: THE AUDITORY SYSTEM

The ear canal, tympanic membrane, bones of the middle ear and cochlea in the inner ear work together to convert sound to electrical signals in the brain.

Sound causes vibration in the air, i.e. a sound wave. It travels through the ear canal and causes vibration of the tympanic membrane. This converts the vibration into mechanical energy transmitted through the malleus, incus and stapes to the oval window. The linkage of these bones causes an increase in amplitude (energy) of the waves. The wave then causes the perilymph in the vestibule of the cochlea to move, leading to transmission of the wave through the endolymph to the tectorial membrane. This causes the hair cells to depolarise and send a signal along the cochlear portion of the vestibulocochlear nerve (CN VIII) to the brain (see *Vestibulocochlear nerve (CN VIII)* in *Section 1.3* for the rest of the pathway).

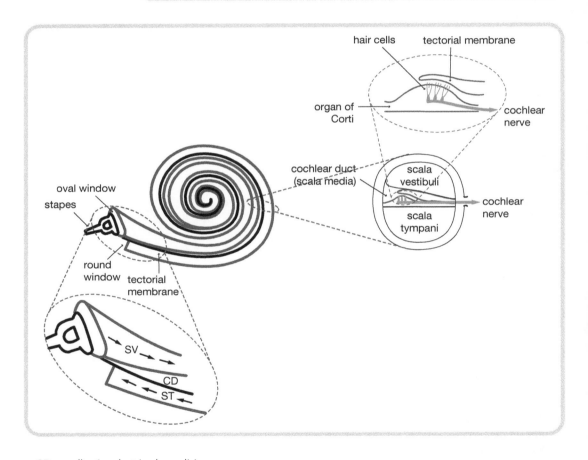

CD collecting duct (scala media)
ST scala tympani
SV scala vestibuli

BALANCE, EQUILIBRIUM AND THE EAR: THE VESTIBULAR ORGANS

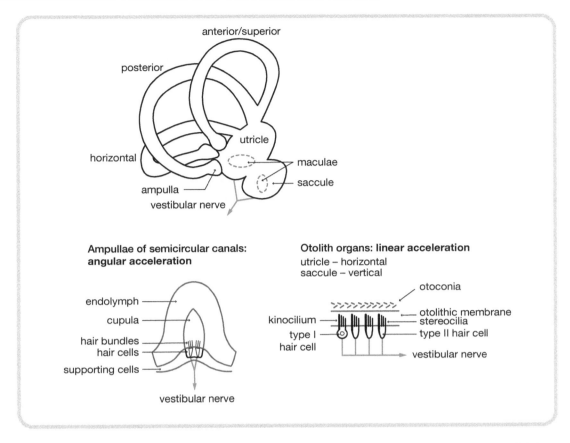

The otolith organs

These consist of 2 membranous sacs called the utricle and saccule. Each sac has a patch of sensory cells called the macula, about 2 mm in diameter. These monitor the position of the head relative to the vertical plane.

- **Utricle:** detects linear acceleration and head tilts in the horizontal plane.
- **Saccule:** detects linear accelerations and head tilts in the vertical plane.

Detection is by hair cells in the maculae. The hair cells have stiff nonmobile projections called stereocilia and flexible mobile projections called kinocilia. Each cell has many stereocilia and only one kinocilium. The stereocilia vary in length; the closer they are to the kinocilium, the longer they are.

The cilia are covered in a gelatinous layer, the otolithic membrane, which has otoconia embedded in it (these are calcium carbonate crystals). Cilia range in length from 1 to 20 μm. If you tilt your head, a time lag in movement of the membrane stimulates the hair cells and the rate of nerve impulses changes.

Semicircular canals

There are 3 semicircular canals with an ampulla in each. They sit in 3 planes:

- **Anterior:** forward and backward motion
- **Posterior:** head tilt, e.g. tipping head forward
- **Horizontal:** swivelling of head.

The ampulla is home to ciliated hair cells; kinocilia projecting from them send signals to sensory epithelium and then the vestibular nerve. The bundles of hair cells lie in a gelatinous mass called the cupula, which is surrounded by endolymph. The kinocilia all lie in the same plane. When the head turns in the plane of the semicircular canal, the endolymph displaces the cupula which causes the cilia to be displaced. Displacement cause all cells to either depolarise or hyperpolarise, depending which direction the head moves. Movements not in plane with that semicircular canal have no effect on its hair cells. As a result, the brain can distinguish the plane and direction of movement.

Each semicircular canal works in alignment with its counterpart on the opposite side of the head. When the head rotates this leads to depolarisation of the semicircular canal on one side and hyperpolarisation of the canal on the other side; this provides information on which way the head rotates and in which direction.

1.4.4 Mouth

THE BLOOD SUPPLY AND SENSORY INNERVATION OF THE LIPS

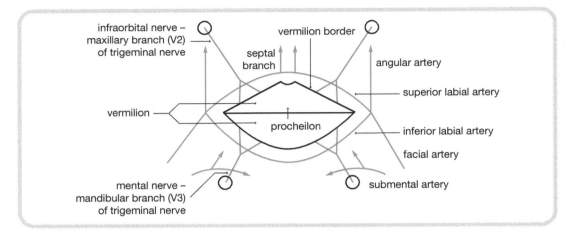

✏️ How to draw

STEP 1

- Draw a simple pair of lips.
- Label the main mass as the vermilion.
- Label the edge of the lip as the vermilion border. The fleshy protuberance in the middle of the top lip is known as the procheilon (or superior labial tubercle).

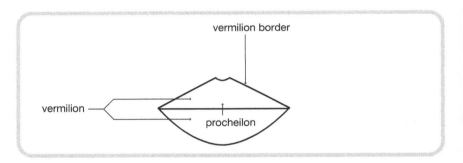

STEP 2

- Starting with the blood supply, encase the lips in a red elliptical shape. The upper half is the superior labial artery and the lower half is the inferior labial artery.
- From the superior aspect draw 2 lines upwards, the septal branches of the superior labial artery.
- Draw a red line up toward the corner of the ellipse on each side. This represents the facial artery which feeds the other arteries.
- Then from the corner of the ellipse draw a line directly upwards on each side to represent the angular artery.

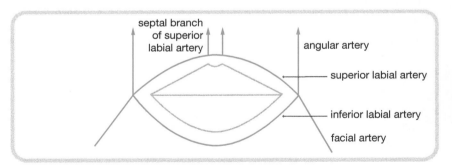

STEP 3

Below the ellipse, draw a snake's tongue shape on each side. These represent the submental arteries (also branches of the facial artery).

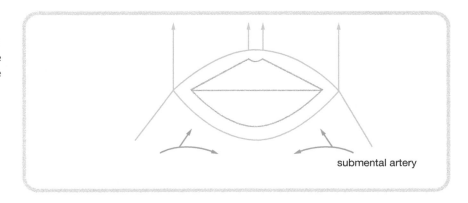

submental artery

STEP 4

- For nerve supply, start by drawing 4 small black circles, 2 above and 2 below; these represent the infraorbital and mental foramina, respectively.
- From each one, draw a snake's tongue to the nearest 1/4 of the lip's edge. Each one supplies the skin in the region it is drawn. The upper ones are the infraorbital nerves, a terminal branch of the maxillary division of the trigeminal nerve. The lower ones are the mental nerves, a terminal branch of the mandibular division of the trigeminal nerve.

Note: motor innervation of orbicularis oris is from the buccal branch and marginal mandibular branches of the facial nerve (CN VII).

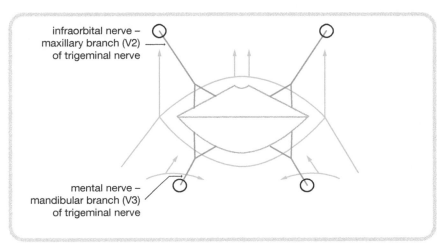

infraorbital nerve – maxillary branch (V2) of trigeminal nerve

mental nerve – mandibular branch (V3) of trigeminal nerve

GROSS ANATOMY OF THE MOUTH

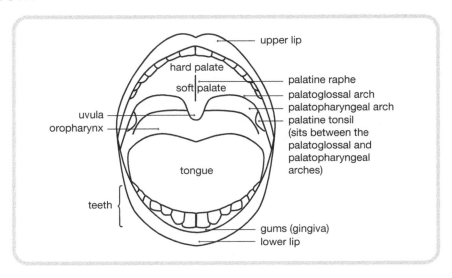

upper lip
hard palate
soft palate
palatine raphe
palatoglossal arch
palatopharyngeal arch
palatine tonsil (sits between the palatoglossal and palatopharyngeal arches)
uvula
oropharynx
tongue
teeth
gums (gingiva)
lower lip

How to draw

STEP 1

- Draw an open mouth by drawing an oval shape with a heart-shaped top.
- Add an inner oval shape that touches the edges of the outer one at the 3 o'clock and 9 o'clock positions; this represents the lips.
- Draw teeth, top and bottom. Try to make them symmetrical. Adults have 8 teeth in each quadrant if their 3rd molars – wisdom teeth – have erupted.

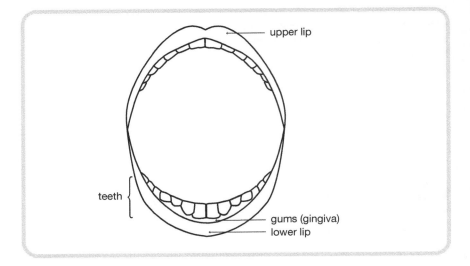

STEP 2

- Draw a rounded M-shaped line from 9 o'clock to 3 o'clock at approximately 1/3 down the open mouth; this represents the hard and soft palate, the uvula and palatoglossal arches. The middle of the M is the uvula.
- Draw a vertical line just above this, the palatine raphe.
- Above the M is the soft palate and then the hard palate anterior to that.

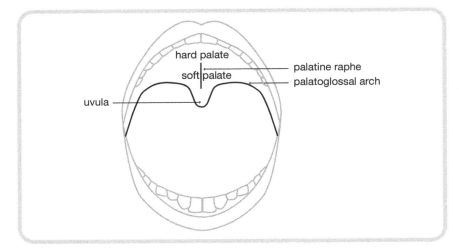

STEP 3

- At 3 o'clock and 9 o'clock draw a semicircle; this represents the palatine tonsils.
- Draw a line below the palatoglossal arch to represent the palatopharyngeal arch; this descends from the soft palate (check out some images online and you'll understand what it actually looks like in reality).
- Finally draw a flattened M from the bottom of the tonsil horizontally; below this is the tongue.

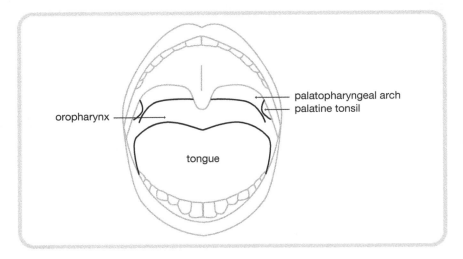

1.5 | Muscles of the face and neck

1.5.1 | Muscles of the face

There are so many muscles in the face that it is hard to learn them. Try to break down the image and follow the step-by-step instructions and diagrams to help you remember even the smallest muscles.

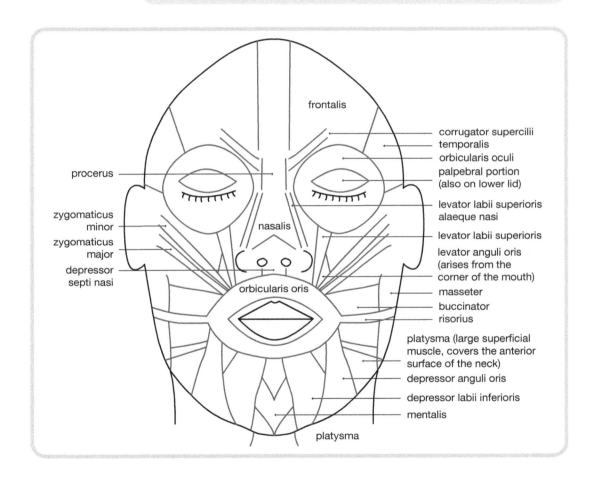

✏️ How to draw

STEP ❶

- Draw the outline of the face and neck.
- Draw the closed eyes and the nose and lips.

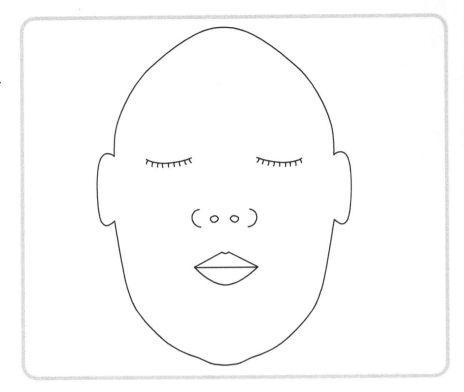

STEP ❷

- Starting with the top of the image draw a large circle around each eye; these are the orbicularis oculi muscles.
- Draw an ellipse in the middle where the upper eyelid would be; this is the palpebral portion of the muscle. There is also a palpebral part where the lower eyelid would be (not shown in image).
- Draw one muscle from the superior aspect of each orbicularis oculi; these are the frontalis muscles.
- Draw a short line from just above each ear to the lateral edge of orbicularis oculi; this marks the lower border of each temporalis muscle (one of the muscles of mastication, see *Section 1.5.2*).

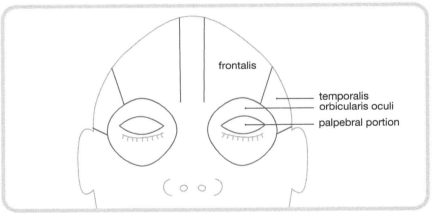

STEP ❸

- Draw a small oblique muscle above the orbicularis oculi on each side as shown. These are the corrugator muscles.
- Between these draw the procerus muscle. These muscles help you frown!

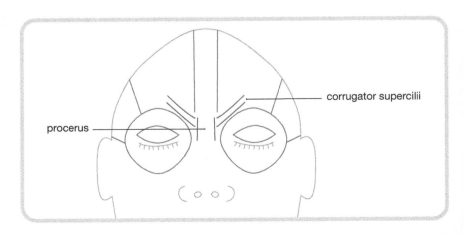

STEP 4

- On the nose the main muscle is the nasalis; draw it across the whole nose as shown.
- Running just lateral to each side of nasalis draw the levator labii superioris alaeque nasi.
- Below the nostrils draw the depressor septi nasi.

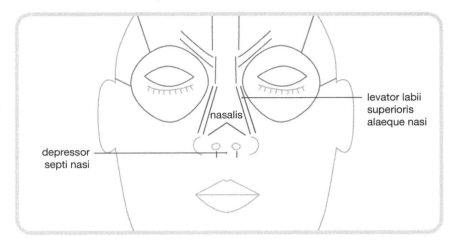

STEP 5

Draw an ellipse around the mouth that has a 'tie' at each corner. The ellipse is the orbicularis oris, the main muscle to purse your lips. The 'tie' is the risorius; this helps you smile.

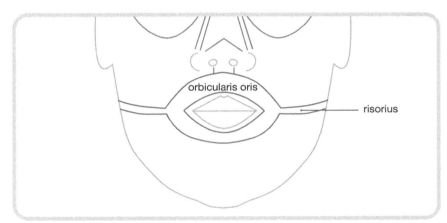

STEP 6

- On each side draw 3 diagonal muscles fanning out from the superior edge of the orbicularis oris. From inner to outer these are: levator labii superioris (LLS), zygomaticus minor (ZMi) and zygomaticus major.
- Between LLS and ZMi draw the small triangular muscle called levator anguli oris, which inserts into the corner of the mouth.

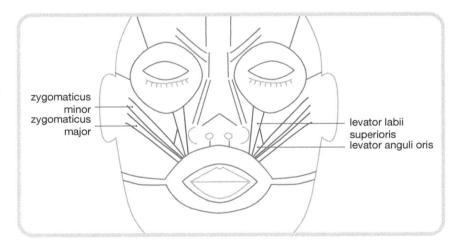

STEP 7

- On each side draw 2 vertical lines, 1 from the corner of the inferior edge of the orbicularis oris muscle and 1 just lateral to its centre.
- Between the 2 lines draw a y shape on the left side of the face and a mirror of y on the right. This demarcates the depressor anguli oris laterally and depressor labii inferioris medially.

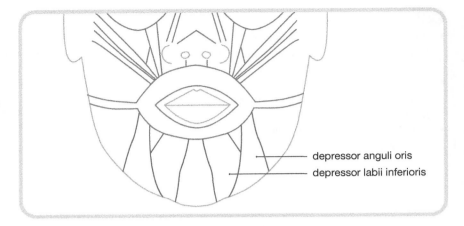

depressor anguli oris
depressor labii inferioris

STEP 8

Draw a V-shaped muscle between the 2 depressor labii inferioris muscles. This is the mentalis.

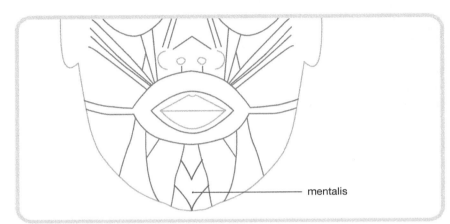

mentalis

STEP 9

Finally, on each side draw the buccinator behind the risorius, the masseter lateral to this and the platysma below and extending into the neck. The masseter is also a muscle of mastication, see *Section 1.5.2*.

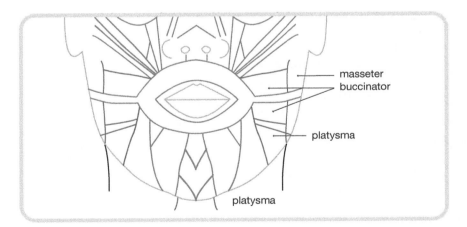

masseter
buccinator
platysma
platysma

1.5.2 Muscles of mastication

The muscles used to elevate, depress and swing the mandible (e.g. for chewing/drinking, etc.) are: temporalis, masseter, and the medial and lateral pterygoid muscles (MP and LP). The MP and LP are termed deep muscles of mastication because they lie behind the zygomatic arch.

Innervation: by branches of trigeminal nerve (V3).

1   coronoid process
2   condylar process
3   angle of mandible
4   ramus of mandible

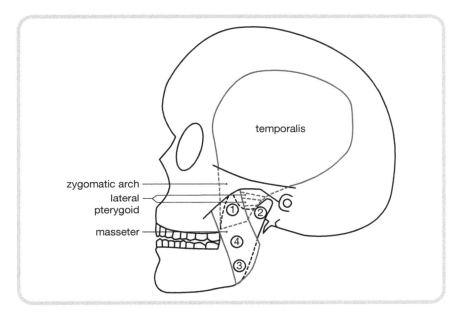

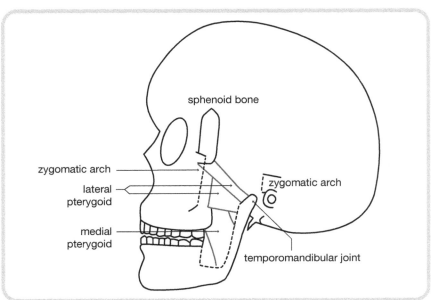

MASSETER AND TEMPORALIS MUSCLES

Masseter muscle

Origin: zygomatic arch.

Insertion: mandible, coronoid process and lateral side of ramus.

Action: contraction causes elevation of the mandible.

(Feel the angle of your mandible and clench teeth: you will feel it here.)

Temporalis muscle

Origin: temporal fossa.

Insertion: medial surface, apex, anterior and posterior borders of the coronoid process.

Action: contraction cause elevation and retraction of mandible.

 How to draw

STEP 1

- Draw a skull, including the zygomatic arch.
- Label the parts of the mandible and use a dashed line to draw its coronoid process and anterior border (muscles will pass in front of these in the next step).

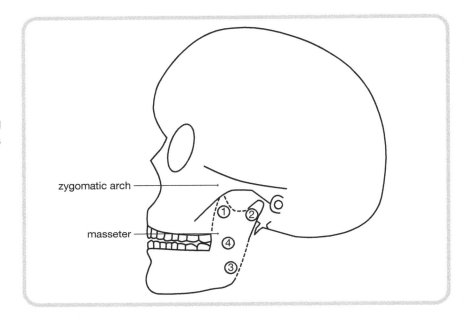

STEP 2

- Draw the masseter muscle from the zygomatic arch and onto the mandible.
- Add the temporalis, using dashed lines to show where it passes under the zygomatic arch and the masseter to insert onto the mandible.
- Return to this figure after drawing the internal muscles of mastication (see below), to add 2 heads of the lateral pterygoid muscle.

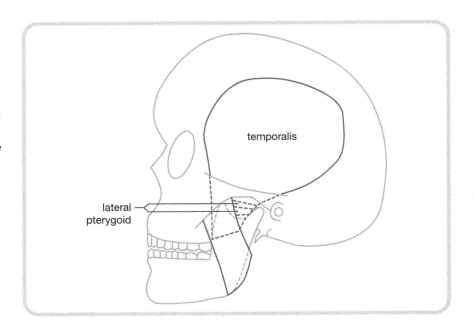

MEDIAL AND LATERAL PTERYGOID MUSCLES

Medial pterygoid muscle

Origin: 2 heads, superficial and deep. Superficial head arises from tuberosity of maxilla. The deep head arises from the medial surface of the lateral pterygoid plate of the sphenoid bone (deep to lower head of lateral pterygoid). The superficial head arises from the tuberosity of the maxilla.

Insertion: medial surface of ramus and angle of mandible.

Action: protrusion and lateral movement of mandible.

Lateral pterygoid muscle

Lies superiorly to medial pterygoid.

Origin: the upper head arises from the infratemporal surface and infratemporal crest of the greater wing of the sphenoid bone. The lower head arises from the lateral surface of the lateral pterygoid plate.

Insertion: upper head inserts into capsule of temporomandibular joint (TMJ). Lower head inserts into condylar process.

Action: the action of the lateral pterygoid muscles is very complicated. The simplified version is that the upper part is responsible for retrusion (pulling mandible inwards) and ipsilateral jaw movement. Lower part responsible for opening mouth, protrusion and contralateral movement of jaw.

 How to draw

STEP 1

- Draw the bottom two-thirds of the same skull but use dashed lines to show parts cut away from the zygomatic arch, the coronoid process and a region of the ramus, and add the sphenoid bone.
- Draw in the posterior border of the maxilla just posterior to the upper teeth.

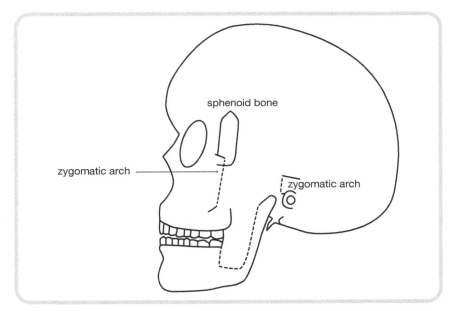

STEP 2

With bone cut away the internal muscles can be drawn.

- Add the 2 heads of the lateral pterygoid muscle, with insertions into the TMJ and condylar process (see text above and *Section 1.5.1* for muscle origins and insertions).
- Add the medial pterygoid. The medial pterygoid muscle has an anteroposterior direction of muscle fibres whereas the lateral pterygoid fibres are horizontally orientated.

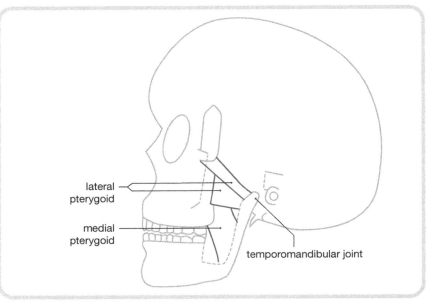

1.5.3   Triangles of the neck

This is a complicated area to learn. Start with the outline (step 1), then the anterior triangle and contents (steps 2–4) and the posterior triangle, then the contents of the posterior triangle (steps 4–5).

The main nerve supply to muscles of the neck are also shown here.

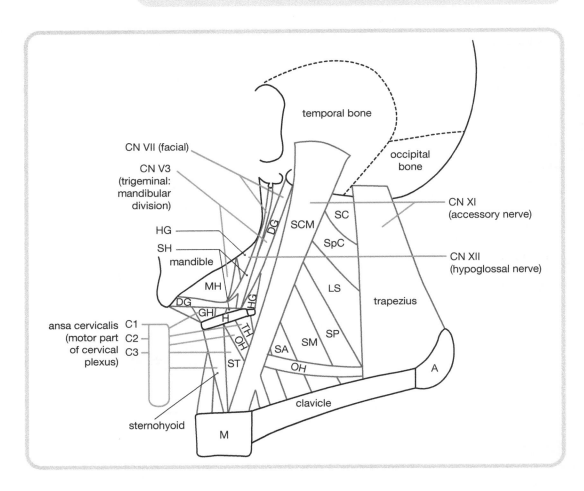

A	acromion	SA	scalenus anterior muscle
DG	digastric muscle	SC	semispinalis capitis muscle
GH	geniohyoid muscle	SCM	sternocleidomastoid muscle
H	hyoid bone	SH	stylohyoid muscle
HG	hyoglossus muscle	SM	scalenus medius muscle
LS	levator scapulae muscle	SP	scalenus posterior muscle
M	manubrium	SpC	splenius capitis muscle
MH	mylohyoid muscle	ST	sternothyroid muscle
OH	omohyoid muscle	TH	thyrohyoid muscle

How to draw

STEP 1

The best approach is to start by drawing the structures that the muscles will attach to.

- Starting at the bottom, draw a square on the left-hand side of the page to represent the manubrium. From here draw a long rectangle heading to the right side of the page, the clavicle. At its end draw a small shape to represent the acromion of the scapula.
- Draw the lower edge of the mandible above the manubrium. As you move backwards draw the lower part of the skull including the temporal bone and occipital bone.
- Draw a hyoid bone as a slim rectangle between the mandible and the manubrium.
- Add dashed lines to delineate the temporal and occipital bones.
- Then draw the left sternocleidomastoid (SCM). This separates the anterior and posterior triangles (see below).
- Add the trapezius, which is the posterior border of the posterior triangle.

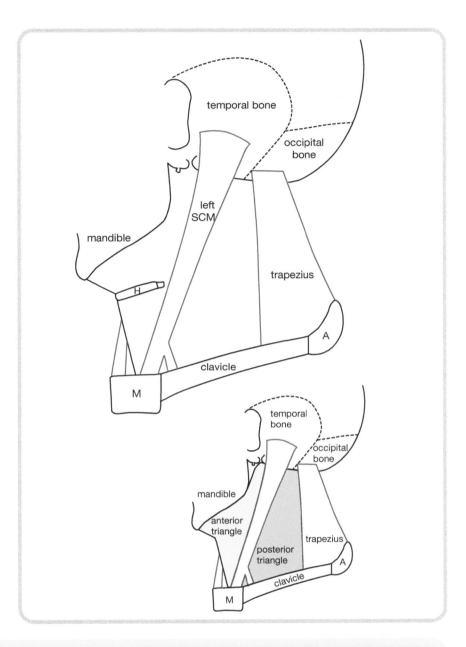

Box 1.3 contents of anterior triangle – part 1

Submental triangle

Submental lymph nodes, submental vein and beginning of anterior jugular vein. Also the geniohyoid and mylohyoid muscles.

Submandibular triangle

Submandibular gland, facial artery and vein, submental artery, mylohyoid artery, mylohyoid muscle, hyoglossus muscle, middle pharyngeal constrictor muscle, external carotid artery, lower part of parotid gland and facial nerve.
More deeply: internal carotid artery, internal jugular vein and vagus nerve. Other nerves include hypoglossal, mylohyoid and glossopharyngeal nerves.

STEP 2

- The digastric muscle has two muscle bellies (di = 2). Draw the digastric muscle from the mental process via the hyoid bone to the mastoid process (like a sling).
- Then draw omohyoid, another muscle with 2 bellies: from the hyoid, under SCM, to the lower edge of trapezius. It attaches to the scapula out of sight.

Now the 4 subdivisions of the anterior triangle and the 2 subdivisions of the posterior triangle become more obvious:

- **Anterior triangle:** divided into the submental, submandibular (sometimes known as digastric), carotid and muscular triangles.
- **Posterior triangle:** divided into 2 triangles, the occipital triangle above the omohyoid and the subclavian (or supraclavicular) triangle below.

The contents of the triangles are listed in Boxes 1.3–1.5.

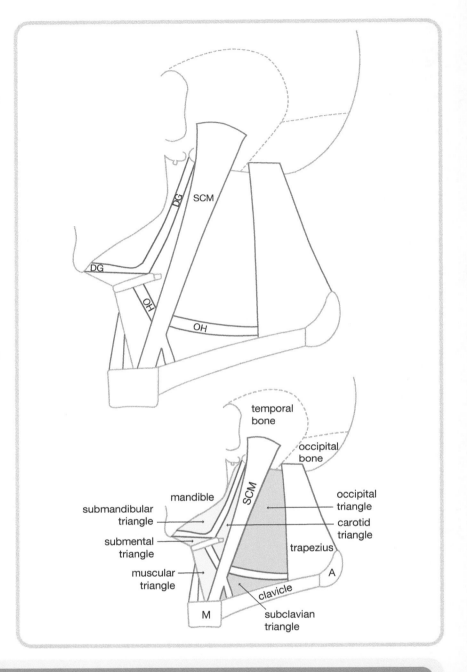

Box 1.4 contents of the subdivisions of the anterior triangle – part 2

Carotid triangle

Arteries: superior thyroid artery, lingual artery, facial artery, occipital artery, ascending pharyngeal artery.
Veins: branches of internal and external jugular veins, e.g. superior thyroid vein, lingual vein.
Nerves: hypoglossal nerve and ansa cervicalis, vagus nerve and accessory nerve.
Other: upper portion of larynx and lower part of pharynx.
Some of the structures are sometimes obscured by SCM and so could be thought of as 'outside' the triangle. I have included all structures that may be seen in it.

Muscular triangle (inferior carotid triangle)

Sternohyoid, sternothyroid and thyrohyoid muscles (collectively they may be called the infrahyoid muscles).
Deep to these structures are: oesophagus, trachea, thyroid gland, lower part of larynx plus inferior thyroid artery and recurrent laryngeal nerve.

STEP 3

- Draw the geniohyoid muscle in the submental triangle. Geniohyoid is deep to mylohyoid and therefore not normally seen in this view.
- Draw the stylohyoid (with DG muscle perforating it), mylohyoid and hyoglossus muscles in the submandibular triangle.

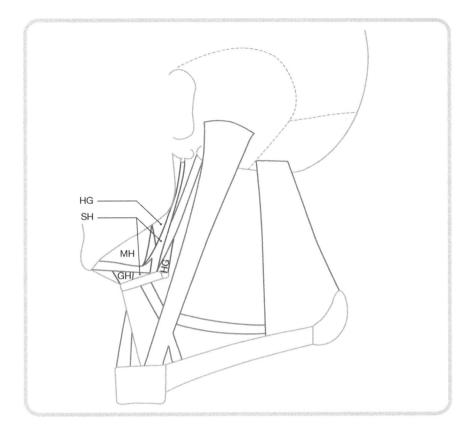

STEP 4

- Draw the thyrohyoid muscle in the carotid triangle.
- Then draw the sternohyoid and sternothyroid muscles in the muscular triangle. Thyrohyoid is superior to sternohyoid, and sternothyroid and thyrohyoid are normally deep to sternohyoid.

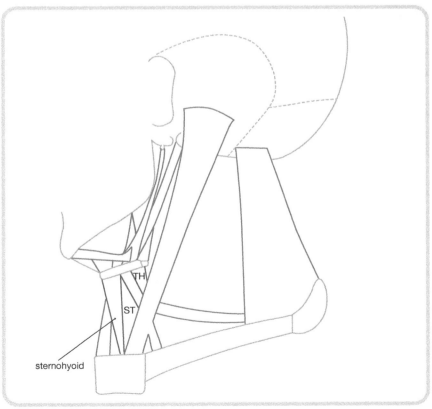

STEP 5

- To draw the muscular contents of the posterior triangle of the neck, draw 6 lines in a fan shape from the SCM.
- Details of muscle origins and insertions in the sections below will help with this.

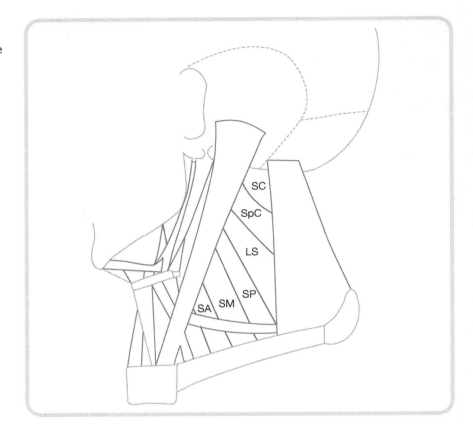

STEP 6

Finally add the nerve supply to the neck, as shown.

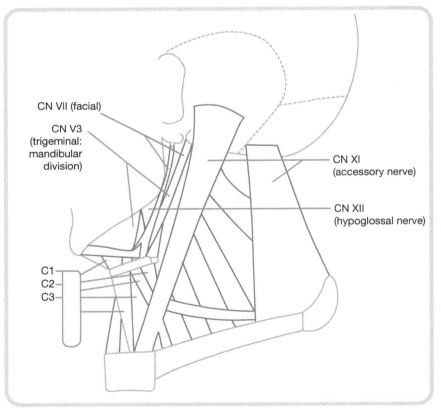

Box 1.5 contents of posterior triangle

Occipital triangle

(Located above inferior belly of omohyoid.)

Nerves and plexuses: spinal accessory nerve (CN XI), branches of cervical plexus.

Vessels: subclavian artery, transverse cervical artery, suprascapular artery and part of external jugular vein.

Lymph nodes: occipital and supraclavicular.

Muscles: inferior belly of omohyoid muscle, semispinalis capitis, splenius capitis, levator scapulae, and scalenus anterior, medius and posterior.

Supraclavicular triangle (subclavian triangle)

(Located below inferior belly of omohyoid.)

Nerves: part of the brachial plexus trunks, nerve to subclavius, and sometimes the phrenic nerve (C5).

Vessels: third part of the subclavian artery.

Muscles: lower parts of the scalene muscles.

MUSCLES DEFINING BOUNDARIES OF ANTERIOR AND POSTERIOR TRIANGLES

Sternocleidomastoid muscle

(Name describes origin and insertion points.)

Origin: manubrium of sternum and medial aspect of clavicle.
Insertion: mastoid process of temporal bone.
Action: rotation of head and lateral flexion of the neck.
Innervation: spinal part (C2–C3) of accessory nerve (CN XI).
Blood supply: upper part: branches of the occipital and posterior auricular arteries; middle part: superior thyroid artery; lower part: suprascapular artery.

Trapezius muscle

Origin: medial third of superior nuchal line, external occipital protuberance, spinous processes of C7 to T12 and the nuchal ligament.
Insertion: lateral third of clavicle, medial aspect of acromion and spine of scapula.
Action: superior fibres draw scapula superomedially, extension of head and neck, lateral flexion of head and neck (ipsilateral), contralateral rotation of head; middle fibres draw scapula medially; inferior fibres draw scapula inferomedially.
Innervation: motor function by accessory nerve (CN XI), sensation via anterior rami of C3 and C4.
Blood supply: upper third: branch from occipital artery; middle third: superficial cervical artery or branch of transverse cervical artery; lower third: dorsal scapular artery.

MUSCLES DEFINING SUBDIVISIONS OF ANTERIOR AND POSTERIOR TRIANGLES

Digastric muscle (suprahyoid muscle)

(Name reflects fact muscle has 2 bellies, anterior and posterior.)

Origin: posterior belly arises from mastoid notch (temporal bone); anterior belly arises from anterior lower mandible.

Insertion: posterior and anterior bellies join as an intermediate tendon which perforates stylohyoid and inserts into hyoid bone.
Action: depresses mandible and elevates hyoid bone; involved in complex jaw action such as speaking, swallowing, chewing and breathing.
Innervation: posterior belly by digastric branch of facial nerve (CN VII); anterior belly by mylohyoid nerve, a branch of inferior alveolar nerve which itself branches from mandibular branch of trigeminal nerve (CN V3).
Blood supply: branches of facial, posterior auricular, occipital and lingual arteries.

Omohyoid muscle (see below)

THE SUPRAHYOID AND INFRAHYOID MUSCLES OF THE ANTERIOR TRIANGLE

Suprahyoid muscles: stylohyoid, digastric, geniohyoid, mylohyoid.
Infrahyoid muscles: omohyoid, thyrohyoid, sternohyoid, sternothyroid.
Other: hyoglossus.

Stylohyoid muscle

Origin: styloid process of temporal bone.
Insertion: perforated by digastric tendon before inserting into hyoid bone.
Action: elevates hyoid bone during deglutition (swallowing).
Innervation: stylohyoid branch of facial nerve (CN VII).
Blood supply: branches of the facial artery, posterior auricular and occipital artery.

Digastric muscle (see above)

Geniohyoid muscle

(Name derived from 'genio', meaning chin.)

Origin: mental spine of mandible.
Insertion: hyoid bone.

Action: moves hyoid bone forward and upwards in deglutition; dilates upper airway in respiration; assists in depressing mandible.
Innervation: fibres of C1 (ansa cervicalis) travelling alongside hypoglossal nerve (CN XII).
Blood supply: branches of lingual artery.

Mylohyoid muscle

Origin: mandible.
Insertion: hyoid bone.
Action: raises floor of oral cavity, elevates hyoid bone and tongue, important in speech and deglutition, depresses mandible.
Innervation: mylohyoid nerve, a branch of inferior alveolar branch of trigeminal nerve (CN V3).
Blood supply: sublingual branch of lingual artery, the mylohyoid artery (a branch of the inferior alveolar artery from the maxillary artery) and the submental branch of the facial artery.

Omohyoid muscle

(Name derived from Greek 'omos', meaning shoulder, and hyoid, its 2 attachments.)

Has 2 muscle bellies separated by an intermediate tendon, superior and inferior. Fascial sheath around intermediate tendon holds muscle in position by anchoring it to clavicle and 1st rib.
Origin: inferior belly arises from upper border of scapula; it then passes behind SCM and becomes tendinous and changes direction to become superior belly of omohyoid.
Insertion: superior belly inserts into lower border of hyoid bone.
Action: depresses hyoid bone.
Innervation: ansa cervicalis of cervical plexus (C1–C3).
Blood supply: branches of superior and inferior thyroid arteries, lingual arteries.

Thyrohyoid muscle

Origin: thyroid cartilage of larynx.
Insertion: hyoid bone.
Action: elevates thyroid, depresses hyoid bone.
Innervation: fibres from the first cervical spinal nerve which branches from the hypoglossal nerve (CN XII).
Blood supply: superior thyroid artery and lingual artery.

Sternohyoid muscle

Origin: medial end of the clavicle, the sternoclavicular ligament and the manubrium of sternum.
Insertion: hyoid bone.
Action: depresses hyoid bone.
Innervation: ansa cervicalis of cervical plexus (C1–C3).
Blood supply: superior thyroid artery.

Sternothyroid muscle

Origin: manubrium of sternum.
Insertion: thyroid cartilage.
Action: depresses thyroid cartilage.

Innervation: ansa cervicalis of cervical plexus (C1–C3).
Blood supply: superior thyroid artery and lingual artery.

Hyoglossus muscle

Origin: whole length of greater cornu of hyoid bone.
Insertion: side of tongue.
Action: depresses and retracts tongue.
Innervation: hypoglossal nerve (CN XII).
Blood supply: sublingual branch of lingual artery and submental branch of facial artery.

MUSCLES OF THE POSTERIOR TRIANGLE

- Omohyoid (see above)
- Semispinalis capitis
- Splenius capitis
- Levator scapulae
- Scalenus anterior
- Scalenus medius
- Scalenus posterior.

Semispinalis capitis

Origin: transverse processes of T1–T6 and cervical spinous processes of C1–C5.
Insertion: occiput.
Action: neck extension, ipsilateral rotation of neck.
Innervation: greater occipital nerve.
Blood supply: descending branches of occipital artery and superior intercostal arteries.

Splenius capitis

Origin: spinous process of C7 to T3.
Insertion: mastoid process of temporal bone and superior nuchal line of occipital bone.
Action: extend, rotate and laterally flex head.
Innervation: lateral branches of posterior ramus of spinal nerves C3/4.
Blood supply: muscular branches of occipital artery.

Levator scapulae

Origin: posterior tubercles of transverse processes of C1–C4.
Insertion: medial border of scapula.
Action: elevates scapula (as the name suggests!).
Innervation: C3, C4 and dorsal scapulae nerve (C5).
Blood supply: transverse cervical and ascending cervical arteries.

Scalenus anterior

Origin: transverse processes of C3–C6.
Insertion: scalene tubercle on 1st rib and ridge of 2nd rib.
Action: lifts 1st rib, rotation and ipsilateral flexion of the neck.
Innervation: anterior ramus of C4–C6.
Blood supply: ascending cervical artery (a branch of the inferior thyroid artery).

Scalenus medius

Origin: posterior tubercles of C2–C7.
Insertion: 1st rib, between tubercle and subclavian groove.

Action: lifts 1st rib, ipsilateral flexion of the neck.
Innervation: anterior ramus of C3–C8.
Blood supply: ascending cervical artery (a branch of the inferior thyroid artery).

Scalenus posterior

Origin: posterior tubercles of the transverse processes of C5–C7 (some books say C4–C6).
Insertion: outer surface of 2nd rib.
Action: lifts 2nd rib, ipsilateral flexion of neck.
Innervation: anterior ramus of C6–C8.
Blood supply: ascending cervical artery (a branch of the inferior thyroid artery).

Chapter 2
Vertebral column and the back

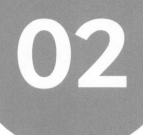

2.1 Classes of vertebrae

Here are a few notes to help. It is also a good idea to research on the internet or in a textbook the differences between the vertebrae. There are some lovely tables that will help you to differentiate between them.

Cervical vertebrae

These are the smallest vertebrae. Each has 3 foramina – 1 vertebral and 2 transverse. A cervical vertebra is fairly flat when you look at it from the side. The first and second cervical vertebrae are atypical (see *Section 2.2: Cervical vertebrae: atlas and axis*).

Thoracic vertebrae

Thoracic vertebrae are bigger than cervical vertebrae but smaller than lumbar vertebrae. The thoracic vertebral body is heart-shaped. Thoracic vertebrae all have 1 vertebral foramen. The spinous processes are longer and thicker than cervical vertebrae and they are directed caudally. The transverse processes are quite large and the costal facets (a key indicator for thoracic vertebrae) sit at each distal point; this is where the ribs meet the vertebrae. The articular facets are oriented vertically. When you look down on the main body and processes it looks a bit like a T-shape.

Lumbar vertebrae

These vertebrae have the largest body. They also all only have 1 vertebral foramen. When you look down on them they look as though they have 5 projections due to the facet joints.

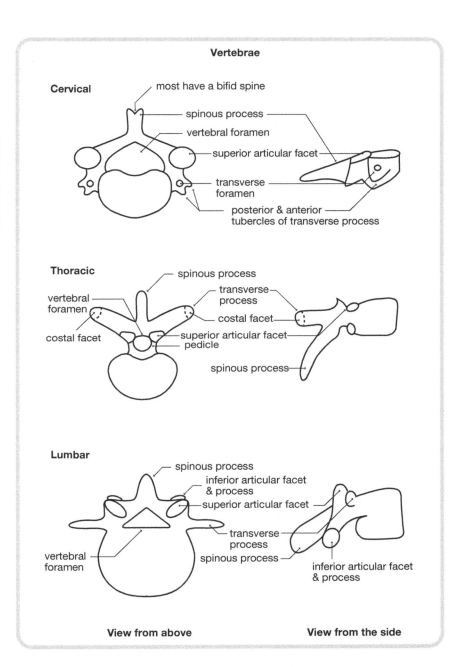

Vertebrae

Cervical
- most have a bifid spine
- spinous process
- vertebral foramen
- superior articular facet
- transverse foramen
- posterior & anterior tubercles of transverse process

Thoracic
- spinous process
- vertebral foramen
- transverse process
- costal facet
- costal facet
- superior articular facet
- pedicle
- spinous process

Lumbar
- spinous process
- inferior articular facet & process
- superior articular facet
- transverse process
- vertebral foramen
- spinous process
- inferior articular facet & process

View from above   **View from the side**

2.2 Cervical vertebrae: the atlas and axis

The atlas is the name for the C1 vertebra. With the axis (C2) it forms the atlanto-axial joints, which together allow axial rotation.

- **Atlanto-occipital joints:** these connect the skull and vertebral column to allow flexion and extension in the sagittal plane (nodding of the head).
- **Atlanto-axial joints:** these allow rotation of the head.

The 3 images of these 2 vertebrae show the articular surfaces (in italic) of these joints. The first image is the superior view of the atlas. The second and third show the axis from an anterior view and a superior view.

The atlas (C1) has no body and is a ring-like shape, it is formed from an anterior and posterior vertebral arch that join at 2 lateral masses. A fracture in C1 is known as a Jefferson fracture.

The axis (C2) is very different from all other vertebrae as it has a distinctive protrusion from the upper surface of the body, known as the odontoid process or dens. Separation of the odontoid process from the vertebral body is known as os odontoideum. This fracture may cause nerve compression. It is not to be confused with a hangman's fracture, which is fracture of the 2 pedicles in C2 and is usually caused by hyperextension injury to the neck. In a hangman's fracture C2 usually lies anterior to C3.

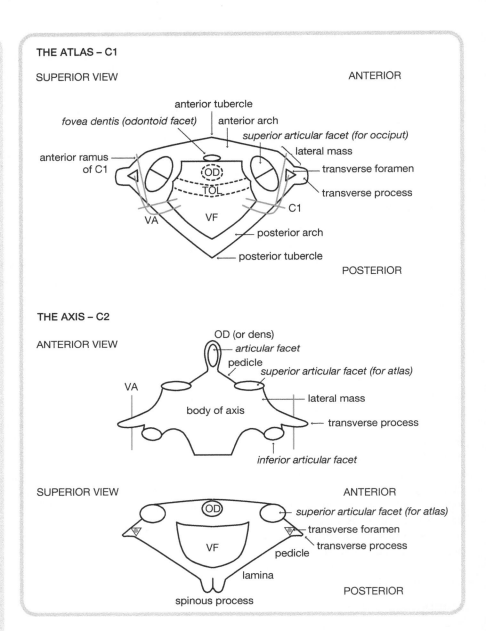

THE ATLAS – C1

SUPERIOR VIEW — ANTERIOR

- anterior tubercle
- *fovea dentis (odontoid facet)*
- anterior arch
- *superior articular facet (for occiput)*
- anterior ramus of C1
- lateral mass
- OD
- transverse foramen
- TOL
- transverse process
- VA — VF — C1
- posterior arch
- posterior tubercle

POSTERIOR

THE AXIS – C2

ANTERIOR VIEW

- OD (or dens)
- *articular facet*
- pedicle
- *superior articular facet (for atlas)*
- VA
- lateral mass
- body of axis
- transverse process
- *inferior articular facet*

SUPERIOR VIEW — ANTERIOR

- OD
- *superior articular facet (for atlas)*
- transverse foramen
- VF
- transverse process
- pedicle
- lamina

POSTERIOR

spinous process

OD	odontoid process
TOL	transverse odontoid ligament
VA	vertebral artery
VF	vertebral foramen

To keep things simple, I have drawn an image showing the spinal tracts, ascending and descending, on one side and the cell body/interneurones/motor neurones on the other side. If you learn the method of drawing this then you will be able to label it easily. If the tract starts with 'spino' it is ascending and if it ends with 'spinal' it is descending. Ascending tracts are solid green and descending tracts are green lines only.

Important points to remember

The arterial supply to the spinal cord is from 2 posterior spinal arteries and 1 anterior spinal artery. The posterior spinal arteries supply the posterior 1/3 of the spinal cord, and the anterior spinal artery supplies the anterior 2/3 of the spinal cord (see *Section 1.2.2: Circle of Willis*).

There are 21 paired radicular arteries from the aorta. Some anatomy textbooks indicate that although the segmental medullary arteries and radicular arteries supply the spinal cord, many radicular arteries are quite small and only supply the nerve roots. The largest radicular artery is the artery of Adamkiewicz, which normally originates from L1 region (see *Section 5.6: Abdominal aorta*). Some sources classify this as one of the segmental medullary arteries.

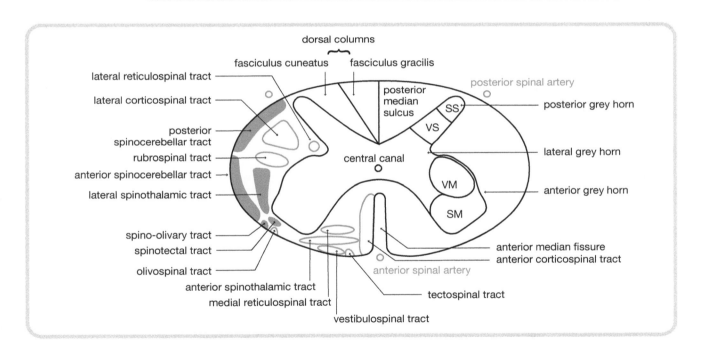

SM   somatic motor – consists of interneurons and lower motor neurons that control motor commands to skeletal muscle.

SS   somatic sensory – represents the location of the interneurons receiving input from somatic sensory neurons.

VM   visceral motor – exists only in the thoracic and upper lumbar region, includes autonomic motor neurons supplying smooth muscle in vessels, viscera and glands. It contains preganglionic visceral motor neurons that project to the sympathetic ganglia.

VS   visceral sensory – represents the location of the interneurons receiving input from visceral sensory neurons.

How to draw

STEP 1

Draw the main structure:

- the spinal cord shape and a 'butterfly', the grey matter in the middle
- a circle in the middle of the butterfly; this is the central canal
- a line from the top of the butterfly posteriorly – this represents the posterior median sulcus.

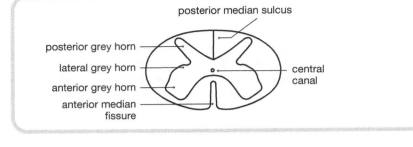

STEP 2

- Draw the 2 posterior spinal arteries and the anterior spinal artery.

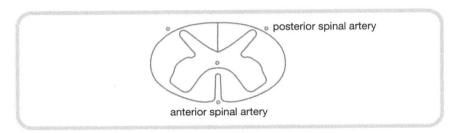

STEP 3

- Draw 4 lines on one side of the grey matter. Label these parts of the grey matter. In the posterior horn are the somatic sensory nuclei and visceral sensory nuclei. In the anterior horn are the visceral motor nuclei and the somatic motor nuclei.

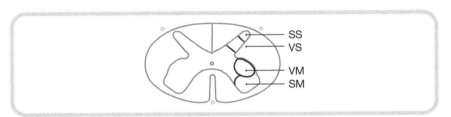

STEP 4

- Draw a line from the centre at the top of the butterfly diagonally. This represents the dorsal columns, the fasciculus cuneatus laterally and fasciculus gracilis medially.

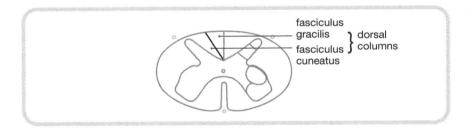

STEP 5

So for the main section.... Start by drawing along the edge, posteriorly to anteriorly. First draw:

- 2 large tracts – these are the posterior spinocerebellar and anterior spinocerebellar tracts
- 2 small tracts – these are the spino-olivary and olivospinal tracts.

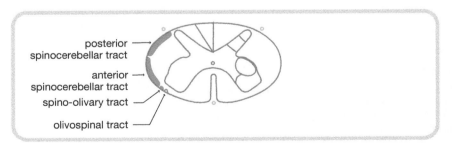

STEP 6

Then draw 3 more tracts finishing just along the anterior median fissure:

- 1 large tract to the right of the olivospinal tract – this is the anterior spinothalamic tract
- 1 small tract – the tectospinal tract
- 1 further large tract – the anterior corticospinal tract.

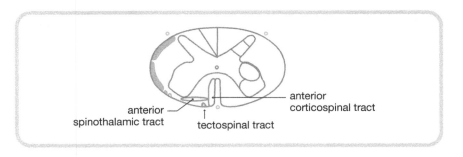

STEP 7

- Add in 2 slightly larger tracts just posteriorly to the tectospinal tract; these are the vestibulospinal and medial reticulospinal tracts.
- Then add in one small tract just behind the olivospinal and spino-olivary tracts; this is the spinotectal tract.

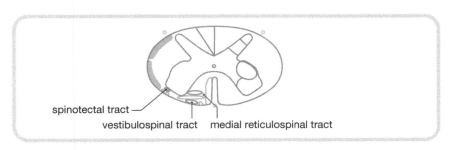

STEP 8

Draw 4 tracts medially to the outer edge, going backwards as shown.

- The most posterior one is the lateral corticospinal tract; this is the biggest.
- The middle one is the rubrospinal tract.
- The one in front of this is the lateral spinothalamic tract.
- In the narrowing of the wing of the butterfly is the lateral reticulospinal tract.

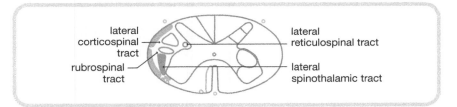

These illustrations simplify the anatomy of the epidural space so you can imagine what it would look like in a sagittal and a horizontal cross-section.

Layers
From the outside to inside: skin, subcutaneous tissue, supraspinous ligament, interspinous ligament and ligamentum flavum.

Contents
Epidural fat, lymphatics, dural sac, spinal nerve roots, and internal vertebral venous plexus.

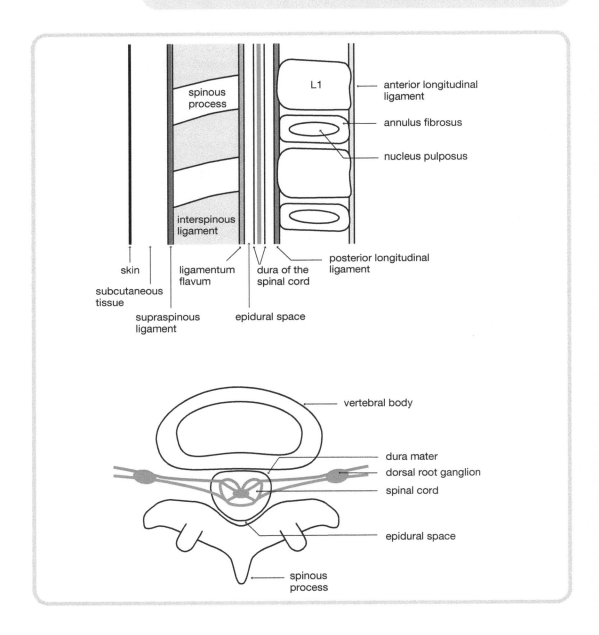

How to draw

STEP 1

- Draw 1 single and 1 pair of longitudinal lines approximately 2 cm apart.
- Draw L1 and L2 vertebrae – in between the vertebrae draw the vertebral discs.

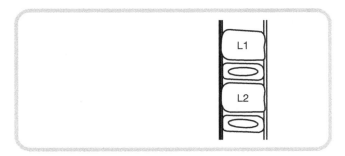

STEP 2

- Draw 3 vertical lines; the middle one is the spinal cord (green).

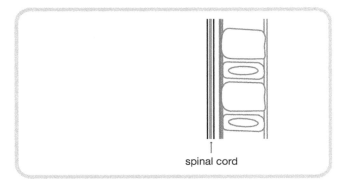

STEP 3

- Draw the ligamentum flavum and then the 2 spinous processes.

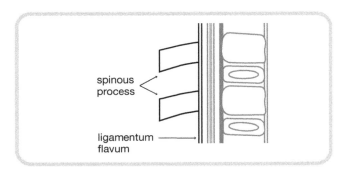

STEP 4

- Draw 4 more vertical lines. The layers are (deep to superficial): interspinous ligament, supraspinous ligament, subcutaneous tissue and skin.

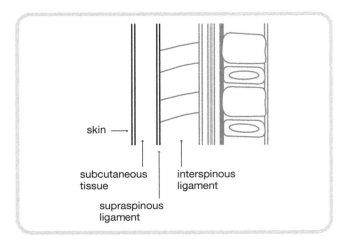

2.5 Paravertebral space

This is a complicated area. I have simplified the image to make it easier to draw and understand (some of the image is representative and not literal). We will draw it as a transverse section viewed from below.

i/c   intercostal

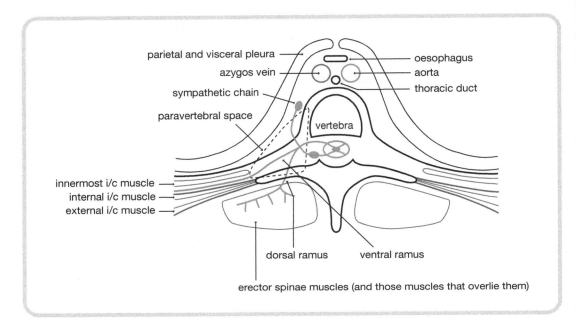

- parietal and visceral pleura
- azygos vein
- sympathetic chain
- paravertebral space
- innermost i/c muscle
- internal i/c muscle
- external i/c muscle
- oesophagus
- aorta
- thoracic duct
- vertebra
- dorsal ramus
- ventral ramus
- erector spinae muscles (and those muscles that overlie them)

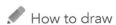 How to draw

 STEP **1**

- Draw the vertebral body as shown.

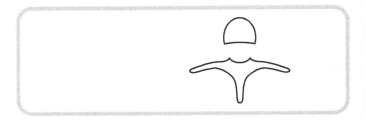

STEP **2**

- Draw 2 oval/square shapes behind the vertebra and lateral to it (as shown). These represent the erector spinae and the latissimus dorsi muscles.
- Draw 4 lines coming out of the transverse process of the vertebrae. These are the external and internal intercostal muscles (at the posterior aspect, the internal intercostal muscles are replaced by the internal intercostal membranes). Draw the innermost intercostal muscle just anterior to these.

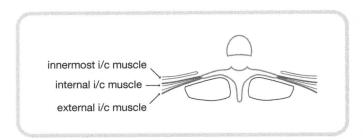

innermost i/c muscle
internal i/c muscle
external i/c muscle

STEP 3

- Draw a line that is anterior to the innermost intercostal muscle and the vertebral body; this is the endothoracic fascia.
- Just in front of this draw the parietal and visceral pleura.

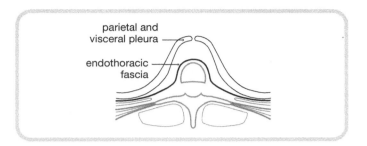

STEP 4

- Draw 1 red circle (aorta), one blue circle (azygos vein), 1 black circle (thoracic duct) and 1 black lozenge (oesophagus) just anterior to the vertebral body.

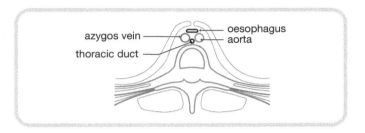

STEP 5

- Draw the simplified version of the spinal cord and branches as shown.
- The dorsal and ventral roots join to form the spinal nerve. The spinal nerve communicates with the sympathetic trunk by the white and grey rami communicantes. The spinal nerve divides into the ventral and dorsal rami. The ventral ramus in the thoracic region is known as the intercostal nerve. The dorsal rami travel to innervate the skin and muscles of the back.

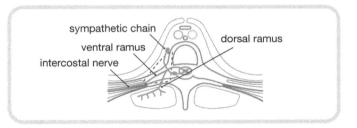

The bony anatomy of the sacrum is fairly simple, but it is important to understand what the sagittal cross-section of the sacral canal looks like, as well as the anterior view. This is for practical purposes, because the sacral hiatus is exploited for caudal epidural injections. The sacral cornua are palpable and are used as landmarks for the procedure.

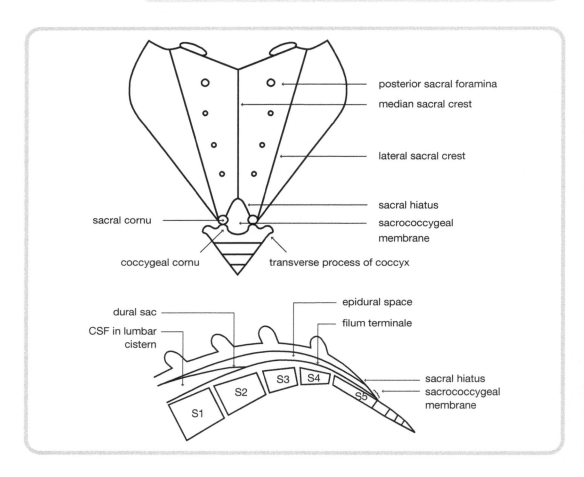

posterior sacral foramina

median sacral crest

lateral sacral crest

sacral hiatus

sacrococcygeal membrane

sacral cornu

coccygeal cornu

transverse process of coccyx

dural sac

CSF in lumbar cistern

epidural space

filum terminale

sacral hiatus

sacrococcygeal membrane

S1 S2 S3 S4 S5

THE CAUDAL SPACE

The volume of the caudal space is normally 30–35 ml in an adult. It contains epidural fat, coccygeal nerves, lymphatics, the filum terminale and the venous plexus.

2.7 Muscles of the back

Table 2.1. Muscles of the back, ordered by depth

Muscles	Depth	Group	Extrinsic or intrinsic
Interspinales, intertransversarii and levator costarum	Deepest	Deep	Intrinsic
Rotatores		Deep	Intrinsic
Multifidus and suboccipital muscles (rectus, obliquus)		Deep	Intrinsic
Semispinalis		Deep	Intrinsic
Erector spinae (iliocostalis, spinalis, longissimus)		Intermediate	Intrinsic
Serratus posterior		Intermediate	Extrinsic
Splenius		Superficial	Intrinsic
Rhomboids		Superficial	Extrinsic
Trapezius	Most superficial	Superficial	Extrinsic

At first sight the muscles of the back may seem easy to learn. However, when you look into the detail the area is a very complicated one. I have tried to simplify it as much as possible without losing detail.

When I think of the muscles of the back, I see them as overlapping layers. Most of the individual muscles span only part of the region from cranium to sacrum. The order in which they are described in the sections below relates to the way the layers overlap. Table 2.1 shows a rough guide of deepest to most superficial.

INTRINSIC MUSCLES

The intrinsic (deep) muscles of the back can be grouped into the superficial, intermediate and deep layers (see Table 2.1).
* The **deep** layer of the intrinsic muscles is the transversospinalis group which consists of the semispinalis (superfical layer of this group), multifidus (middle layer) and rotatores (deepest layer).
* The **intermediate** layer of the intrinsic muscles consists of the erector spinae which are divided into the iliocostalis, longissimus and spinalis.
* The **superficial** layer of the intrinsic muscles consists of the splenius muscles.

EXTRINSIC MUSCLES

Extrinsic muscles of the back are the posterior axio-appendicular muscles that connect the axial skeleton with the proximal appendicular skeleton.
* The **superficial** extrinsic back muscles are trapezius, rhomboid, latissimus dorsi and levator scapulae.
* The **intermediate** extrinsic back muscles consist of the serratus posterior superior and serratus posterior inferior.

The suboccipital muscles are a separate group from those mentioned above because they are the muscles of the suboccipital region found deep to the upper part of the posterior neck.

See *Section 2.7.8* for further information.

Blood supply to most deep muscles of the back is from the deep cervical, posterior intercostal, subcostal and lumbar arteries. It varies between people. Blood supply to more superficial muscles is illustrated in *Section 2.7.8: Intermediate and superficial muscles of the back.*

2.7.1 Interspinales and intertransversarii

These are the deepest muscles of the back. They are well developed in the cervical and lumbar regions, but relatively sparse in the thoracic region. They lie between pairs of adjacent vertebrae the whole length of the spine:

- **an interspinales muscle** joins the spinous processes of adjacent vertebrae
- **intertransversarii** on each side join their transverse processes.

Action:
- **Interspinales:** extension and rotation of the spine
- **Intertransversarii:** lateral flexion of trunk.

Innervation:
- **Interspinales:** posterior rami of spinal nerves
- **Intertransversarii:** anterior and posterior rami of spinal nerves.

Levatores costarum (not shown)
Levatores costarum are 2 groups of 12 small triangular muscles connecting the vertebrae to the lower adjacent ribs. The muscles originate from the end of the transverse processes of vertebrae C7 to T11 and pass obliquely outward to insert onto the rib directly below.

Action: elevates thoracic cage.
Innervation: posterior rami of spinal nerves.

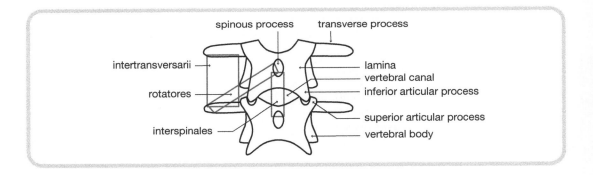

How to draw

STEP 1

Start by drawing a posterior view of 2 simplified vertebrae:

- Draw an almost butterfly-like shape with a central oval to represent the spinous process coming out of the page. Then add 2 small triangular shapes 'behind' the butterfly to represent the parts of the vertebral body that are seen in this view.
- Draw 2 processes out of the top of the 'wings', 1 each side. These are the transverse processes.
- Draw an identical shape below, labelling the articular processes and other structures.

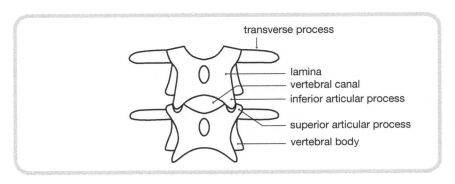

STEP 2

Draw a vertical rectangle from the lower edge of the upper transverse process to the upper edge of the lower transverse process. There is one of these on each side; they are the intertransversarii.

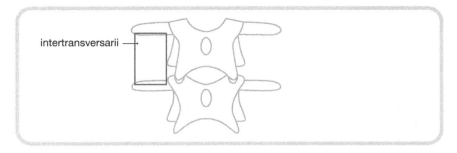

STEP 3

Draw a vertical rectangle from the upper spinous process to the lower spinous process. This is the interspinales muscle.

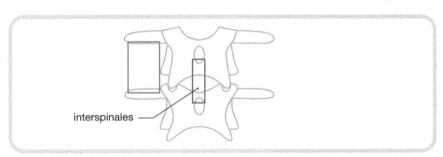

STEP 4

Draw a slanted rectangle from the lateral edge of the lower transverse process to the spinous process of the vertebra above. This is a rotatores muscle (see also *Section 2.7.2: Rotatores and multifidus*). Rotatores are best developed in the thoracic region.

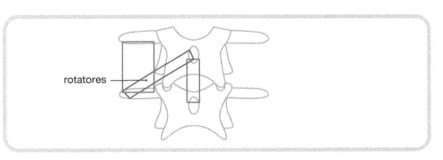

2.7.2 Rotatores and multifidus

ROTATORES

Are best developed in the thoracic region. 11 paired muscles on each side. Each has its origin on the transverse process of a lower vertebra and inserts into the spinous process of the vertebra above, spanning 1–2 segments. They are deep to multifidus.

Action: proprioception and postural control (by stabilising vertebrae). They also aid extension and rotational movements of the vertebral column.

Innervation: posterior rami of spinal nerves.

MULTIFIDUS

Spans from the sacral region to C2. It fills the depression on either side of the spinous processes and is very thin. Its actions stabilise the vertebral column. Each segment of muscle spans 2–4 segments.

Action: stabilise vertebrae during local movements of the vertebral column, lateral flexion of the vertebral column (ipsilateral) and rotation of the vertebral column (contralateral).

Innervation: posterior rami of spinal nerves, and medial branches of posterior rami.

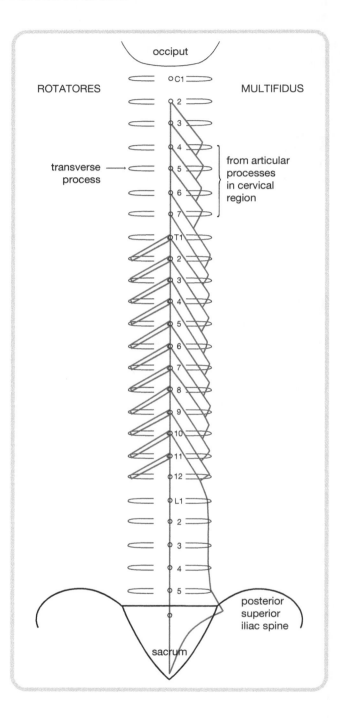

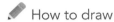 How to draw

STEP 1

- Draw the occiput at the top of the page.
- Label C1 down to L5 down the page and finish with a triangle to represent the sacrum at the bottom.
- Draw each vertebra as a small circle to represent the spinous process.
- Draw the transverse process for each vertebra down both sides.

STEP 2

- Draw a slim rectangle to represent each rotatores muscle. Start on the lateral edge of the left transverse process of T12 and draw the rectangle diagonally up to join the spinous process of the vertebra above, i.e. T11. Do this for all 11 muscles. To keep things simple, don't draw their counterparts on the right side.

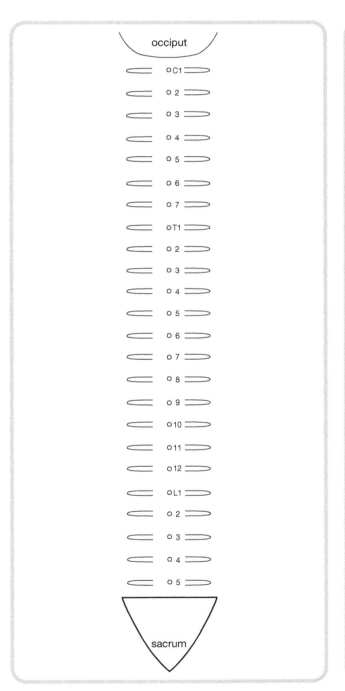

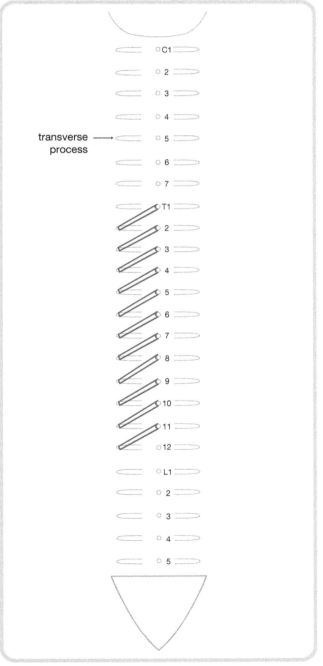

STEP 3

Multifidus is superficial to the rotatores; for simplicity we will draw it only on the right side.

- Add the posterior superior iliac spine on both sides.
- Start drawing the muscle from the origin in the sacrum and posterior superior iliac spine (it also originates in the erector spinae aponeurosis, but this is hard to draw).
- Draw a line joining all spinous processes from the sacrum to C2. This is the insertion point of the muscles.
- In the cervical region, start from C2 working your way down the spine drawing a diagonal downward slanting line from each spinous process to the articular process of the vertebra 2 levels below. For example, join a slanting line from the spinous process of C2 to the articular process of C4. We have drawn multifidus spanning 2 segments but it can span up to 4 segments.
- In the thoracic region, draw from the spinous processes in a similar way but this time take the line further out, to the transverse process of the vertebra 2 below, as shown.
- Note: although we have drawn the lines from the spinous process of the upper vertebra to the transverse process/ articular process of the lower vertebra, the muscle originates at the articular process in the cervical region and transverse process in all other regions. They insert into the spinous processes throughout the spinal column. This is why the multifidus, rotatores and semispinalis are classified as the 'transversospinalis group'. I have drawn it this way to make it easier to draw.
- Do the same all the way down to join the origin of multifidus.

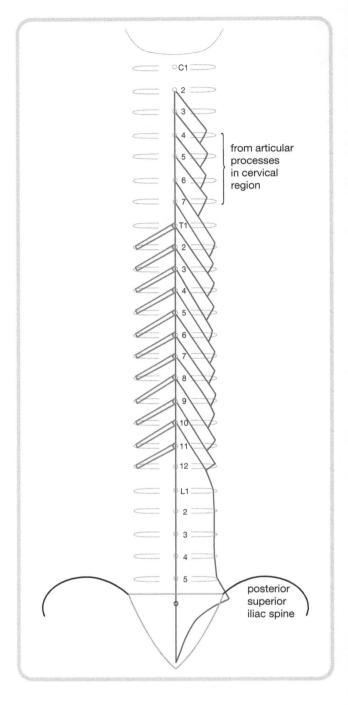

from articular processes in cervical region

posterior superior iliac spine

2.7.3 Erector spinae muscles

Erector spinae is a collective term for the muscle group; it does not refer to one muscle. There are 3 divisions (or columns) on each side; spinalis, longissimus and iliocostalis. These are depicted in slightly different shades of colour to help you distinguish which column is which. Each column has 3 parts. From lateral to medial the 3 columns of muscles are (parts in brackets):

- iliocostalis (cervicis, thoracis and lumborum)
- longissimus (capitis, cervicis and thoracis)
- spinalis (capitis, cervicis and thoracis).

As the erector spinae is complicated we will draw each of the 3 parts for each column separately. The common origin for these muscles is a broad tendon which would be more difficult to show.

Action: extension of the vertebral column and head when acting bilaterally. When acting on one side contraction causes lateral flexion of the vertebral column. They also help maintain the correct posture and curvature of the spine.

Innervation: dorsal rami of the spinal nerves.

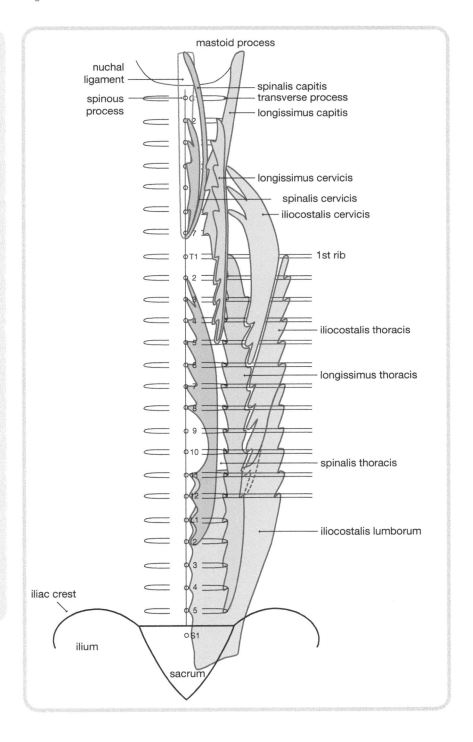

How to draw

STEP 1

- Draw the base of the occiput at the top of the page.
- Draw a circle to represent each spinous process, going down the middle of the page from C1 to L5.
- Draw the sacrum at the bottom of the page and both iliac crests.
- Draw the transverse processes on both sides from C1 down to L5.
- With a less heavy pen or in pencil draw the transverse processes and the ribs from T1 to T12 on the right side.

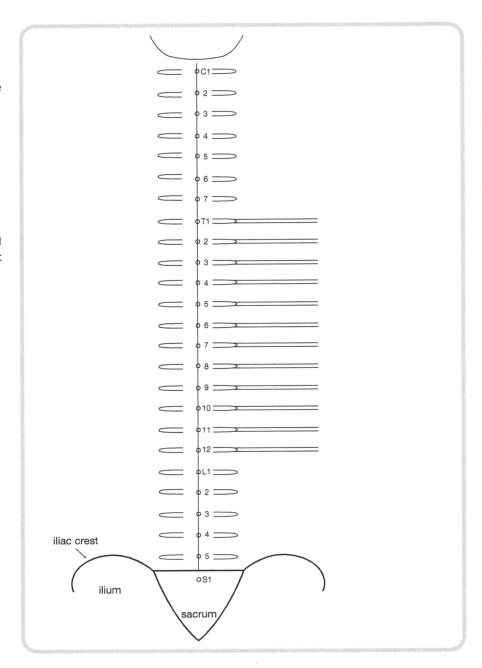

ILIOCOSTALIS MUSCLES

STEP 2

- The erector spinae originates from a broad tendon on the posterior part of the iliac crest, posterior surface of the sacrum, sacral and inferior lumbar spinous processes and supraspinous ligament.
- For iliocostalis lumborum, draw a line from the spinous process of T11 down to S3 just medial to the sacral foramina. Continue the line laterally to the ilium and then head upward over the medial edge of the iliac crest to under the 12th rib.
- Continue the muscle by drawing insertion points on the angle of the ribs 12 to 7. Join the line to the origin at the spinous process of T11. I think it looks a bit like an 'angel wing'.

STEP 3

Draw the iliocostalis thoracis. It arises from tendons on the upper borders of the angle of the rib that the iliocostalis lumborum is inserted into. It then inserts into the upper border of the angle of ribs 1 to 6.

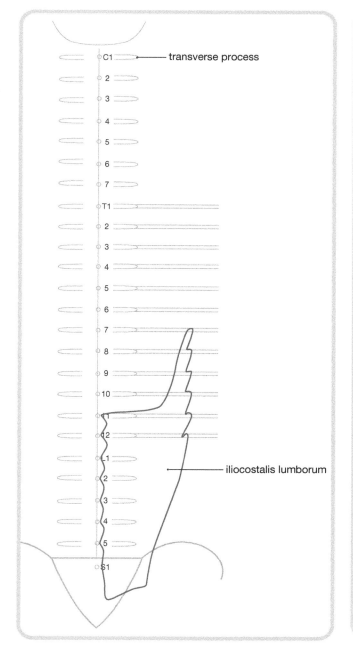

transverse process

iliocostalis lumborum

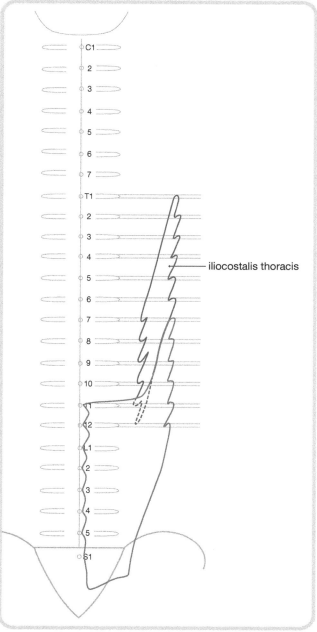

iliocostalis thoracis

STEP 4

- Draw the iliocostalis cervicis with its origin from the angle of ribs 3 to 6 (similar to iliocostalis thoracis) and its insertion into the transverse processes of C4 to C6.
- In reality the 3 parts of iliocostalis can appear as though they are joined, as a result of their overlapping origin and insertion points.

LONGISSIMUS MUSCLES

STEP 5

- The longissimus muscle group (the longest of the erector spinae) has a common origin shared with the erector spinae. The longissimus group lies between the iliocostalis and the spinalis muscle groups.
- Starting from the top, draw the longissimus capitis. Draw a line from the transverse processes of T1 to T5 and the articular processes of C4 to C7 as shown. It is a thin muscle that inserts into the mastoid process of the temporal bone.

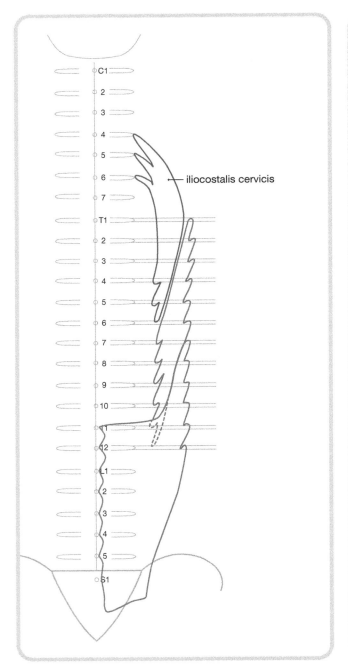

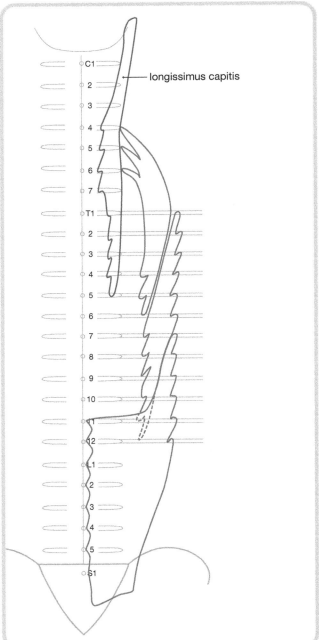

STEP 6

Draw the longissimus cervicis as a thin muscle that runs from the transverse processes of T1 to T5 (part of the broad tendon) and inserts into the transverse processes of C2 to C6. It has a smooth outer edge.

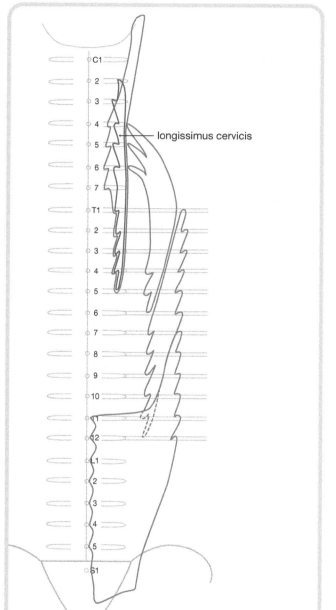
longissimus cervicis

STEP 7

Draw the longissimus thoracis running from the transverse processes of L1 to L5 (part of the broad tendon) and inserting into the transverse processes of T1 to T12 and also ribs 3 to 12. It looks a bit like a 'feather'.

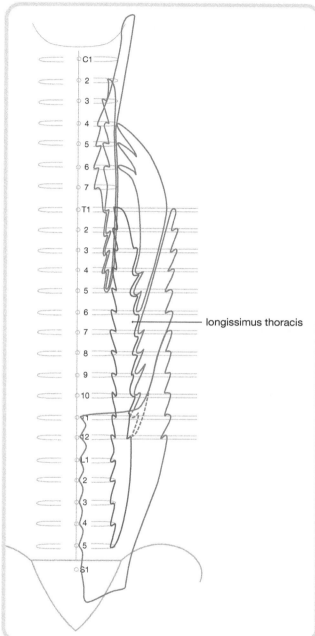
longissimus thoracis

SPINALIS MUSCLES

STEP 8

- Draw the nuchal ligament in grey, from the external occipital crest to the spinous process of C7.
- Draw the spinalis thoracis starting from the spinous processes of T11 to L2 (part of the broad tendon) and extending to the insertion into the spinous processes of T2 to T8.

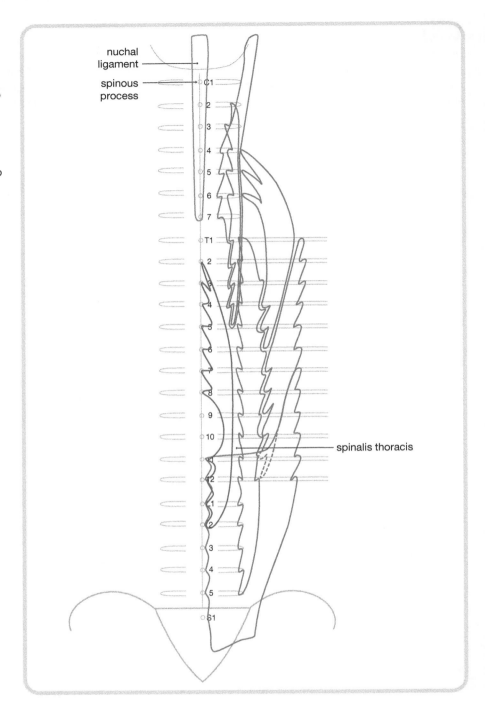

nuchal ligament

spinous process

spinalis thoracis

STEP 9

Draw the spinalis cervicis from the spinous processes of C6 and C7 to the spinous processes of C2–C4. It lies in a similar shape to the spinalis thoracis.

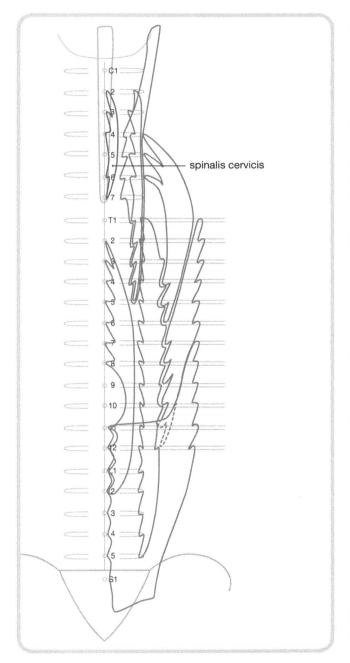

spinalis cervicis

 STEP 10

Draw the spinalis capitis as it runs from the nuchal ligament and the spinous process of C7 to the occipital bone. It is a thin curved muscle.

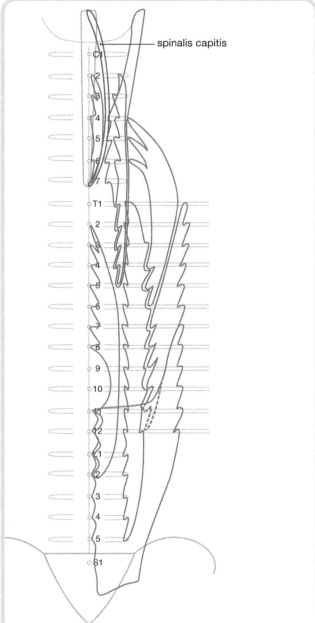

spinalis capitis

2.7.4 Semispinalis muscles

The semispinalis has 3 parts on each side:

- semispinalis capitis
- semispinalis cervicis
- semispinalis thoracis.

Semispinalis capitis originates on the transverse processes of C7–T6 and inserts between the superior and inferior nuchal lines of the skull. Semispinalis cervicis originates on the transverse processes of T6–T12 and inserts onto the spinous processes of C1–C5.

Semispinalis is the superfiical group of the transversospinalis (as per its name, it originates from the transverse processes and then inserts onto the spinal processes of the vertebrae). The semispinalis is divided into 3 parts according to the superior attachments (semispinalis thoracis, semispinalis cervicis and semispinalis capitis). It spans 4–6 vertebral segments.

Sometimes if you bend your neck back and feel for the cervical spinous processes and then straighten your neck, you will feel a tubular muscle on each side of the processes. This is the semispinalis muscle.

Action: extends head and the cervical and thoracic region of the vertebral column, and rotates the cervical and thoracic vertebrae contralaterally.

Innervation: posterior rami of spinal nerves.

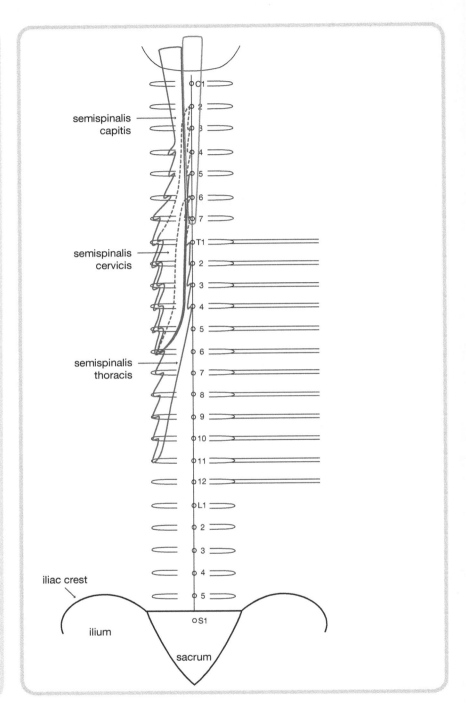

✏️ How to draw

STEP 1

- Start by drawing Step 1 of the erector spinae muscles (*Section 2.7.3*) drawing.
- Draw semispinalis thoracis, with its origin at the transverse processes of T6 to T10, 11 or 12 (varying between people) and insertion into the spinous processes of C6 to T4.
- Use broken lines where shown: the semispinalis thoracis lies deep to the semispinalis cervicis in this region.

STEP 2

- Draw the semispinalis cervicis, with its origin at the transverse processes of T1 to T6 and insertion into the spinous processes of C2 to C5.
- Again, use broken lines where shown: the semispinalis cervicis lies deep to the semispinalis capitis in this region.

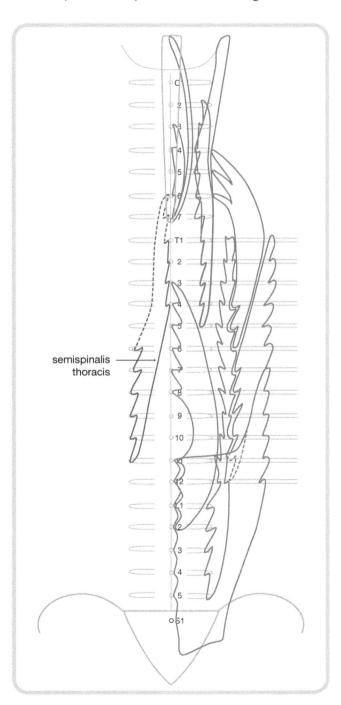

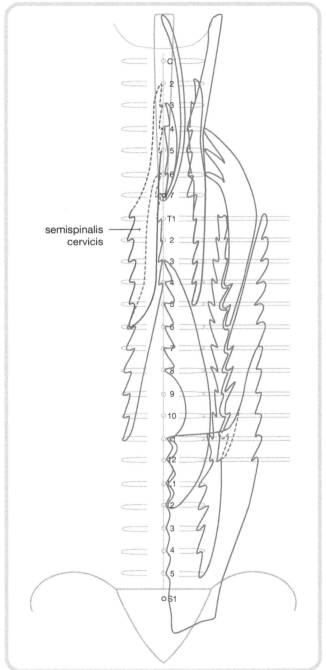

STEP 3

- Draw the semispinalis capitis, starting with the lower part of its origin, on the transverse processes of C7 to T6. This is difficult to show because most of it is the same as the origin of the semispinalis cervicis.
- Continue upwards showing the upper part of the origin, on the articular processes of C4 to C6.
- The semispinalis capitis inserts into the occipital bone between the superior and inferior nuchal lines.

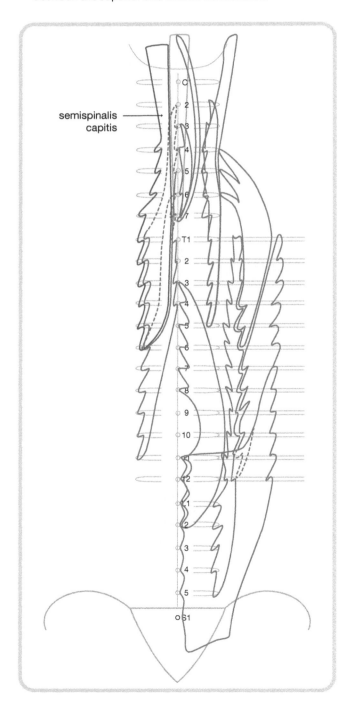

semispinalis capitis

2.7.5　Splenius muscles

There are 2 splenius muscles on each side:

- splenius capitis
- splenius cervicis.

Action: extension of the head and neck (when acting together) and lateral flexion and rotation of the head (when acting alone).

Innervation: posterior rami of spinal nerves.

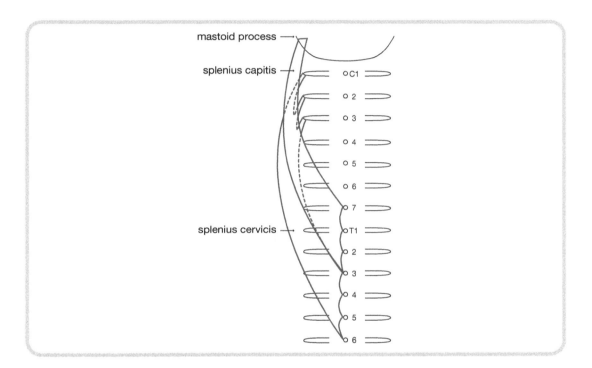

✏️ How to draw

STEP 1

- Draw the occipital bone and spinous processes of C1 to T6. Add the transverse processes to each side. Label the mastoid process (bony projection on the temporal bone).
- Draw the splenius cervicis by starting from the spinous processes of T3 to T6. Draw its insertion into the transverse processes of C1 to C3.

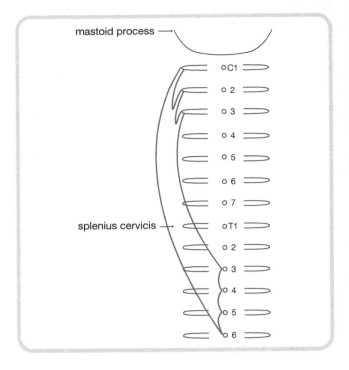

STEP 2

- Draw the splenius capitis by drawing its origin from the spinous processes of C7 to T3 and nuchal ligament and then insertion into the mastoid process of the temporal bone, and the lateral third of the superior nuchal line of the occipital bone. Part of the splenius capitis lies superior to the splenius cervicis.

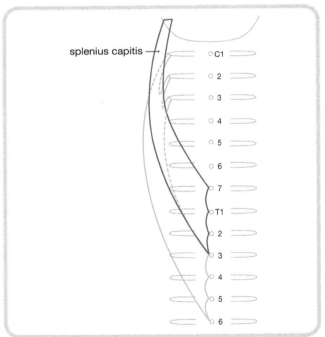

2.7.6 Extrinsic back muscles and muscles of the posterior abdominal wall

Now we will learn to draw the superficial layers of the muscles of the back. The extrinsic back muscles can be divided into 2 groups: the superficial extrinsic back muscles (latissimus dorsi, trapezius, levator scapulae and rhomboids) and intermediate extrinsic back muscles (serratus posterior superior and serratus posterior inferior). The left side of the drawing shows:

- trapezius
- latissimus dorsi.

The right side of the drawing shows

- Extrinsic back muscles
  - levator scapulae
  - rhomboid major and minor
- Muscles of the upper limb
  - supraspinatus, infraspinatus, subscapularis and teres minor (muscles of the scapula, rotator cuff muscles)
- Posterior abdominal wall muscles
  - psoas major and minor
  - quadratus lumborum.

Action: described in tables in drawing steps.

Innervation: described in tables in drawing steps and illustrated in Step 7.

Blood supply: described and illustrated in Step 8.

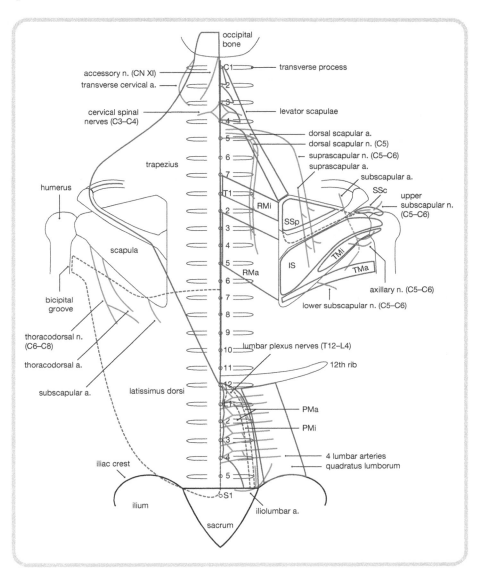

IS	infraspinatus
PMa	psoas major
PMi	psoas minor
RMa	rhomboid major
RMi	rhomboid minor
SSc	subscapularis
SSp	supraspinatus
TMa	teres major
TMi	teres minor

How to draw

SUPERFICIAL EXTRINSIC BACK MUSCLES (TABLE 2.2)

Table 2.2. Superficial extrinsic back muscles (see text for origins and insertions)

Muscle	Action	Innervation
Trapezius	Descending part of the trapezius elevates the scapula. Ascending part depresses the scapula. Middle part (or all parts together) retract the scapula. Ascending and descending parts act together to rotate the glenoid cavity superiorly	Spinal accessory nerve (CN XI) (motor) and C3, C4 spinal nerves (pain and proprioceptive fibres)
Latissimus dorsi	Adducts, medially rotates and extends arm	Thoracodorsal nerve (C6–C8)
Levator scapulae	Elevates the scapula and rotates the glenoid cavity inferiorly	Dorsal scapular nerve (C5) and anterior rami of C3 and C4
Rhomboid major	Retracts the scapula and rotates the glenoid cavity inferiorly; fixes the scapula to the thoracic wall	Dorsal scapular nerve (C5)
Rhomboid minor	Retracts the scapula and rotates the glenoid cavity inferiorly; fixes the scapula to the thoracic wall	Dorsal scapular nerve (C5)

STEP 1

- Draw the occipital bone at the top and a line down the middle of the page.
- At equal spaces label from C1 down to L5.
- At the bottom draw the sacrum and 2 iliac crests.
- Draw the transverse processes on both sides from C1 to L5.

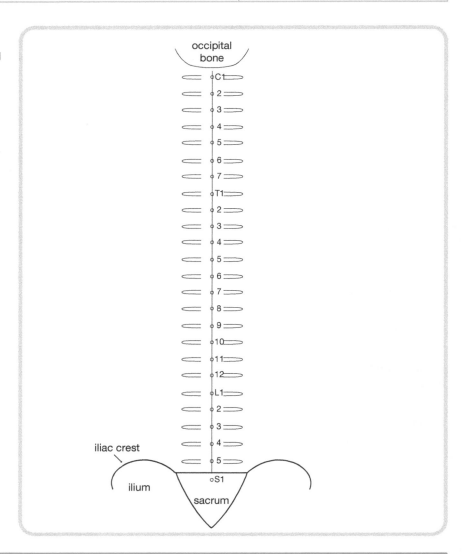

STEP 2

- Draw the outline of the scapula, clavicle and top one-third of humerus on each side. The scapula's inferior angle is normally in line with approximately T7 spinous process. The superior angle of the scapula is around T2. The acromioclavicular joint lies above the outer edge of the scapula. The shape of the scapula is a triangle with a diagonal rectangle from the middle of the medial side up to above the lateral end to represent the spine of the scapula.
- Drawing the trapezius at the same time will help with positioning and size of these bones, as follows.
- The origin of trapezius is the medial third of the superior nuchal line and external protuberance of the occipital bone, nuchal ligament and spinous processes of C7 to T12. Draw this by drawing a line along the occipital bone horizontally from left to right. At the end of this line, turn 90° and draw a line vertically down the spine from here to T12.
- The trapezius then inserts into the spine of the scapula, the acromion and the lateral one-third of the clavicle. Draw a diagonal line from T12 to the start of this insertion into the spine of scapula. Continue the line along the spine of scapula so it curves around the acromion and then runs diagonally to join the outer end of the origin on the occipital bone. Draw a small line from the edge of the trapezius along the lateral one-third of the clavicle to show it inserts here too.

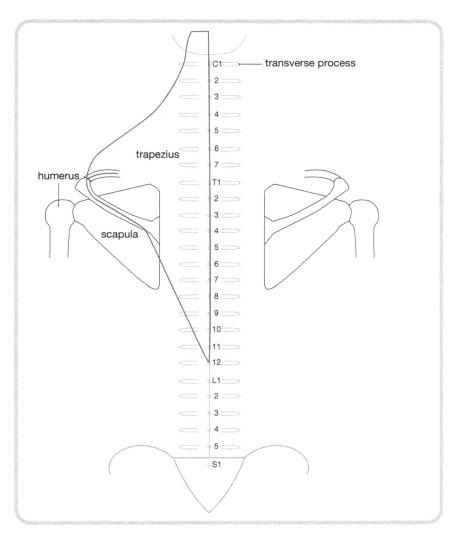

STEP 3

Next, we will draw the latissimus dorsi, a large triangular, flat muscle, with a large origin and small insertion. Where they overlap, the trapezius overlies it.

- Start by drawing a line directly down from the spinous process of T7 to the top of the sacrum (this description and image do not present an accurate point of origin of the latissimus dorsi in this area because here it arises from the thoracolumbar fascia, which is not shown).
- Then draw a curved line along the iliac crest and then upwards to the bicipital groove of the humerus as shown.
- Draw a short line up the medial edge of the humerus; this represents the insertion into the bicipital groove of the humerus. Continue the line passing through the inferior tip of the scapula and joining the start point at T7. The origin of this muscle is also from the inferior angle of the scapula and the lower 3 or 4 ribs.

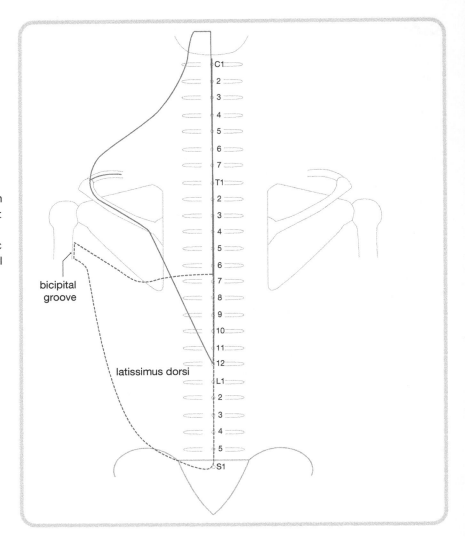

STEP 4

- To draw the levator scapulae, start by drawing its origins from the transverse processes of C1 to C4.
- Draw the rest of the levator scapulae as an elongated rectangle with its base on the medial border of the scapula superior to the root of the spine of the scapula (its insertion).
- Add the 2 rhomboid muscles as follows.
- Draw the origin of the rhomboid minor from the lower part of the nuchal ligament and the spinous processes of C7 and T1. Draw its insertion into the medial border of the scapula around the level of the spine of the scapula.
- Draw the rhomboid major in the same way but slightly bigger. Draw the origin from the spinous processes of T2 to T5, then the insertion into the medial border of the scapula from the level of the spine to the inferior angle; finally complete the rhomboid shape.

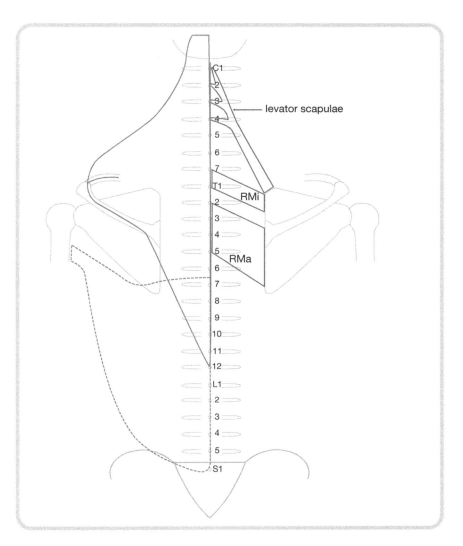

INTRINSIC SHOULDER MUSCLES (TABLE 2.3)

Table 2.3. Intrinsic shoulder muscles (see *Section 7.7.1*)

Muscle	Origin	Insertion	Action	Innervation
Supraspinatus	Supraspinous fossa of scapula	Superior facet of greater tubercle of humerus	Initiates and helps deltoid to abduct the arm; stabilises humerus	Suprascapular nerve (C5–C6)
Infraspinatus	Infraspinous fossa of scapula	Middle facet of the greater tubercle of humerus	Externally rotates arm; stabilises shoulder joint	Suprascapular nerve (C5–C6)
Subscapularis	Subscapular fossa	Lesser tubercle of humerus	Internally rotates and adducts humerus; stabilises shoulder joint	Upper subscapular nerve and lower subscapular nerve (C5–C6) (see Step 7)
Teres minor	Middle part of lateral border of scapula	Inferior facet of greater tubercle of humerus	Laterally rotates arm; stabilises shoulder joint	Axillary nerve (C5–C6) (see Step 7)
Teres major	Posterior surface of the inferior angle of scapula	Crest of the lesser tubercle of humerus (aka the medial lip of the intertubercular sulcus)	Rotates arm medially and adducts arm	Lower subscapular nerve C5/6 (see Step 7)

STEP 5

The 4 muscles that make up the rotator cuff are supraspinatus, infraspinatus, subscapularis and teres minor. As a group they are often referred to as the rotator cuff muscles; they stabilise the shoulder joint by holding the head of the humerus in the glenoid cavity.

- Draw a soft-edged triangle above the spine of scapula; this is the supraspinatus. It passes under the acromion and inserts into the superior facet of the greater tubercle.
- Draw the infraspinatus under the spine of the scapula; include its insertion onto the middle facet of the greater tubercle.
- Starting at the inner edge of the the scapula, draw the subscapularis joining onto the lesser tubercle on the head of the humerus. The subscapularis actually inserts more on the anterior side of the humerus, but is shown here like this so that it is easier to imagine how the rotator cuff lies.
- Finally draw the teres minor just below the infraspinatus, ending on the inferior facet of the greater tubercle on the humeral head.

After drawing the rotator cuff muscles, add the teres major. Show its origin from below the medial end of infraspinatus on the posterior surface of the inferior angle of the scapula and its insertion onto the lesser tubercle of the humerus.

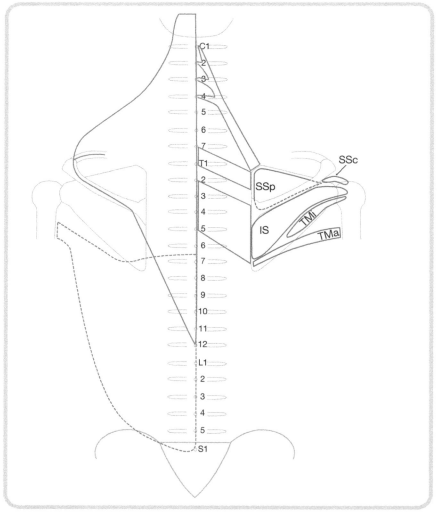

MUSCLES OF THE POSTERIOR ABDOMINAL WALL (TABLE 2.4)

Table 2.4. Muscles of the posterior abdominal wall (see text for origins and insertions)

Muscle	Action	Innervation
Psoas minor	Weak flexor of trunk	Anterior ramus of L1 (see Step 7)
Psoas major	Acting inferiorly, it flexes the thigh; acting superiorly, it flexes the vertebral column laterally	Anterior rami of L1–L3 (some textbooks say L2–L4) (see Step 7)
Quadratus lumborum	Unilateral contraction causes lateral flexion of the trunk Bilateral contraction extends the trunk and fixes 12th rib during inspiration	Anterior rami of T12–L4 (see Step 7)

STEP 6

- Draw the 12th rib.
- Draw the psoas minor in broken lines: draw its origin from the vertebral bodies of T12 and L1, and show it going downwards and anterior to the iliac crest. It inserts into the iliopubic eminence and the pectineal line of the pubic bone (not shown).
- Draw the origin of the psoas major from the sides of the bodies of T12 to L4 vertebrae to the superior edge of the sacrum. It inserts into the lesser trochanter of femur (not shown).
- For the quadratus lumborum, draw a line along the posterior iliac crest (origin) and then turn 90° up to the inferior border of the 12th rib (insertion). The muscle also inserts into the tips of the transverse processes of L1 to L4 (not shown). Finish the rectangle by joining the lines together. The quadratus lumborum lies superficial to the psoas major, overlapping it (not shown).

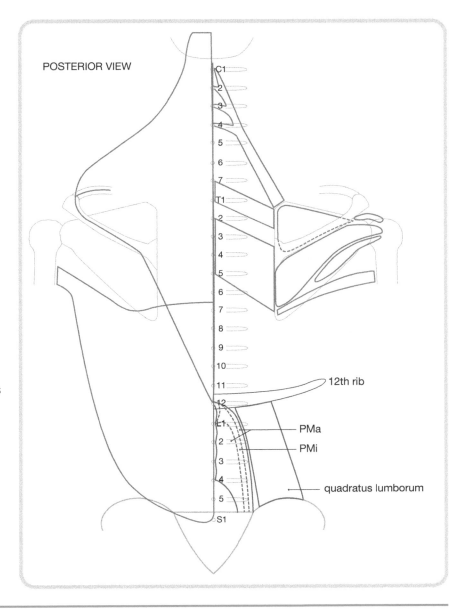

POSTERIOR VIEW

12th rib

PMa

PMi

quadratus lumborum

NERVE SUPPLY

STEP 7

- Starting with the trapezius draw a nerve from the base of the occiput down towards the main part of the muscle; this is the accessory nerve (CN XI; motor). Then draw a nerve in the shape of a snake's tongue from C3 and C4 into the trapezius to represent the cervical spinal nerves (sensory).
- Staying on the left side, from behind the scapula draw a nerve descending into the latissimus dorsi; this is the thoracodorsal nerve (C6–8).
- On the right side draw a nerve from C5 to supply the levator scapulae and both rhomboid muscles; this is the dorsal scapular nerve.
- Draw a nerve from C3–C4 to innervate the levator scapulae (anterior rami of C3/4).
- Draw a nerve from near C5 to innervate the supraspinatus and infraspinatus. This is the suprascapular nerve (C5–C6).
- Add the axillary nerve (C5–C6), which supplies the teres minor, and 2 subscapular nerves (C5/6), upper and lower, that supply subscapularis and teres major, respectively.
- In the lumbar area, draw 4 linked forks or snakes' tongues to innervate the psoas major and quadratus lumborum. These represent nerves from the lumbar plexus (T12–L4).
- Finally draw a short branch from L1, innervating the psoas minor.

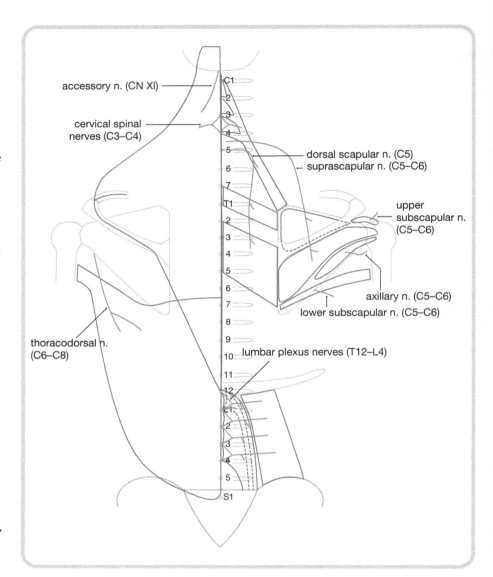

accessory n. (CN XI)

cervical spinal nerves (C3–C4)

dorsal scapular n. (C5)
suprascapular n. (C5–C6)

upper subscapular n. (C5–C6)

axillary n. (C5–C6)
lower subscapular n. (C5–C6)

thoracodorsal n. (C6–C8)

lumbar plexus nerves (T12–L4)

BLOOD SUPPLY

STEP 8

- Draw the transverse cervical artery supplying the trapezius.
- Draw the thoracodorsal branch of the subscapular artery supplying the latissimus dorsi.
- Draw the dorsal scapular artery supplying the levator scapulae and the rhomboid muscles.
- Draw the suprascapular artery for the supraspinatus and infraspinatus.
- On the right side draw the subscapular artery and circumflex scapular branch, using a broken line where it courses anterior to the scapula, and show branches supplying the subscapularis, teres minor and teres major.
- Finally, show supply to the psoas major, psoas minor and quadratus lumborum by 4 lumbar arteries. Add the iliolumbar artery, a branch of the internal iliac artery, coming from below to supply the psoas major and quadratus lumborum.

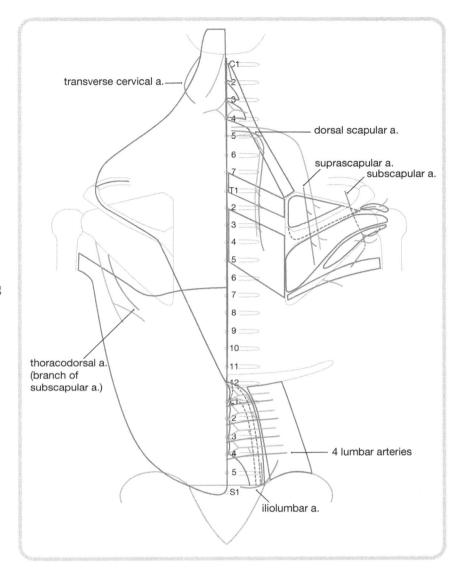

transverse cervical a.

dorsal scapular a.

suprascapular a.
subscapular a.

thoracodorsal a.
(branch of
subscapular a.)

4 lumbar arteries

iliolumbar a.

2.7.7 Serratus posterior muscles

There are 2 serratus posterior muscles, inferior and superior. Serratus posterior muscles are intermediate extrinsic back muscles. The layering of muscles makes them hard to include in illustrations of nearby muscles, but drawing them in isolation is useful to demonstrate their shapes:

- Serratus posterior superior is an upside-down V shape.
- Serratus posterior inferior is a V shape.

SERRATUS POSTERIOR SUPERIOR

Lies deep to the rhomboid muscles and arises from spinous processes of C7, the upper 2 or 3 thoracic vertebrae and the ligamentum nuchae. It passes downwards and laterally and inserts onto the 2nd to 5th ribs.

Action: raises 2nd to 5th ribs and helps with inspiration.

Innervation: the first 4 intercostal nerves.

SERRATUS POSTERIOR INFERIOR

Originates on the spinous processes of T11 to L2 and the supraspinal ligament. It is inserted into the lower 4 ribs in finger-like projections. It lies superficial to the erector spinae and deep to the latissimmus dorsi.

Action: draws lower ribs downward.

Innervation: intercostal nerves 9 to 12.

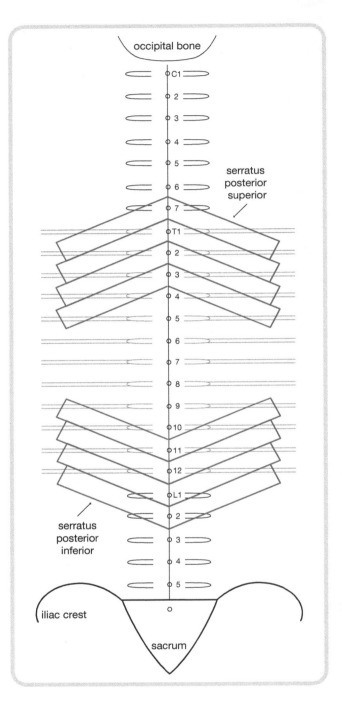

2.7.8 Suboccipital muscles

The suboccipital muscles are in a separate group from the extrinsic and intrinsic back muscles because they are the muscles of the suboccipital region, found deep to the upper part of the posterior neck.

The suboccipital muscles originate on the C1 and C2 vertebrae and all but the obliquus capitis inferior attach to the skull. The obliquus capitis inferior inserts onto the transverse process of C1. There are 4 on each side:

- obliquus capitis inferior
- obliquus capitis superior
- rectus capitis posterior major
- rectus capitis posterior minor.

Action: overall they work together for extension and rotation of the head.
- Obliquus capitis inferior: bilateral contraction of the atlanto-occipital joint causes head extension and unilateral contraction leads to ipsilateral head rotation.
- Obliquus capitis superior: bilateral contraction of the atlanto-occipital joint causes head extension and unilateral contraction leads to ipsilateral lateral flexion of the head.
- Rectus capitis posterior major: bilateral contraction at the atlanto-occipital joint leads to head extension and unilateral contraction at the atlanto-axial joint leads to ipsilateral head rotation.
- Rectus capitis posterior minor: bilateral contraction of the atlanto-occipital joint leads to head extension.

Innervation: suboccipital nerve (posterior ramus of C1).

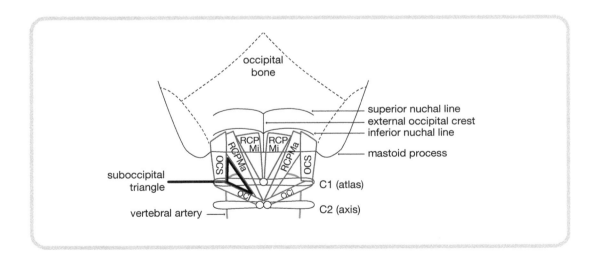

OCI	obliquus capitis inferior
OCS	obliquus capitis superior
RCPMa	rectus capitis posterior major
RCPMi	rectus capitis posterior minor

✎ How to draw

STEP 1

As usual we will start by drawing the framework for the muscles.

- Draw the occipital bone as a W shape with a flattened middle; this is the back of the skull.
- Add dashed lines from the inner edge of the mastoid process up towards where the ear would be; this defines the temporal bone.
- Add a dotted arrowhead from the upper 1/3 of the temporal bone, using dashed lines. This defines the occipital bone below.
- In the centre of the lower half of the occiput, draw an 'aerial antenna shape'. This represents the superior and inferior nuchal lines, and the external occipital crest.
- Centrally, below the skull draw a small circle to represent the spinous process of C1 and two for C2's spinous process. Then draw transverse processes on each side.

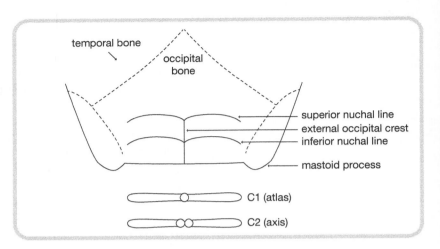

STEP 2

Draw a pair of obliquus capitis inferior muscles as slanted rectangles on each side, originating from the posterior tubercle of the posterior arch of C2 to the lateral edge of the transverse processes of C1 above (producing a V shape).

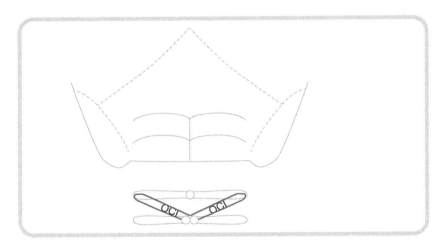

STEP 3

Draw the two obliquus capitis superior muscles: show each one as a trapezoid shape from the lateral end of the transverse process of C1 to the occipital bone between the superior and inferior nuchal lines.

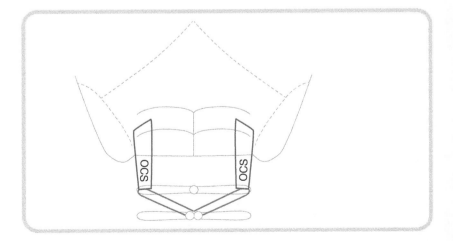

STEP 4

Draw rectus capitis posterior major muscles as trapezoid shapes starting from the spinous process of C2 and ending in the lateral part of the inferior nuchal line of the occipital bone on each side.

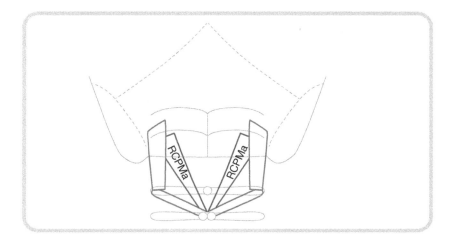

STEP 5

Draw the final pair, the rectus capitis posterior minor muscles: each one is a triangular muscle from the posterior tubercle of the posterior arch of C1 to the medial part of the inferior nuchal line of the occipital bone.

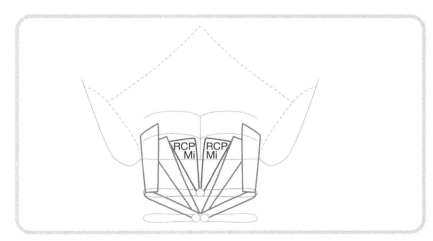

STEP 6

- Draw the outline of a triangle from the lower medial edge of obliquus capitis superior, the lateral edge of rectus capitis posterior major and the upper edge of obliquus capitis inferior. This is the suboccipital triangle; its roof is semispinalis capitis. The suboccipital triangle is a useful anatomical landmark to locate the vertebral artery.
- Add the vertebral artery.

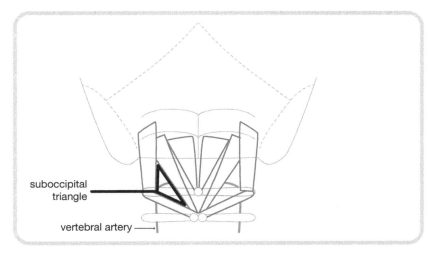

Chapter 3
Cardiac anatomy

03

Gross anatomy of the heart

The heart may seem simple but on closer examination its structure and function are difficult to learn and remember. It is a muscular structure that pumps deoxygenated blood to the lungs to be oxygenated and then returns it to the heart to be pumped around the body, providing oxygen to body tissues. Circulation through the heart changes at birth, with closure of the foramen ovale. This leads to formation of a depression called the fossa ovalis.

There are 4 valves:

- **2 atrioventricular valves**: tricuspid and mitral (bicuspid)
- **2 semilunar valves**: pulmonary and aortic.

Valves ensure the unidirectional flow of blood through different heart chambers and prevent back flow of blood (regurgitation). The atrioventricular valves open during diastole to allow the ventricles to fill with blood. During systole the atrioventricular valves are forced closed as the blood is pushed into the aorta and pulmonary arteries via the semilunar valves, the aortic and pulmonary valves respectively. The chordae tendineae prevent the tricuspid and mitral valves from prolapsing into the atria as a result of the high pressure of systole.

Remember to break the usual convention when colouring pulmonary vessels: use red for pulmonary veins delivering oxygenated blood from the lungs, and blue for pulmonary arteries transporting deoxygenated blood to the lungs.

ELECTRICAL ACTIVITY

The electrical activity of the heart is depicted by green arrows in the image. The electrical impulse starts in the sinoatrial node (SAN), a group of specialised myocardial cells that spontaneously produce an electrical action potential. It passes through the atria to the atrioventricular node (AVN). The impulse slows as it passes through the AVN, and then continues down through the ventricles via the bundle of His and Purkinje fibres. The impulse also travels via Bachmann's bundle (the interatrial tract), a branch of the anterior internodal tract that lies in the left atrium (as shown).

This cycle repeats itself after each impulse generated by the SAN. The rate is controlled by sympathetic and parasympathetic innervation. This is discussed separately in *Section 3.3: Innervation of the heart*.

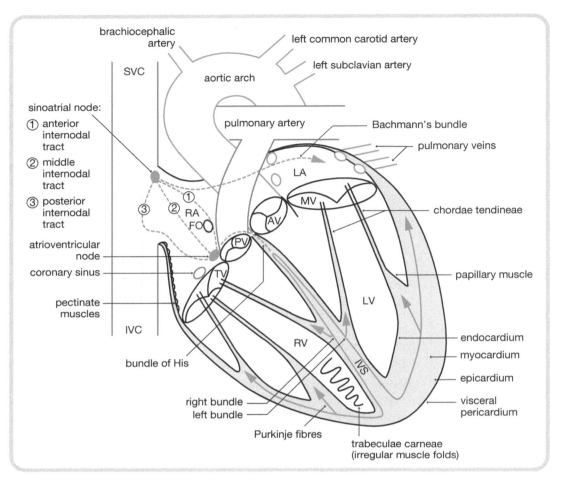

AV	aortic valve	MV	mitral valve (bicuspid valve)
FO	fossa ovalis (site of foramen ovale in the fetus, now covered and closed)	PV	pulmonary valve
		RA	right atrium
IVC	inferior vena cava	RV	right ventricle
IVS	interventricular septum	SVC	superior vena cava
LA	left atrium	TV	tricuspid valve
LV	left ventricle		

The pericardium is a double-layered membrane enclosing the heart and roots of the great vessels. It holds the heart in position in the mediastinum and provides lubrication while pumping.

It consists of an outer fibrous layer and an inner double, serous layer. The outer layer is called the fibrous pericardium. Going inwards, the serous layers are called the parietal and visceral layer, respectively; they have pericardial fluid between them. The visceral layer is also known as the epicardium. These layers cover the fatty connective tissue layer that contains the coronary blood vessels, the myocardium and endocardium.

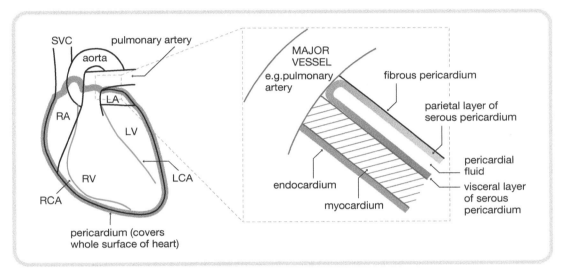

LA	left atrium	RCA	right coronary artery
LCA	left coronary artery	RV	right ventricle
LV	left ventricle	SVC	superior vena cava
RA	right atrium		

Innervation of the heart

This is very complicated because many things affect heart rate. I'll try and simplify it as best I can.

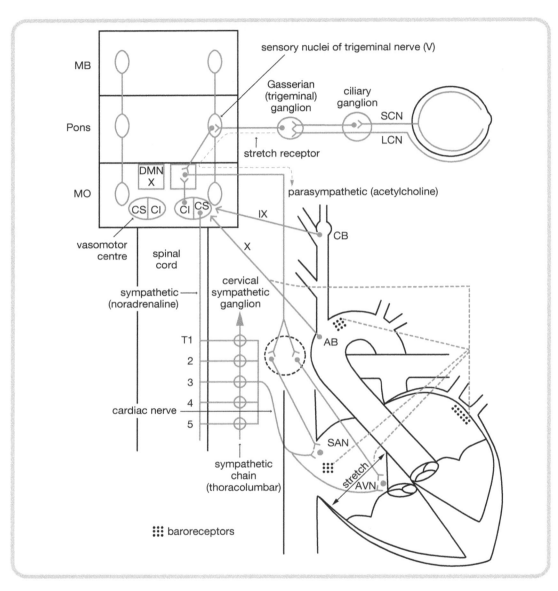

AB	aortic body	**LCN**	long ciliary nerve
AVN	atrioventricular node	**MB**	midbrain
CB	carotid body	**MO**	medulla oblongata
CI	cardioinhibitory centre	**SAN**	sinoatrial node
CS	cardiostimulatory centre	**SCN**	short ciliary nerve
DMN X	dorsal motor nucleus of vagus nerve (X)		

3.3.1 Autonomic control of heart rate

Heart rate is mainly controlled from within the medulla oblongata in the brainstem. The cardioregulatory (vasomotor) centre comprises the cardioaccelerary or cardiostimulatory (CS) centre and the cardioinhibitory (CI) centre.

The nervous supply is autonomic:

- sympathetic fibres arise from the CS centre
- parasympathetic fibres arise from the CI centre

Sympathetic innervation is mainly from the vagus nerve. The right vagus nerve primarily innervates the sinoatrial node (SAN) and the left vagus nerve innervates the atrioventricular node (AVN). This can vary between people.

Sympathetic stimulation leads to an increase in heart rate (positive chronotropy), increase in contraction strength (inotropy) and increase in conduction velocity. Parasympathetic stimulation causes an opposite effect.

The SAN is a natural pacemaker; if you cut all nerves to the heart it would continue to beat but at a faster than normal rate. Usually, parasympathetic innervation slows down this innate heart rate.

3.3.2 Other receptors that cause a change in heart rate

CAROTID BODIES

- 2 in number.
- 2 mg in weight.
- Present at the bifurcation of each common carotid artery.
- Innervated by glossopharyngeal nerve (IX) and carotid sinus nerve.
- Sensitive to changes in PaO_2, $PaCO_2$ and pH.
- Also stimulate respiratory centres.

AORTIC BODIES

- 1–3 in number.
- Adjacent to aorta.
- Innervated by vagus nerve (X).
- Sensitive to changes in PaO_2, $PaCO_2$ and pH.
- Also stimulate respiratory centres.
- Directly stimulate sympathetic system.

CENTRAL CHEMORECEPTORS IN MEDULLA

- Sensitive to acidosis (H^+ only).
- Monitor blood CO_2 and pH.
- Also stimulate respiratory centres.

A decrease in blood O_2 and/or increased CO_2 and/or decreased pH leads to decreased parasympathetic stimulation, causing an increase in heart rate. These stimuli also lead to an increase in sympathetic stimulation, leading to an increase in heart rate and stroke volume, and vasoconstriction of blood vessels.

DIRECT CARDIAC RECEPTORS AND THE BAINBRIDGE REFLEX (ATRIAL REFLEX)

An increase in right atrial pressure due to an increase in central venous pressure/blood volume leads to stretching of the SAN, causing a direct increase in firing and hence increased heart rate. It also causes a signal to pass via the vagus nerve to the vasomotor centre in the medulla oblongata. This in turn leads to stimulation of sympathetic activity, which leads to an increase in heart rate despite the lack of change in parasympathetic activity.

The reflex is abolished by atropine or cutting the vagus nerve.

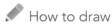

How to draw

STEP 1

- Draw a rectangle in the upper left quarter of the page. Label the midbrain above, then the pons and then the medulla oblongata.
- Draw 2 lines down from the MO to represent the spinal cord and label T1–T5.
- Draw a sagittal cross-section of the eye in the upper right quarter of the page.
- Draw the outlines of the heart and vessels in the lower right quarter of the page.

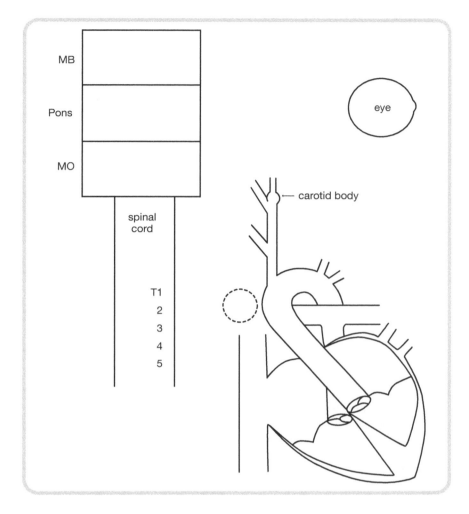

STEP 2

- Draw 2 small green ovals in each of the brainstem areas and on either side link them with a vertical line. These represent the sensory nuclei of the trigeminal nerves.
- Draw 2 squares in the medulla to represent the dorsal motor nuclei of the vagus nerves (CN X).
- Draw 2 ovals below the squares and divide them in two. These represent the vasomotor centres, each divided into a CS centre and a CI centre.

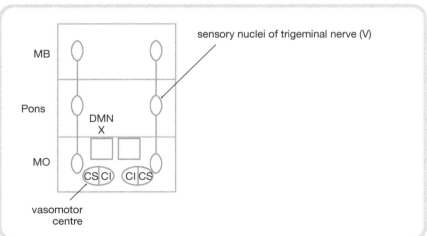

STEP ③

- Draw a green line down from the right side's vasomotor centre, from the CS centre to level T1–T5 in the spinal cord. Draw a horizontal line at each level with a circle about 3/4 of the way along it. Join the circles with a line. The circles represent the left sympathetic chain (for simplicity the right sympathetic chain is not shown; it too supplies the heart).
- Draw an arrow upwards from the upper circle and label it as going to the cervical sympathetic ganglion.
- Draw 2 green circles in the right atrium to represent the SAN in the upper part and the AVN in the lower part near the tricuspid valve.
- From the middle of the sympathetic chain draw the cardiac nerve and a branch to each of the nodes.

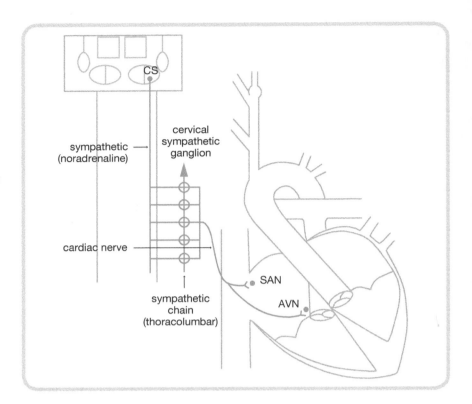

STEP ④

- Draw a nerve from the CI centre on the right side to its DMN above.
- Draw a nerve from the DMN across and then down to approximately in line with the arch of aorta. Here it divides into two sides, as a snake's tongue shape. These represent the parasympathetic nerves.
- From the right side draw a branch to the AVN.
- From the left side draw a branch to the SAN.

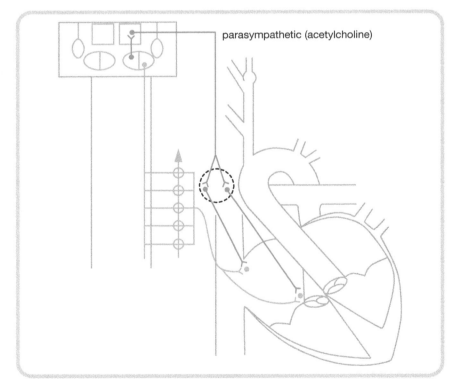

STEP 5

- Draw a green circle in the carotid artery to represent the carotid body. From here draw a nerve to the CS centre. This is the glossopharyngeal nerve (CN IX).
- Draw a green circle in the arch of aorta to represent the aortic body. From here draw a nerve to the CS centre. This is the vagus nerve (CN X).

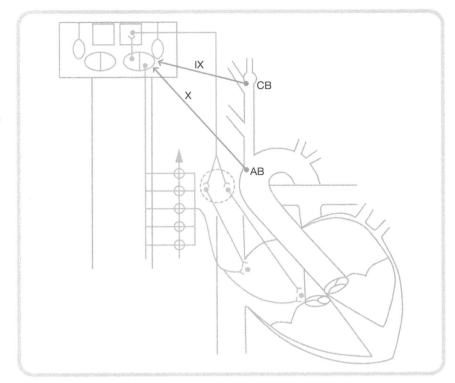

STEP 6

- From the vagus nerve draw a dotted line horizontally to the right side of the page. Continue the line down to the upper part of the left atrium. Draw some black dots here to represent the baroreceptors. When these are stimulated, they send a signal to the CS centre via the vagus nerve.
- Draw some black dots to represent baroreceptors in the right atrium just below the SAN. From here draw a green dotted line to join the vagus nerve.
- Draw black dots to represent baroreceptors in the arch of aorta. From here draw a green dotted line to join the vagus nerve.

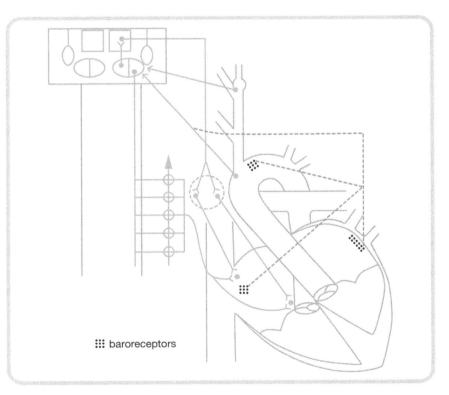

⠿ baroreceptors

STEP 7

- Draw a black arrow across the right atrium; this represents the stretch receptors.
- From here draw a green dotted line to the vagus nerve to show that stretch receptors also give signals to stimulate the heart via the vagus nerve.

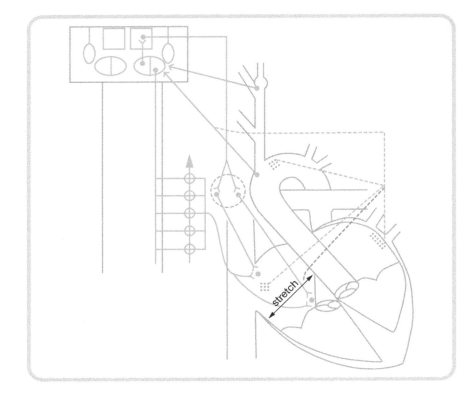

STEP 8

- Draw a green line from the dorsal motor nucleus to the middle oval of the trigeminal nucleus. Draw a second green line horizontally for about an inch, ending in a circle. Around this synapse draw a circle and label it as the Gasserian ganglion (GG, also called the trigeminal ganglion). Draw another line starting in the GG and ending in a small circle an inch further to the right. Draw a circle around this to represent the ciliary ganglion (CG).

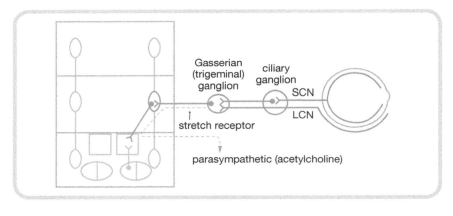

- Draw a green C shape at the back of the eye and a line back to the CG. This is the short ciliary nerve.
- Draw a green curve around the lower part of the outside of the eye, and from here draw a straight line to the GG. This is the long ciliary nerve.
- Draw a dotted grey line alongside the nerve from the GG to the parasympathetic nerve. This shows that when stretch receptors in the eye are stimulated, they lead to parasympathetic activity, a decrease in heart rate and blood pressure. This is why people sometimes have vagal episodes when the eye is being instrumented.

- The two coronary ostia arise from the sinuses of Valsalva (also known as the aortic sinus) just above the aortic valve.
- The left coronary artery starts as the left main stem. It then divides into the left anterior descending (LAD) artery, also called the left interventricular artery, and circumflex artery. The LAD has diagonal arteries coming off it and supplies the interventricular septum and the lateral and anterior walls of the left ventricle.
- The circumflex artery winds around the back of the heart. The posterior descending artery comes from the right coronary artery in 85% of people (right dominant) and from the circumflex artery in 15% of people (left dominant). The circumflex artery supplies the posterior and lateral side of the left ventricle. The left marginal (or obtuse) artery branches from the circumflex.
- The right coronary artery starts as the right main stem and divides into the acute marginal artery (anteriorly) and the posterior descending artery (posteriorly). These supply the right ventricle.
- The sinoatrial (nodal) artery arises from the right coronary artery in 60% of the population; this is the main artery that supplies the sinoatrial node.

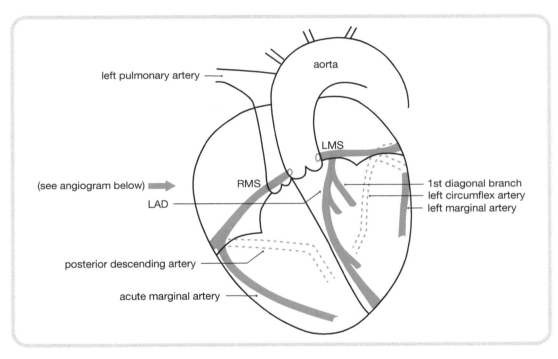

LAD	left anterior descending artery	LMS	left main stem	
		RMS	right main stem	

COMMON QUESTION

When you look at an angiogram it is normally shown as a sagittal cross-section through the heart (see arrow in image above). Hence the LAD is along the top of the image.

Angiogram
Looks from RIGHT lateral, see red arrow in main drawing

LMS   LAD

1st diagonal

circumflex artery

- Most cardiac veins follow the course of the coronary arteries. They mainly drain into the coronary sinus located in the right atrium between the IVC and the tricuspid valve.
- There are 2–5 anterior cardiac veins that receive blood from the right ventricle and pass the coronary sinus to empty directly into the right atrium (one drawn in the image below as an example).
- Thebesian veins are small and directly drain into the chambers of the heart. They account for true shunt.

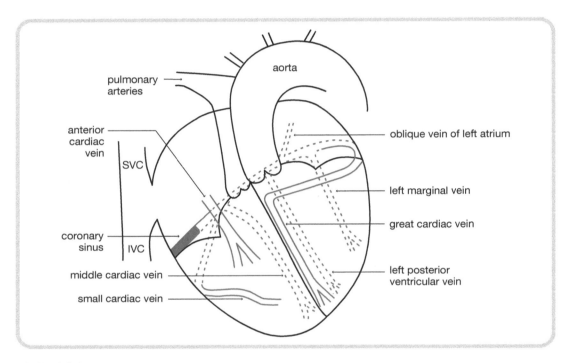

IVC   inferior vena cava
SVC   superior vena cava

Chapter 4
Airway and respiratory system

4.1 Airway sensation

CN V   trigeminal nerve
     CN V1 – anterior ethmoidal nerve
     CN V2 – sphenopalatine nerve
     CN V3 – lingual nerve
CN IX   glossopharyngeal nerve
CN X   vagus nerve
     CN X RLN – recurrent laryngeal nerve
     CN X SLN – superior laryngeal nerve

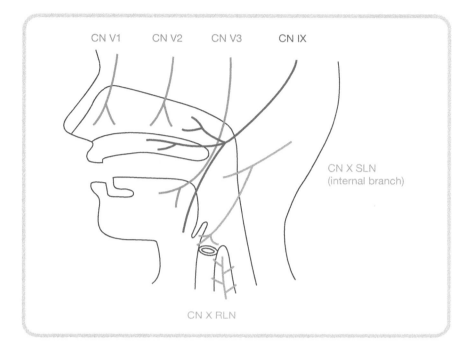

Airway sensation is from the trigeminal (CN V), glossopharyngeal (CN IX) and vagus (CN X) nerves.

TRIGEMINAL NERVE, CN V

- V1 branch: the anterior ethmoidal nerve; innervates the septum and nasal cavity.
- V2 branch: the sphenopalatine, greater and lesser palatine nerves. The greater palatine nerve supplies general sensation to the gingiva (gums) and the mucous membrane of the hard palate. The lesser palatine nerve innervates the nasal cavity, the soft palate, the tonsils and the uvula.
- V3 branch: the lingual nerve; general sensation of the anterior 2/3 of the tongue (special taste sensation is supplied by CN VII).

GLOSSOPHARYNGEAL NERVE, CN IX

- General sensory innervation to oropharynx and posterior 1/3 of the tongue. Special sensation to posterior 1/3 of the tongue.

VAGUS NERVE, CN X

- Superior laryngeal nerve: sensory innervation to the lower pharynx, epiglottis, vallecula and piriform fossa.
- Recurrent laryngeal nerve: sensation to vocal cord and subglottic mucosa.

4.2 Larynx

4.2.1 Anatomy of the larynx

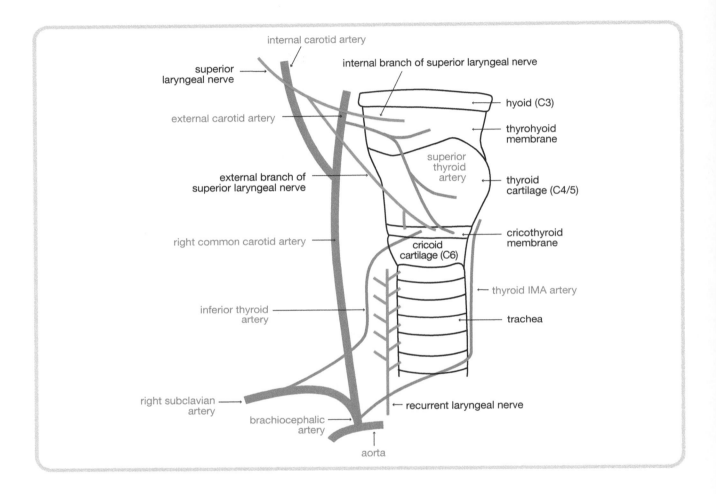

✏️ How to draw

STEP 1

Draw the main structures in black pen.

- Start with the trachea, a rectangle shape with lines to represent the cartilage rings (c-shaped).
- Then add in the cricoid cartilage by drawing a trapezium above the trachea (see image). The cricoid cartilage is actually slightly larger at the back than the front, in the shape of a signet ring.
- Next draw an irregular polygon to represent the thyrohyoid membrane, thyroid cartilage and cricothyroid membrane.
- Draw 2 lines inside this to separate the 3 structures.
- Draw the hyoid bone as a rounded rectangle above the thyrohyoid membrane.

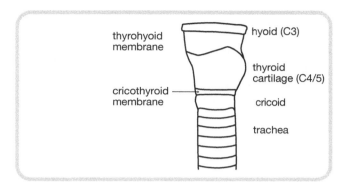

STEP 2

- Draw the superior laryngeal nerve (SLN), a branch of the vagus nerve (CN X). The SLN branches from the vagus nerve at approximately C2. It then divides into the internal branch and external branch at the level of hyoid (C3).
- The internal branch pierces the thyrohyoid membrane with the superior laryngeal artery. It supplies sensation to the mucosa above the vocal cords.
- The external branch supplies the cricothyroid muscle (see where it ends on the diagram).

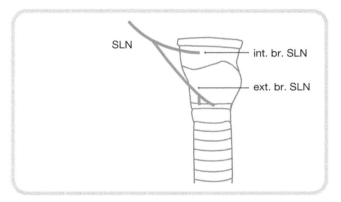

STEP 3

- Draw in the recurrent laryngeal nerve, a branch of the vagus nerve. It runs in the groove between the oesophagus and the trachea and supplies sensation to the mucosa of the larynx below the vocal cords. It also innervates the remainder of the intrinsic muscles of the pharynx.

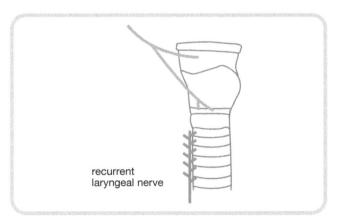

STEP 4

- Draw in the arch of the aorta inferiorly. The brachiocephalic artery arises here and then divides into the right subclavian artery and the right common carotid artery.
- The common carotid artery ascends and divides into the internal and external carotid arteries at the level of the thyroid cartilage (approximately C4).
- The left carotid and left subclavian arteries arise directly from the aortic arch (not shown here).

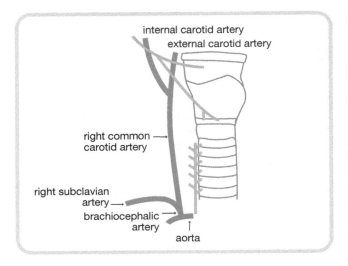

STEP 5

- Draw in the inferior thyroid artery, a branch of the thyrocervical trunk which arises in the subclavian.
- Draw in the superior thyroid artery, a branch of the external carotid artery (at approximately C3). Finally draw in the thyroid IMA artery, a variable branch of the brachiocephalic artery. This artery is only present in 3–10% of the population. It can be the reason for bleeding during a tracheostomy.

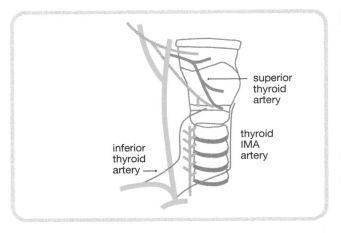

4.2.2 Laryngoscopic view of the vocal cords

G   glottis

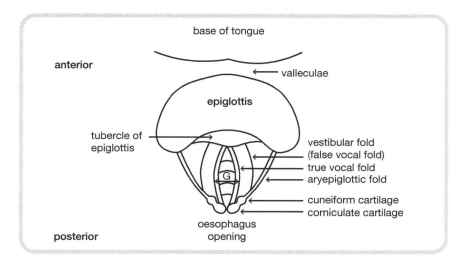

Looking through the mouth at the larynx with a laryngoscope is an essential skill for an anaesthetist. The first image shows exactly what you will see, the tongue base superiorly and the corniculate cartilage (in front of the oesophagus) posteriorly.

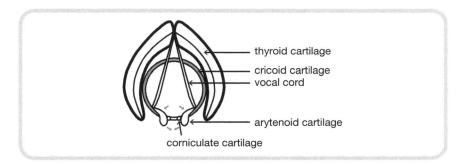

The second image shows what the view would look like with no soft tissue and shows how the cartilage is moved to open and close the vocal cords.

NERVE SUPPLY TO THE LARYNX

The nervous supply to the larynx is by the internal branch of the superior laryngeal nerve above the vocal folds and the recurrent (inferior) laryngeal nerve below the folds. Both are branches of the vagus nerve (CN X).

The external branch of the superior laryngeal nerve only supplies the cricothyroid muscle and the recurrent laryngeal nerve supplies all other intrinsic muscles of the larynx. Damage to the recurrent laryngeal nerve can lead to vocal fold palsy (see next page for more detail).

The vocal cords are used to generate sound by vibration of air passing between the adducted cords. Abducted cords are for breathing/breathy sounds and whispering. The vocal cords oscillate due to increased pressure beneath the vocal folds. The lower part of the vocal cords move before the upper part and this creates a wave-like motion. The pitch of a person's voice depends on length, size and tension of their vocal cords.

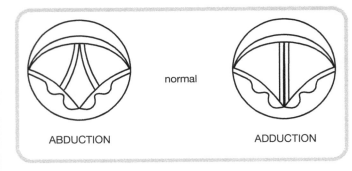

normal

ABDUCTION   ADDUCTION

SUPERIOR LARYNGEAL NERVE DAMAGE

- The external branch of the superior laryngeal nerve may be damaged during thyroid surgery.
- It supplies cricothyroid muscle.
- Damage leads to a loss of vocal cord tension and hence a hoarse voice.
- If unilateral the other side often compensates.

RECURRENT LARYNGEAL NERVE DAMAGE

This causes vocal fold palsy / paresis which results in a hoarse voice, and this can cause bilateral and unilateral paralysis as shown in the following images.

Bilateral damage

Complete transection of the recurrent laryngeal nerve causes complete paralysis of most muscles except cricothyroid (innervated by the external branch of the superior laryngeal nerve). This leads to a half abducted, half adducted position—the cadaveric position.

Symptoms: patient cannot speak or cough.

Trauma/partial transection leads to partial paralysis. This leaves the cords in an adducted position.

Symptoms: respiratory distress, stridor, life threatening.

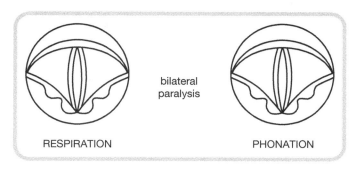

RESPIRATION   bilateral paralysis   PHONATION

Unilateral damage

Image shows right-sided recurrent laryngeal nerve palsy; note that the left cord moves in the image and the right cord stays still.

If one cord is damaged then the other cord will partially compensate. The damaged cord will sit in an adducted position and the cricothyroid muscle should still work (due to innervation by the superior laryngeal nerve).

Symptoms: breathy voice, weak cough, sensation of shortness of breath and sometimes swallowing difficulties.

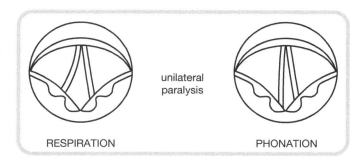

RESPIRATION   unilateral paralysis   PHONATION

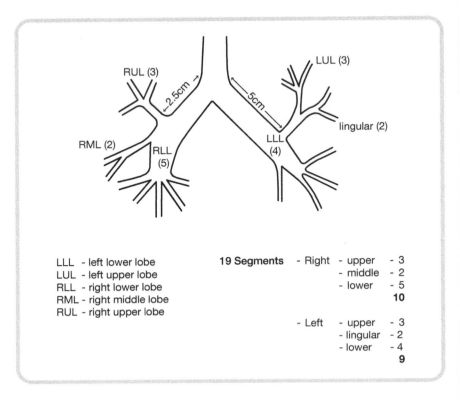

LLL - left lower lobe
LUL - left upper lobe
RLL - right lower lobe
RML - right middle lobe
RUL - right upper lobe

19 Segments - Right - upper - 3
                      - middle - 2
                      - lower - 5
                               10

            - Left - upper - 3
                   - lingular - 2
                   - lower - 4
                            9

Knowing the number of segments and their names is useful. I remember it as '325, 324'. This adds up to 19 segments in total, 10 on the right and 9 on the left.

The right main bronchus is approximately 2.5 cm long and straight, about 25° off the midline.

The left main bronchus is approximately 5 cm long and lies more horizontally over the heart, about 45° off the midline.

RIGHT SIDE

- 3: APA – Apical, Posterior, Anterior
- 2: LM: Lateral, Medial
- 5: APALM: Apical, Posterior, Anterior, Lateral, Medial

LEFT SIDE

- 3: APA – Apical, Posterior, Anterior
- 2: IS – Inferior, Superior
- 4: APAL – Apical, Posterior, Anterior, Lateral (there is no medial one – this can be remembered by thinking that the heart lies where it would have been!)

4.4 Lungs and lung pleurae

4.4.1 Pleurae

The pleurae comprise two distinct layers: visceral and parietal. These are continuous with each other around the root of the lung, forming a loose cuff called the pulmonary ligament.

The space between the layers is the pleural space and contains approximately 10 ml of pleural fluid.

VISCERAL PLEURA

Sensitive to stretch only; supplied by autonomic nervous system. Covers the lung.

PARIETAL PLEURA

Sensitive to pain, pressure, temperature and touch.

4 areas:

1. **Cervical**: projects into neck about an inch above medial 1/3 of clavicle.
2. **Costal**: lines back of sternum, ribs, costal cartilages, intercostal spaces and sides of vertebral bodies. Innervated by intercostal nerves.
3. **Mediastinal**: covers mediastinum. Reflects onto bronchi and vessels entering lungs. Continuous with visceral pleura. Innervate by phrenic nerve.
4. **Diaphragmatic**: covers diaphragm. Innervated by phrenic nerve over dome and intercostal nerves around edge.

B   bronchus
PA   pulmonary artery
PV   pulmonary vein

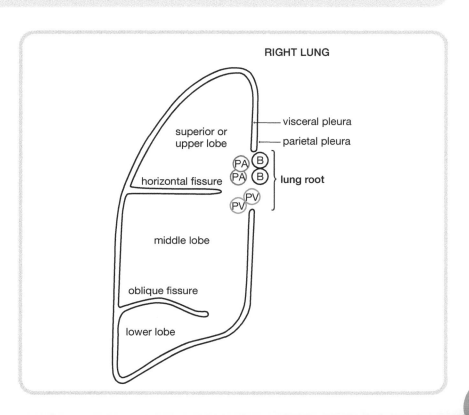

RIGHT LUNG

superior or upper lobe

visceral pleura

parietal pleura

horizontal fissure

lung root

middle lobe

oblique fissure

lower lobe

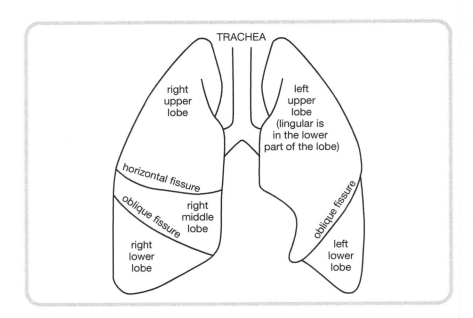

4.4.2 Lungs

 How to draw

STEP 1

- Draw the left and right upper lobes and the trachea. In the left lobe, use a concave shape for the lower part of the medial border, where the heart sits; this is the cardiac impression.
- The inferior border on the right side is the horizontal fissure and the inferior border on the left side is the oblique fissure.

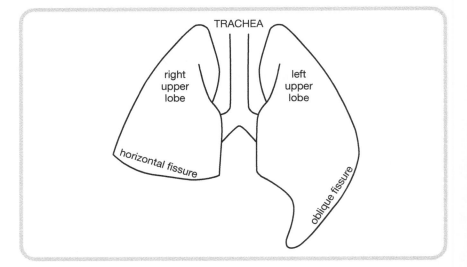

STEP 2

- Draw the middle lobe on the right only. Its inferior border is the oblique fissure.
- The left does not have a middle lobe.

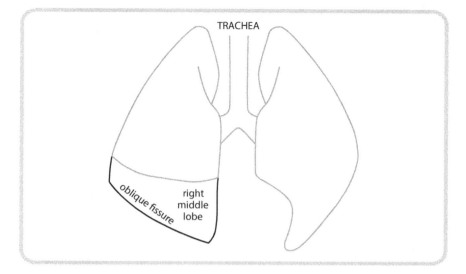

STEP 3

Draw the left and right lower lobes.

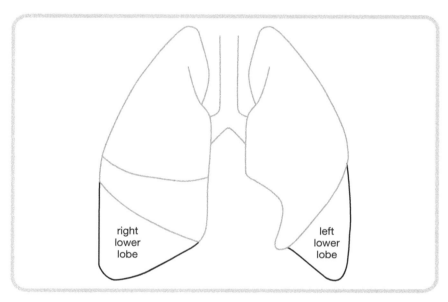

4.5 Thoracic inlet

The thoracic inlet is at the level of the 1st rib. It is a complicated area and drawing it will help you visualise and remember it.

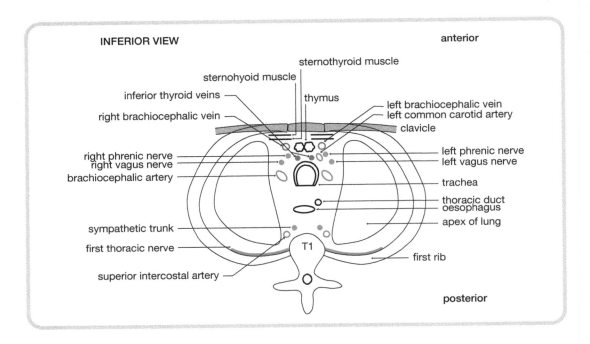

INFERIOR VIEW — anterior

- sternothyroid muscle
- sternohyoid muscle
- inferior thyroid veins
- thymus
- right brachiocephalic vein
- left brachiocephalic vein
- left common carotid artery
- clavicle
- right phrenic nerve
- right vagus nerve
- brachiocephalic artery
- left phrenic nerve
- left vagus nerve
- trachea
- thoracic duct
- oesophagus
- apex of lung
- sympathetic trunk
- first thoracic nerve
- superior intercostal artery
- T1
- first rib
- posterior

 ## How to draw

STEP 1

- Draw an oval shape with T1 in the centre at the back.
- Draw a second oval inside this; the outer area is the first rib.
- Draw a straight line at the front that represents the manubrium and the clavicle.

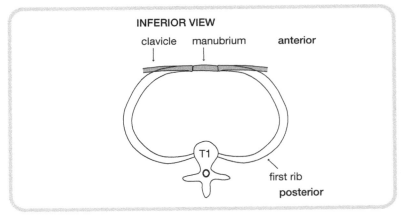

INFERIOR VIEW

- clavicle
- manubrium
- anterior
- T1
- first rib
- posterior

STEP 2

Draw an enclosed semicircle on each side to represent the apex of each lung. Draw 2 sets of small parallel lines at the front just behind the manubrium. These are the sternohyoid and sternothyroid muscles. Just behind these draw two little fluffy cloud shapes to represent the thymus.

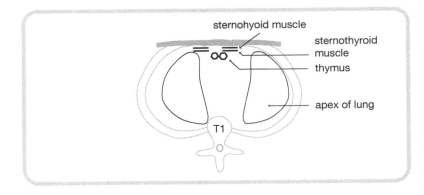

- sternohyoid muscle
- sternothyroid muscle
- thymus
- apex of lung
- T1

STEP 3

Add in a trachea behind the thymus and then draw the oesophagus and thoracic duct behind the trachea.

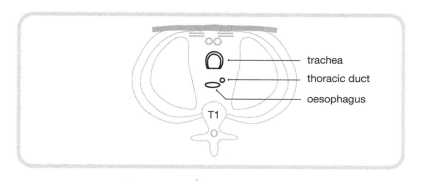

STEP 4

- Draw 2 green lines from T1 to just in front of the posterior first rib; these represent the first thoracic nerves.
- Draw 2 green dots anterior to T1 body; these are the sympathetic trunks.
- Draw 2 green dots just in front of and lateral to the trachea; these are the right and left vagus nerves.
- Draw 2 green dots just in front of the vagus nerves; these are the phrenic nerves.

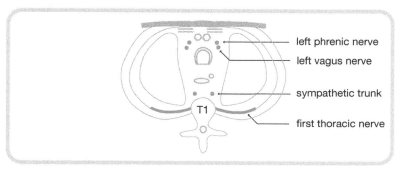

STEP 5

- Draw 2 red circles just lateral and behind the sympathetic trunks; these are the superior intercostal arteries.
- Draw 2 red ovals lateral to the trachea; these represent the brachiocephalic artery and the left subclavian artery.
- Draw a red circle just anterior to the left subclavian artery and medial to the phrenic and vagus nerves; this is the left common carotid artery.

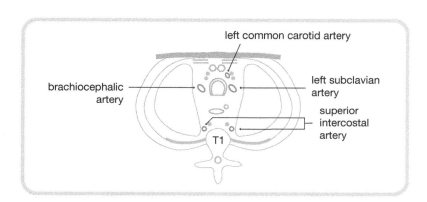

STEP 6

- Draw 2 blue dots just in front of the trachea; these are the inferior thyroid veins.
- Draw 2 blue circles anterior to these and lateral to the thymus; these are the brachiocephalic veins.

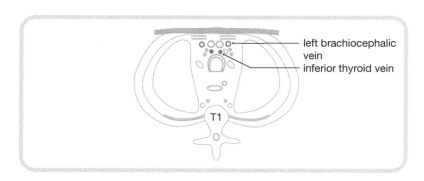

4.6 First rib

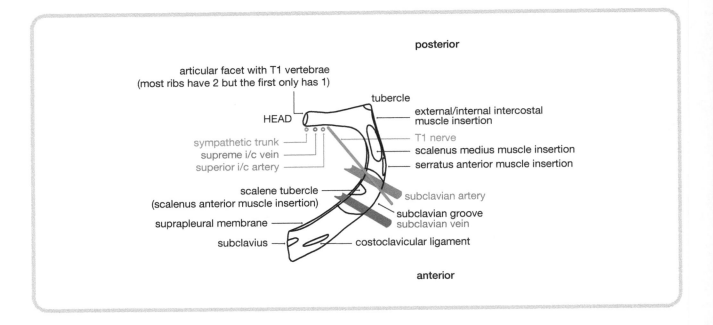

The inferior surface of the first rib is smoother than the upper surface. If you lay the rib on the table you can see it is the correct way up as the head will touch the surface.

The image shows the superior surface of the first rib. It is important to know where the vessels run over the rib.

If you find the scalenus tubercle (for scalenus anterior) then you will find the subclavian groove.

- The subclavian artery runs posteriorly to this and the subclavian vein runs anteriorly.
- The T1 nerve root runs under the subclavian artery.

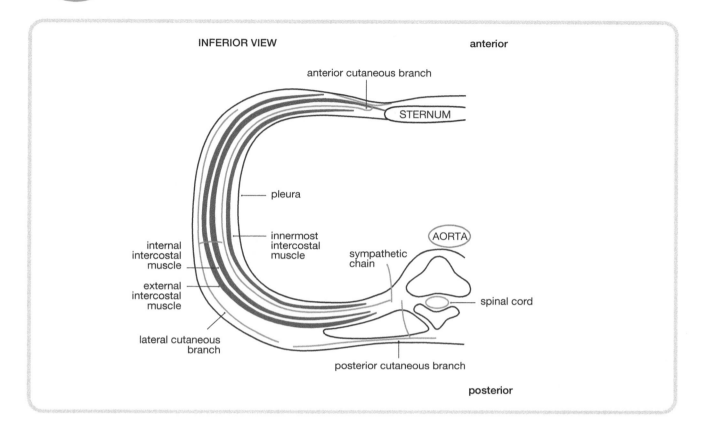

INFERIOR VIEW — anterior

anterior cutaneous branch

STERNUM

pleura

innermost intercostal muscle

AORTA

internal intercostal muscle

sympathetic chain

external intercostal muscle

spinal cord

lateral cutaneous branch

posterior cutaneous branch

posterior

The intercostal nerves arise from the anterior rami of the thoracic nerves T1 to T11. The upper two nerves supply the upper limb and the thorax. The next 4 nerves supply the thorax, and the lower five nerves supply the thorax and abdominal walls. The 7th intercostal nerve terminates at the xiphoid process and the 10th intercostal nerve terminates at the navel.

How to draw

STEP 1

- Draw an approximate semicircle to represent the thorax and then draw one of the thoracic vertebrae (in two halves, the body and the spinous processes).

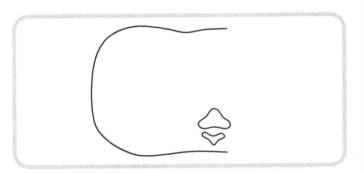

STEP 2

- Add in the external intercostal muscle by drawing a red semicircle from the transverse process anteriorly. Draw the erector spinae muscle.
- Draw the pleura, anterior to the thoracic vertebral body and ending by drawing the sternum. Add the aorta anterior to the pleura.

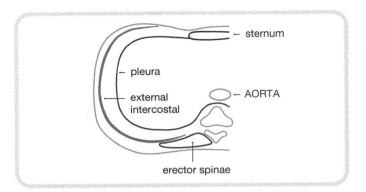

STEP 3

- Draw the internal intercostal muscle by drawing a semicircular line from the transverse process to the sternum.

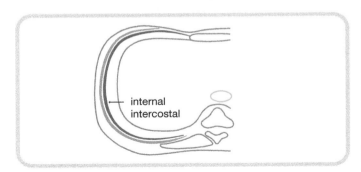

STEP 4

- Draw the innermost intercostal muscle by drawing a semicircular line just inside the pleura.

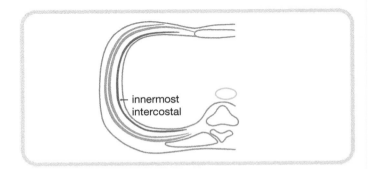

STEP 5

- Draw the spinal cord in between the body of the vertebrae and the spinous process.
- Draw the sympathetic chain anteriorly and the posterior cutaneous nerve posteriorly.

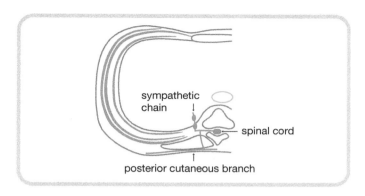

STEP 6

- As a new branch from the spinal nerve, draw a semi-circular nerve between the innermost and internal intercostal muscles. Finish it anteriorly with an anterior cutaneous branch.
- Draw a lateral cutaneous branch from the anterior branch as shown.

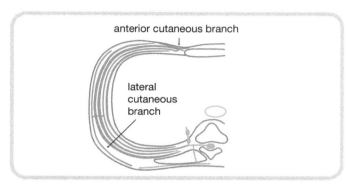

Mediastinum

The mediastinum is divided into superior and inferior:

- superior mediastinum
- inferior mediastinum
  - anterior mediastinum
  - middle mediastinum
  - posterior mediastinum.

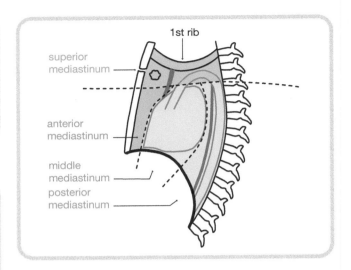

SUPERIOR MEDIASTINUM

- Major blood vessels are in this part of the mediastinum, including the arch of the aorta and branches (brachiocephalic, left common carotid, left subclavian artery), the superior vena cava, left and right brachiocephalic veins, supreme intercostal vein and azygos vein.
- Nerves here are the right and left vagus nerves, phrenic nerves, cardiac nerves and sympathetic trunk.
- Other structures include the thymus, trachea and thoracic duct.

ANTERIOR MEDIASTINUM

- This contains loose connective tissue, fat, lymphatic vessels, lymph nodes and branches of internal thoracic vessels.
- The thymus sometimes extends inferiorly into the anterior mediastinum.

MIDDLE MEDIASTINUM

- This contains the heart and the pericardium along with vessels including the ascending aorta, pulmonary trunk, superior vena cava, tracheal bifurcation and left and right main bronchi.
- There are also tracheobronchial lymph nodes.

POSTERIOR MEDIASTINUM

- This is where the thoracic descending aorta lies. Branches that come off the aorta here are the posterior intercostal arteries, bronchial arteries, oesophageal arteries and superior phrenic arteries.
- The oesophagus, thoracic duct, azygos vein, hemiazygos vein and sympathetic trunks lie here.

4.9 Diaphragm

A   right phrenic nerve
B   vagal trunks
C   left gastric vessels
D   aorta
E   thoracic duct
F   hemiazygos vein

IVC   inferior vena cava

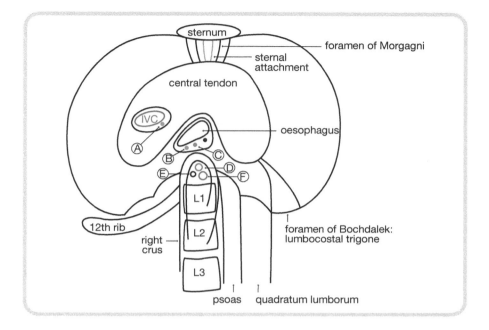

This is an awkward area to draw. This is the simplest version I could come up with. It shows the abdominal aspect looking upwards and slightly posteriorly. The main things to learn are what passes through the diaphragm and where, along with the nerve supply.

The motor supply of the diaphragm is from the left and right phrenic nerves (C3, 4 and 5). The phrenic nerve also supplies sensation to the central tendon. The sensation at the edge of the diaphragm is from the intercostal nerves T5 to T12.

The right crus of the diaphragm arises from L1 to L3. The left crus arises from L1 to L2.

Caval opening: **T8**

- Vena cava (8 letters)
- R phrenic (8 letters) nerve (R = right)

Oesophageal opening: **T10**

- Oesophagus (**10** letters)
- Vagal trunk (cranial nerve **10**)
- Left gastric vessels

Aortic hiatus (**12** letters): **T12**

- Aorta
- Thoracic duct (12 letters)
- Azygos vein

Congenital hernias into the thorax can occur at diaphragmatic foramina:

- foramina of Bochdalek, spaces between the diaphragm's lumbar and costal regions (shown on one side only in the image)
- foramina of Morgagni (sternocostal triangle), a space between the diaphragm's sternal and costal attachments.

4.10 Muscles of the thorax

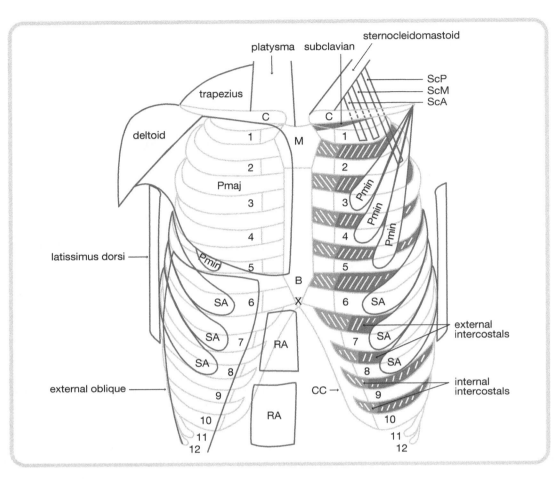

B	body of sternum	**RA**	rectus abdominis
C	clavicle	**SA**	serratus anterior
CC	costal cartilage	**ScA**	scalenus anterior
M	manubrium of sternum	**ScM**	scalenus medius
Pmaj	pectorals major	**ScP**	scalenus posterior
Pmin	pectorals minor	**X**	xiphisternum

How to draw

STEP 1

- In black pen draw the sternum as 2 irregular hexagons, as shown, with a quadrilateral xiphisternum most inferiorly.
- Then add the clavicle and 12 ribs on each side. Show ribs 7 to 10 being joined by the costal cartilage.

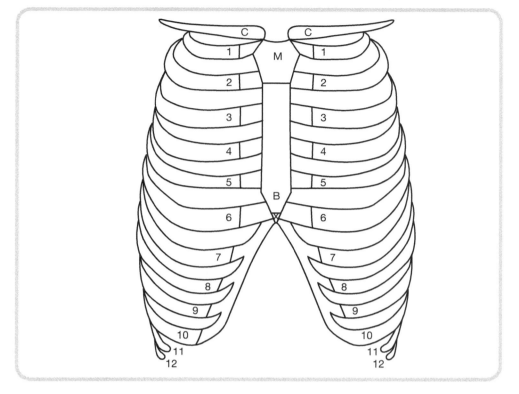

STEP 2

- The muscles are the same on each side of the thorax. To be able to show all of them, we will draw all of the muscles, but not all on both sides. Hopefully it will help you to learn the anterior view of the thorax and upper abdomen.
- On the right side of the body, draw the platysma and trapezius muscle in the 'neck' then the deltoid on the shoulder.

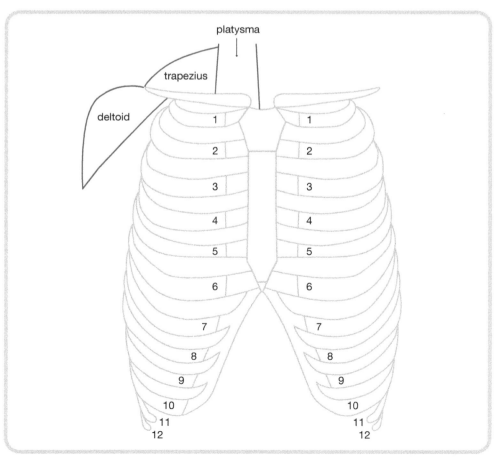

STEP 3

On the right side draw a quadrilateral shape over ribs 1 to 5, to represent the pectoralis major.

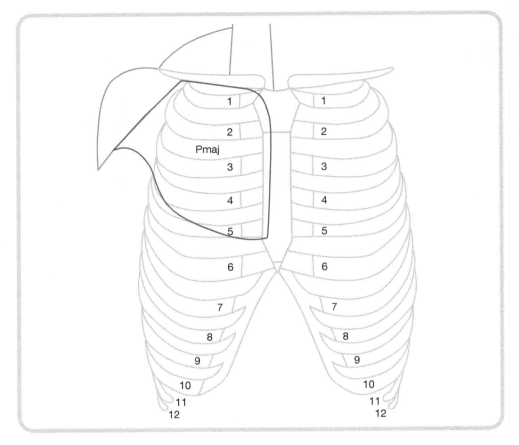

STEP 4

- Draw the bottom end of the pectoralis minor coming out from beneath the pectoralis major, ending on the 5th rib (see step 10 for the pectoralis minor).
- Inferior to the pectoralis minor draw 3 'finger' shapes (called digitations).
- This is the serratus anterior, attaching to ribs 6, 7 and 8. It also has digitations attaching to ribs 1–5 deep to the pectoralis major and minor (not shown here).

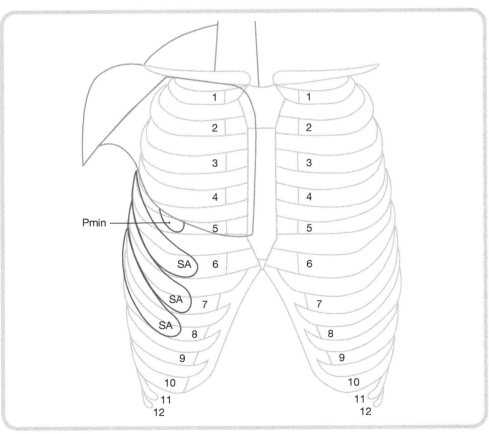

STEP 5

- Lateral to this, a small area of the latissimus dorsi (LD) is visible in an anterior view; draw it on both sides.
- It continues upwards to insert into the humerus (insertion not shown).

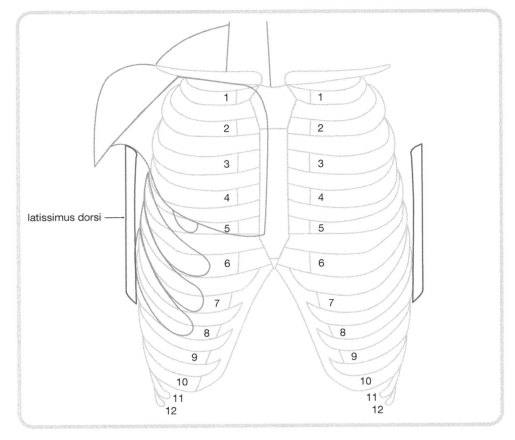

latissimus dorsi

STEP 6

- Add the external oblique on the right side of the body.
- It arises from the inferior, external surface of ribs 5 to 12.

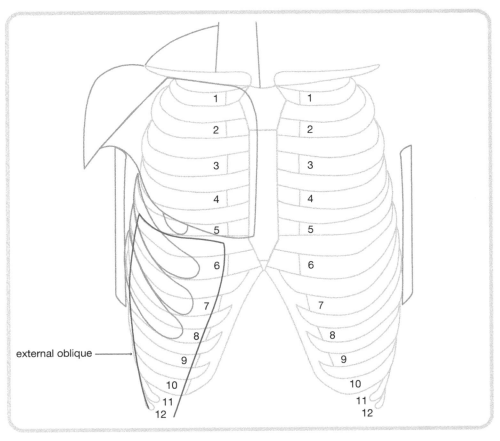

external oblique

STEP 7

Draw 2 roughly rectangular shapes to represent the right rectus abdominis muscle.

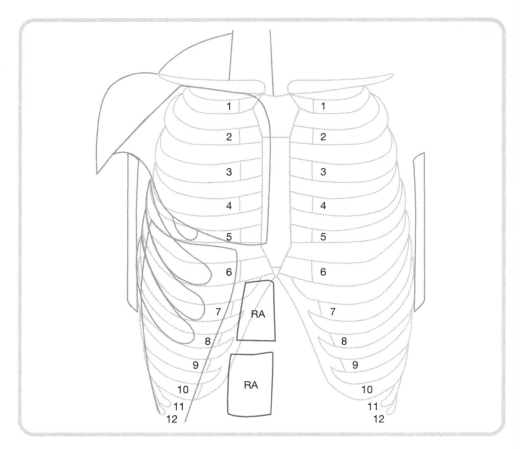

STEP 8

- Starting at the medial upper surface of the left clavicle, draw the diagonal sternocleidomastoid muscle.
- Approximately perpendicular to this draw 3 smaller diagonal muscles. These are the scalene muscles: scalenus anterior, medius and posterior (also see *Section 1.5.3: Triangles of the neck*). These pass deep to the clavicle.

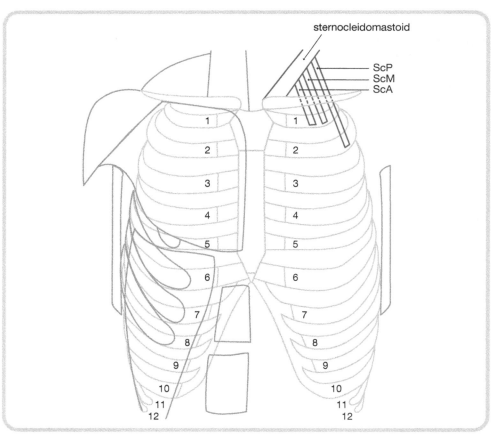

STEP 9

Draw the subclavian muscle (subclavius) below the clavicle; this is superficial to the scalene muscles.

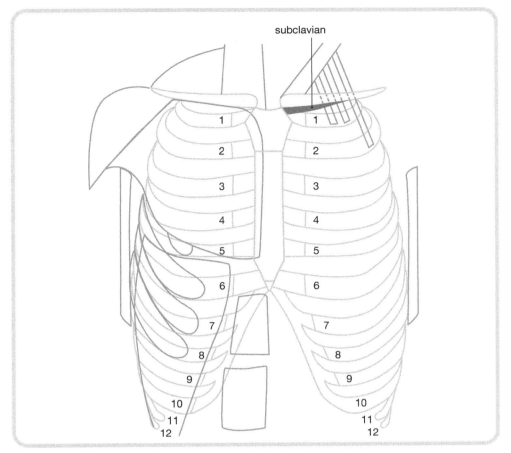

STEP 10

- Draw 6 teardrop-shaped muscles.
- The upper 3 are digitations of the pectoralis minor, inserting onto ribs 3, 4 and 5 as shown. The lower 3 are parts of the serratus anterior and insert, as they do on the other side, into ribs 6, 7 and 8.

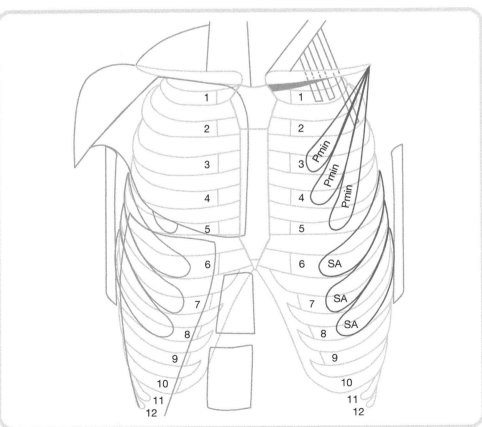

STEP 11

- We will now add the internal and external intercostal muscles between each set of ribs as shown.
- Draw the fibres of the external intercostal muscles running inferiorly and medially. Their medial borders represent the muscles being cut to reveal the internal intercostal muscles.
- Draw the internal intercostals with fibres in the opposite orientation.

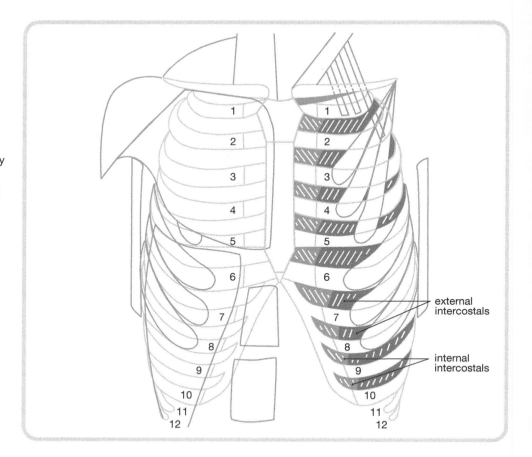

MUSCLES OF THE THORAX

Pectoralis major

2 heads: clavicular head from medial half of clavicle and sternocostal head from sternum, 6 intercostal cartilages and aponeurosis of external oblique. Inserts into bicipital groove of humerus.

Action: clavicular head flexes humerus and sternocostal head adducts humerus. Also draws scapula forwards and down.
Innervation: medial and lateral pectoral nerves (see *Section 7.2: Brachial plexus*).
Blood supply: pectoral artery.

Pectoralis minor

Lies beneath pectoralis major. Origin on ribs 3 to 5, near to costochondral junction; inserts into coracoid process of scapula.

Action: stabilises scapula against thoracic wall. Raises ribs in inspiration.
Innervation: medial and lateral pectoral nerves.
Blood supply: pectoral artery.

Latissimus dorsi

Origin is spinous processes of T7 to L5, thoracolumbar fascia, iliac crest, inferior 3–4 ribs and scapula. Inserts into humerus.

Action: adducts, extends and internally rotates arm. Also is a strong rotator of the trunk.
Innervation: thoracodorsal nerve, roots C6–C8 (see *Section 7.2: Brachial plexus*).
Blood supply: thoracodorsal branch of subscapular artery.

Serratus anterior

Originates from upper 8 or 9 ribs and inserts into medial side of scapula.

Action: stabilises scapula and assists in upward rotation.
Innervation: Long thoracic nerve, C5–C7 (see *Section 7.2: Brachial plexus*).
Blood supply: thoracic artery (lateral and superior).

External oblique muscle

Middle and upper parts become aponeurotic to form anterior layer of rectus muscle. Lowest part inserts into iliac crest; aponeurosis forms inguinal ligament.

Action: flexion and contralateral rotation of torso.
Innervation: lower 6 thoracoabdominal nerves and subcostal nerve on each side.
Blood supply: from intercostal arteries to upper half; deep circumflex iliac artery or iliolumbar artery to lower half.

Rectus abdominus muscle

2 parallel muscles run from superior to inferior, joined medially by connective tissue known as the linea alba. Extend from pubic crest and pubic symphysis to xiphoid process and costal cartilages of ribs 5 to 7. Tendinous intersections subdivide muscle into 'false' muscle bellies – the 6 pack!

Action: flexion of lumbar spine.

Innervation: thoracoabdominal nerves, continuation of T7–T11 intercostal nerves.

Blood supply: superior and inferior epigastric arteries and lower 6 intercostal arteries.

Scalene muscles, sternocleidomastoid and trapezius

See *Section 1.5.3: Triangles of the neck.*

Chapter 5

Abdomen and abdominal cavity

5.1 Organs and systems

5.1.1 Oesophagus and stomach

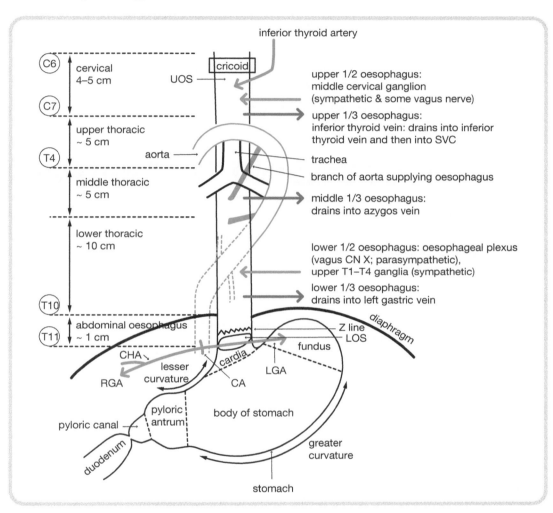

inferior thyroid artery

cricoid

C6 | cervical 4–5 cm

UOS

C7

upper thoracic ~ 5 cm

aorta

T4

middle thoracic ~ 5 cm

lower thoracic ~ 10 cm

T10

T11 | abdominal oesophagus ~ 1 cm

upper 1/2 oesophagus: middle cervical ganglion (sympathetic & some vagus nerve)

upper 1/3 oesophagus: inferior thyroid vein: drains into inferior thyroid vein and then into SVC

trachea

branch of aorta supplying oesophagus

middle 1/3 oesophagus: drains into azygos vein

lower 1/2 oesophagus: oesophageal plexus (vagus CN X; parasympathetic), upper T1–T4 ganglia (sympathetic)

lower 1/3 oesophagus: drains into left gastric vein

diaphragm

Z line

LOS

fundus

CHA

lesser curvature

cardia

CA

LGA

RGA

pyloric antrum

pyloric canal

body of stomach

duodenum

greater curvature

stomach

CA   coeliac artery
CHA   common hepatic artery
LGA   left gastric artery
LOS   lower oesophageal sphincter
RGA   right gastric artery
SVC   superior vena cava
UOS   upper oesophageal sphincter

OESOPHAGUS

The oesophagus is 20–25 cm long, running from about C6 to T11. At rest the oesophagus is normally collapsed and flattish in the upper 2/3 and rounded in the lower 1/3 in transverse section. It passes through the diaphragm at approximately T10 (*aide mémoire*: oesophagus has 10 letters). It has 2 sphincters:

- **Lower oesophageal sphincter**, at approximately T11 with 2 components: the inner part is a thickening of oesophageal muscle and the external part is the diaphragm.
- **Upper oesophageal sphincter**, at approximately C5 to C6; made of musculocartilaginous cricopharyngeal fibres which encircle it. This is the "cricopharyngeal" part of the inferior pharyngeal constrictor muscle.

The oesophagus has two layers of muscle, an outer longitudinal layer and an inner circular layer. Its mucosa is described in Box 5.1.

Box 5.1: Gastric and oesophageal mucosa and the Z line

Oesophageal mucosa (squamous) is pink and smooth in comparison to gastric mucosa, which is red, mammillated and secretory. Gastric mucosa consists of simple columnar epithelium, the lamina propria, and the muscularis mucosae.

The Z line is the junction between the 2 types of mucosa (aka squamo-columnar junction). Normally it is <3 cm from the lower oesophageal sphincter. In Barrett's oesophagus, a pathological condition arising from chronic gastro-oesophageal reflux, the distance is >3 cm.

Blood supply

- The cervical portion is supplied by branches from the inferior thyroid artery.
- The thoracic portion feeds from branches directly from the aorta.
- Some additional supply to the thoracic portion comes from branches from the bronchial arteries, and ascending branches from the left gastric artery.
- Venous drainage is shown in the image.

Innervation

Oesophageal innervation is very complex (see major anatomy textbooks), but I have just shown the basics in the image, plus plexi:

- **Myenteric plexus** (Auerbach's plexus): ganglia lie between the 2 muscle layers of the oesophagus; it causes the outer muscle layer to contract.
- **Submucosal plexus** (Meissner's plexus): lies within the submucosa; it regulates secretion and peristaltic contraction of the smooth muscle.

STOMACH

The stomach is located between the oesophagus and duodenum. It has a 'J' shape, with the smaller side superiorly (the lesser curvature) and longer side inferiorly (greater curvature). It mostly lies in the epigastric and umbilical region and has 4 main anatomical divisions.

- **Cardia:** at the opening of the stomach, at approximately T11 level
- **Fundus:** superior and to the left of the cardia, rounded in shape and often containing gas (because it's the highest region)
- **Body:** main, central part of the stomach
- **Pylorus:** area connecting the stomach to the duodenum, divided into the pyloric antrum, canal and sphincter (approximately at L1 level). In pyloric stenosis the sphincter is narrowed due to hypertrophy of the pylorus.

The stomach has two sphincters, the lower oesophageal sphincter (LOS, see *Oesophagus* section, above) and pyloric sphincter. Neither is under voluntary control. The pyloric sphincter lies between the pylorus and the first part of the duodenum. It controls the exit of chyme (food and gastric acid) from the stomach into the duodenum. It works as an anatomical sphincter: when intragastric pressure is higher than the resistance of the pylorus then the sphincter opens. Gastric peristalsis pushes chyme into the duodenum.

Aide mémoire:

- The LESSER omentum attaches to the LESSER curvature of the stomach.
- The GREATER omentum attaches to the GREATER curvature of the stomach.

Blood supply

See later for steps in drawing blood supply to the stomach.

Innervation

- **Parasympathetic:** from the anterior and posterior vagal trunks (derived from the vagus nerve, CN X)
- **Sympathetic:** from spinal cord segments T6 to T9 (some say T5–T12). Fibres pass to the coeliac plexus via the greater splanchnic nerve.

  How to draw

STEP 1

- Use a whole page and draw a line down its left side, approximately 2/3 of the page depth, representing the length of the oesophagus (which is approximately 26 cm).
- Draw horizontal broken lines at the top and corresponding to 5, 10, 15 and 25 cm down the line's length and at its base. These divide the sections of the oesophagus as labelled in the image.

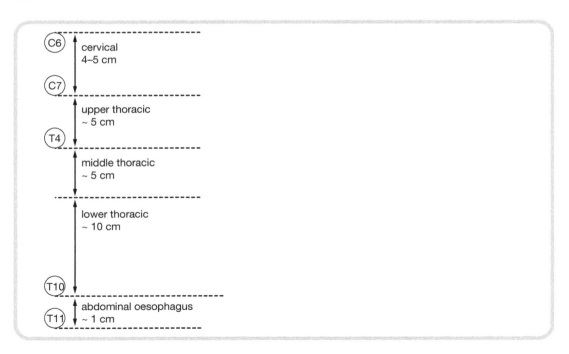

STEP 2

- Draw in the diaphragm at approximately T10.
- Add the oesophagus as a tube from the uppermost horizontal line to just below the diaphragm.
- Add in the cricoid cartilage as a horizontal rectangle at approximately C6.
- Draw the stomach and part of the duodenum as shown.

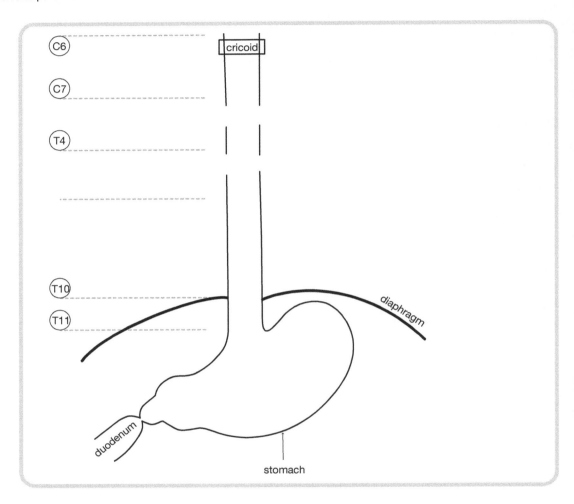

STEP 3

- Draw the junction of the trachea and two bronchi at approximately the level of T4.
- To draw the blood supply, start with the arch of the aorta at approximately T3 and show it curving back towards the left side of the base of the oesophagus.
- Draw a short artery down the middle of the aorta below the diaphragm; this is the coeliac artery (also called the coeliac trunk and coeliac axis). Draw a curved line crossing it from above the right side of the stomach to the top left part of the stomach; this represents the left gastric artery and the common hepatic artery (which feeds the right gastric artery). For further details, see *Blood supply to the stomach*, below.
- Draw a few branches from the aorta towards the oesophagus.

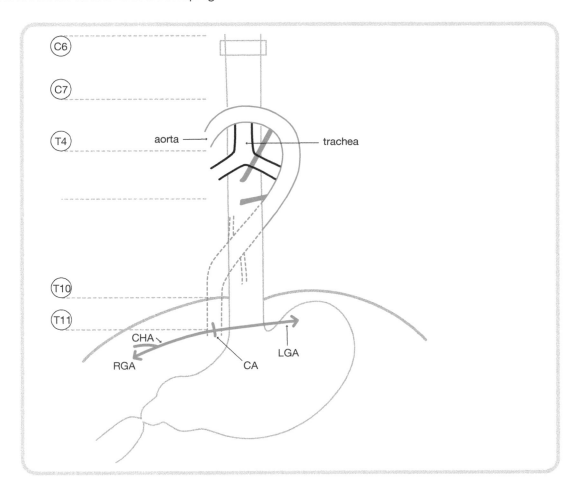

STEP 4

- Label the areas of the stomach as shown. Draw a zigzag black line across the oesophagus at approximately T10/11; this represents the Z line.
- Below the Z line, draw an oval to represent the lower oesophageal sphincter.
- Label the greater curvature of the stomach on the lower border and the lesser curvature on the upper border.

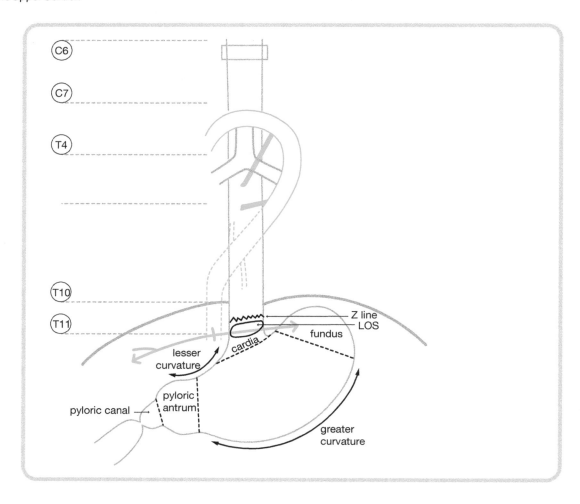

STEP 5

- Add a red arrow to the upper part of the oesophagus, to represent a branch of the inferior thyroid artery.
- Draw one green arrow to the cervical section of the oesophagus and a second one to the lower thoracic section. These represent the middle cervical ganglion (sympathetic) above and the upper T1–T4 ganglia (sympathetic) and oesophageal plexus (vagus CN X, parasympathetic) below.
- Draw 3 blue arrows from the upper, middle and the lower third of the oesophagus. These represent the inferior thyroid, azygos and left gastric veins, respectively.

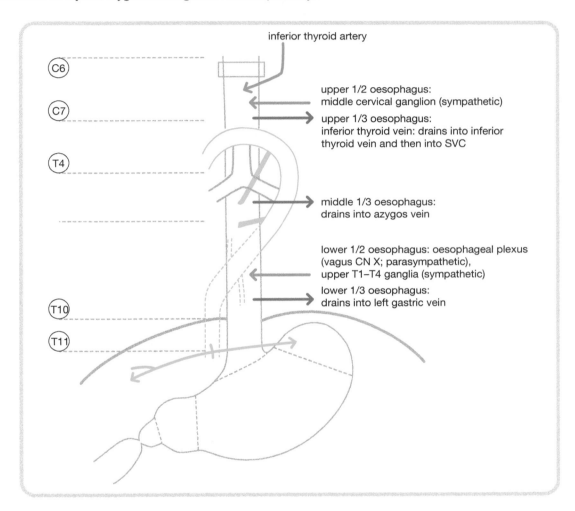

BLOOD SUPPLY TO THE STOMACH

Blood supply to the stomach is mainly from the arteries supplied by the coeliac artery, as follows.

- **Tissues near to the lesser curvature** of the stomach are supplied by the right gastric artery inferiorly and the left gastric artery superiorly, which also supplies the cardiac region.
- **Tissues near to the greater curvature** are supplied by the right gastroepiploic artery inferiorly and the left gastroepiploic artery superiorly.
- **The fundus** is supplied by short gastric arteries (branches of the splenic artery) and the left gastroepiploic artery.

CA	coeliac artery
CHA	common hepatic artery
GDA	gastroduodenal artery
LGA	left gastric artery
LGEA	left gastroepiploic artery
LGEV	left gastroepiploic vein
LGV	left gastric vein
RGA	right gastric artery
RGEA	right gastroepiploic artery
RGEV	right gastroepiploic vein
RGV	right gastric vein
SA	splenic artery
SMV	superior mesenteric vein
SV	splenic vein

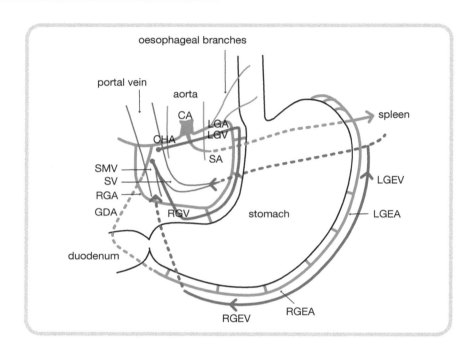

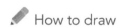 How to draw

STEP 1

- Draw the outline of the stomach as shown.

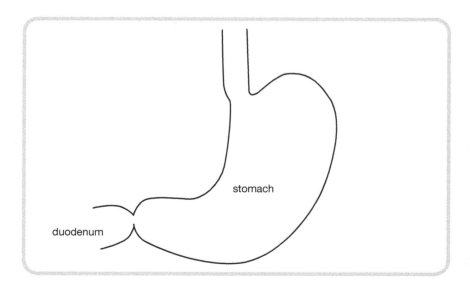

STEP 2

- Draw the lower part of the aorta.
- Draw the coeliac artery in the middle. From here draw the left gastric artery, the splenic artery and the common hepatic artery as shown.

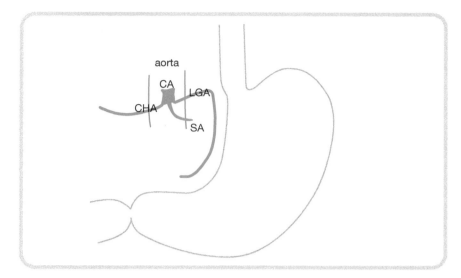

STEP 3

- From the CHA draw a line downwards to represent the right gastric artery. Join the left and right gastric arteries in a loop along the upper edge of the stomach. Draw a few branches from here to the lesser curvature of the stomach. Draw 2 oesophageal branches from the left gastric artery to the oesophagus.
- Draw a dotted line behind the stomach to represent the splenic artery.
- Draw a 2nd 'loop' from the splenic artery around the greater curvature of the stomach to the gastroduodenal artery (from the CHA). Draw multiple branches to the greater curvature of the stomach. Label the left and right gastroepiploic arteries as shown (also called gastro-omental arteries).
- Draw branches from the splenic artery to the fundus; these are the short gastric arteries.

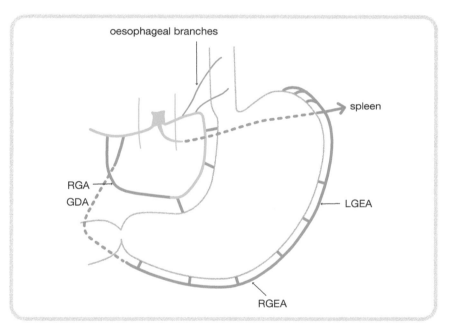

STEP 4

- Draw 'trouser legs' above the CHA, to represent the portal, splenic and superior mesenteric veins.
- Using a dotted line extend the splenic vein, to show it drains from the spleen.

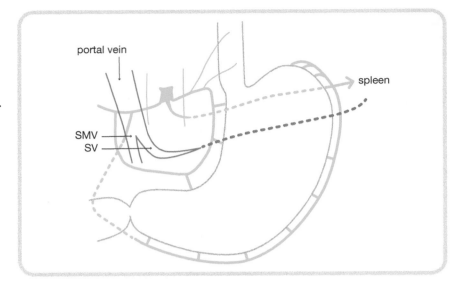

STEP 5

- Draw a branch off the portal vein to loop around from above the splenic vein, down the lesser curvature of the stomach and back into the portal vein. This represents the left and right gastric veins.
- Draw a vein along the greater curvature of the stomach, draining to the splenic vein on the right side of the page and the SMV on the left. This represents the left and right gastroepiploic veins.

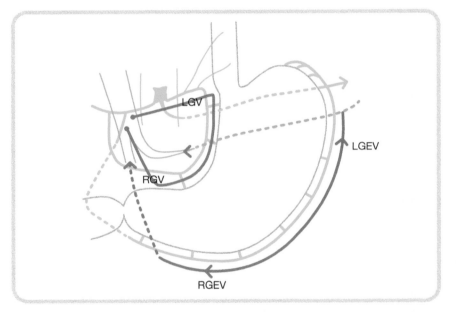

5.1.2 Small and large intestines

The small intestine is approximately 6 metres long and the large intestine is approximately 1.5 metres long.

Blood supply

Arterial supply is as follows:

- Coeliac trunk: down to junction of 2nd/3rd parts of duodenum (called 'the foregut').
- Superior mesenteric artery: from this to 2/3 of the way along the transverse colon (includes parts 3 and 4 of duodenum, all of jejunum, ileum, caecum, ascending colon, plus 1/3 of transverse colon) (called 'the midgut').
- Inferior mesenteric artery: from this to the upper anal canal (includes distal 1/3 of transverse colon, descending colon, sigmoid colon, rectum and upper portion of anus) (called 'the hindgut').

Section 5.3: Abdominal aorta shows the origins of these arteries. Venous drainage is described and illustrated in *Section 5.7.1: Hepatic portal venous system*.

Innervation

The intestines are innervated by two plexi:

- **Superior mesenteric plexus:** this has parasympathetic (right vagus nerve), sympathetic (thoracic splanchnic nerves) and sensory input, and is a continuation of the coeliac plexus. It travels with the superior mesenteric artery and supplies the midgut.
- **Inferior mesenteric plexus**: this has parasympathetic input from pelvic splanchnic nerves and sympathetic input from lumbar splanchnic nerves. It follows the inferior mesenteric artery and supplies the hindgut. It joins with the pelvic plexi.

AC ascending colon
DC descending colon
GB gallbladder
SC sigmoid colon
TC transverse colon

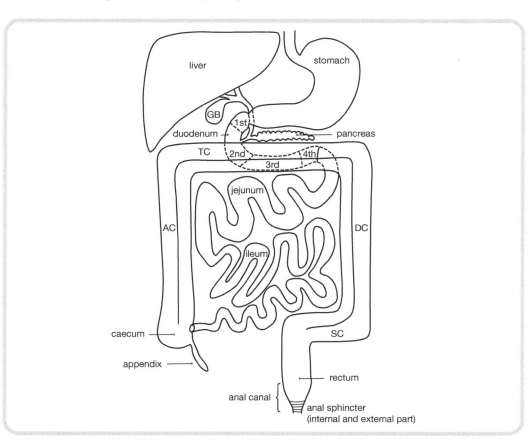

How to draw

STEP 1

- Draw 2 sides and the top of a square. Inside it, draw the same shape twice, smaller each time. This creates the outline of the large intestine, with a central line representing the taeniae coli (longitudinal bands of smooth muscle).
- At the bottom, on the left side of the page, draw a curved line to complete the base of the caecum, and draw a little 'tail' to represent the appendix.
- Label the ascending, transverse and descending colon. The transverse colon is at the level of approximately L2.
- At the bottom, on the right side of the page, draw a bend and continue the 3 lines horizontally; this area represents the sigmoid colon. Continue the inner and outer lines down and towards each other (not touching), as the outlines of the rectum and anal canal.

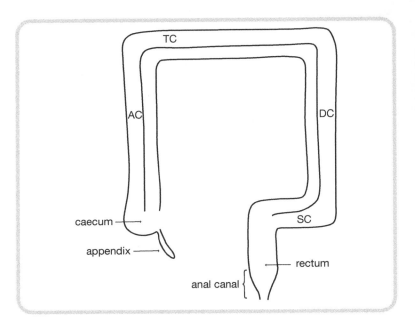

STEP 2

- Draw a triangular shaped liver on the left side of the page.
- Draw a stomach on the right side of the page, leaving space between it and the liver and transverse colon.

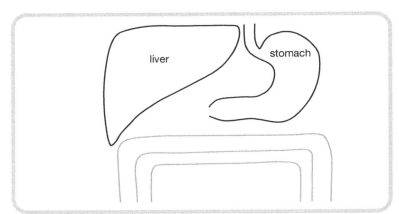

STEP 3

- Now we will start to draw the small intestine, which joins the stomach to the caecum. There are 3 main parts, first the duodenum, then the jejunum and finally the ileum.
- Draw the duodenum as half a C shape, dividing it into 4 parts: the 1st part is superior, the 2nd is descending, the 3rd is horizontal and the 4th is ascending. The 2nd, 3rd and 4th parts lie behind the TC.
- Show the parts are different lengths: from 1st to 4th, they are approximately 5, 7.5, 10 and 2.5 cm long, totalling 25 cm.

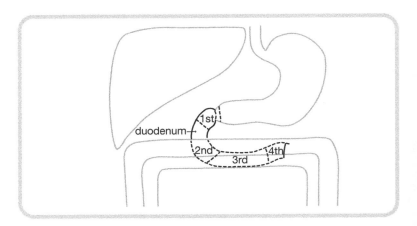

STEP 4

- From the end of the duodenum continue the outlines in a snake-like fashion across the page as shown. This represents the jejunum; it is approximately 2.5 metres in length.

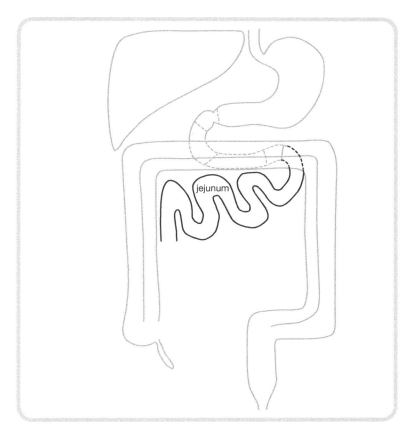

STEP 5

- Continue the outlines, drawing them closer together, in a long wiggly path to join the caecum at the iliocaecal valve. This is the ileum; it is approximately 3 metres in length. It is thinner and longer than the jejunum.

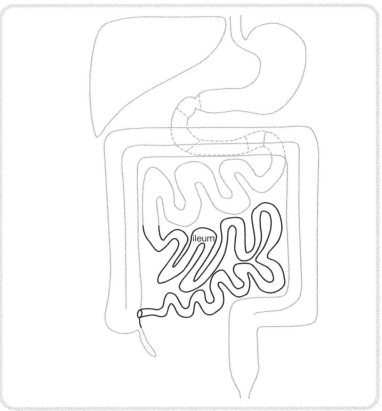

STEP 6

- Draw a Y-shaped duct from the liver to the left side of the 2nd part of the duodenum; use broken lines where it runs behind the stomach.
- At its top, draw it connecting to the gallbladder as shown.
- At its base draw a bumpy leaf shape to represent the pancreas.
- Show the ducts from the liver and pancreas joining and entering the duodenum (see *Section 5.1.3: Pancreas* for details).
- Draw a few lines across the anal opening; this is the anal sphincter.

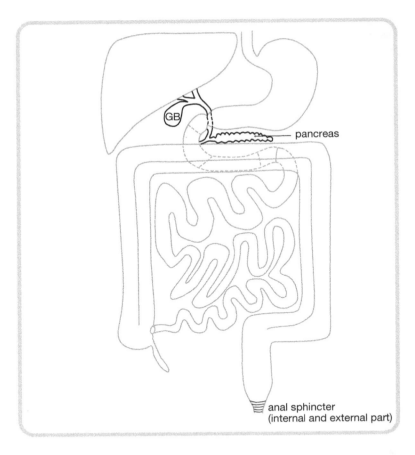

GB

pancreas

anal sphincter
(internal and external part)

5.1.3 Pancreas

We will look at the pancreas and biliary tree in more detail. It is 12–15 cm in length and has two types of function:

- exocrine
- endocrine.

Its exocrine function involves the production and release of pancreatic secretions. These contain bicarbonate, which neutralises stomach acid. In addition, it secretes digestive enzymes to help break down the protein, fat and carbohydrate ingested.

The endocrine function of the pancreas is mainly to regulate blood sugar levels. It secretes the hormones insulin, glucagon, somatostatin, and pancreatic polypeptide.

Innervation

Pancreatic plexus, coeliac ganglion and vagus nerve (CN X).

Blood supply

See Step 3.

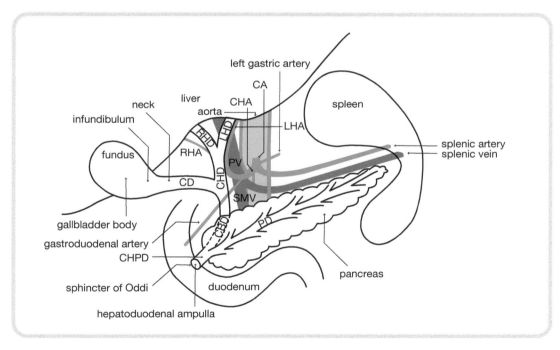

CA	coeliac artery	**LHD**	left hepatic duct
CBD	common bile duct	**PD**	pancreatic duct
CD	cystic duct	**PV**	portal vein
CHA	common hepatic artery	**RHA**	right hepatic artery
CHD	common hepatic duct	**RHD**	right hepatic duct
CHPD	common hepatopancreatic duct	**SMV**	superior mesenteric vein
LHA	left hepatic artery		

How to draw

STEP ①

- Draw a Y-shaped tube to represent the left and right hepatic ducts joining to form the common hepatic duct (CHD).
- Branching from the CHD draw a balloon shape to represent the gallbladder. Label its fundus, body, infundibulum and neck, and the cystic duct which joins it to the CHD.
- At the bottom of the Y, draw a leaf shape; this is the pancreas. Along its central axis draw the pancreatic duct as a stalk with smaller ducts feeding into it, like the centre of a leaf. Draw the common bile duct in broken lines behind the pancreas; join it to the pancreatic duct to form the slightly bigger common hepatopancreatic duct.
- Draw a circle at the end of this duct to represent the hepatoduodenal ampulla (ampulla of Vater); this is surrounded by a sphincter of muscle, the sphincter of Oddi. It opens into the duodenum.

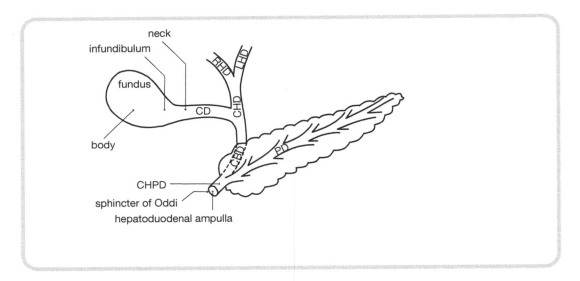

STEP ②

- Draw a line diagonally across the page from top right to bottom left. The upper side of this line represents the liver.
- Draw a distorted backward C shape around the end of the pancreas; this is the spleen.
- Draw the duodenum as a flattened C shape.

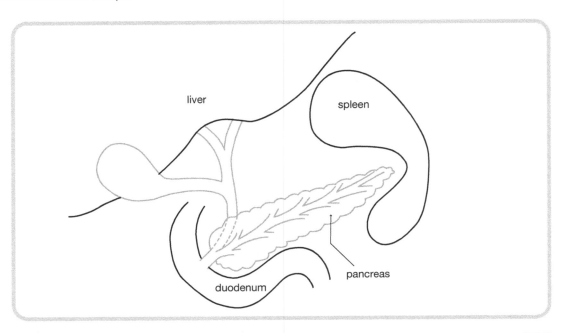

STEP 3

- Draw the abdominal aorta (AA) just medial to the CHD.
- From here draw the coeliac artery (also called coeliac trunk and coeliac axis). Draw branches off this: left gastric (to the stomach), splenic (to the spleen, along the top of the pancreas), common hepatic branching to form the gastroduodenal artery (to stomach and duodenum) and hepatic (to the liver). The pancreas also receives some blood supply from the superior mesenteric artery (not shown).
- Draw the portal vein just between the CHD and the AA. This is fed by the superior mesenteric vein and splenic vein as shown. The pancreas drains into the splenic vein and the superior mesenteric vein which in turn drain into the portal vein.

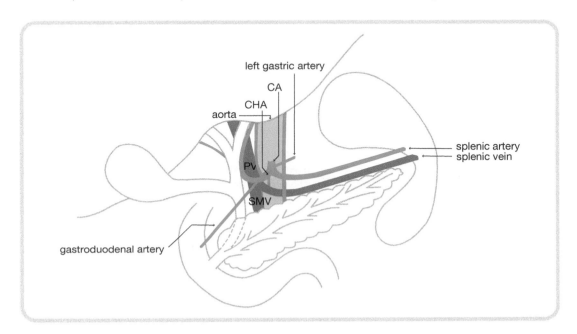

5.1.4 Biliary system

Bile is green/yellow in colour. It consists of bile salts, electrolytes, bile pigments, cholesterol and lipids. It helps aid digestion and eliminates excess haemoglobin and cholesterol from the body. Bilirubin is the main pigment. It is a waste product of haemoglobin from old or damaged red blood cells.

About half the bile secreted between meals is diverted to the gallbladder for storage. Water is absorbed there, so the bile becomes very concentrated. When food enters the small intestine, hormonal and nervous signals cause the gallbladder to contract and the sphincter of Oddi to open. This releases the concentrated bile to help aid digestion. However, we can live without a gallbladder.

About 90% of bile salts are reabsorbed in the ileum; the liver extracts the bile salts and re-secretes them. This happens every 2–3 hours.

Gall stones are hard masses, mainly, but not always, cholesterol-based. They are generally asymptomatic but can cause pain or jaundice if they block the cystic or common bile duct; jaundice is less likely if they only block the cystic duct because the bile still has a drainage route.

Blood supply (to gallbladder)

Cystic artery which is a branch of the right hepatic artery. So blood flows in this order: abdominal aorta → coeliac trunk → common hepatic artery → hepatic artery proper → right hepatic artery → cystic artery.

Innervation

Coeliac plexus and vagus nerve (CN X) for parasympathetic stimulation. Parasympathetic stimulation causes contraction of the gallbladder.

CBD	common bile duct
CD	cystic duct
CHD	common hepatic duct
LHD	left hepatic duct
PD	pancreatic duct
RHD	right hepatic duct

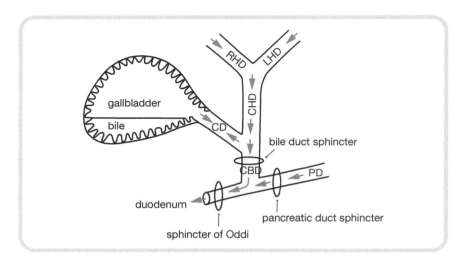

How to draw

STEP 1

- Draw a 'Y' shape. Label the left hepatic duct, right hepatic duct and common hepatic duct (CHD).
- On the left side of the page draw a duct and 'balloon' coming off the common hepatic duct at about 45° – the gallbladder and cystic duct. Draw the lining of the gallbladder as a squiggly line and show bile collecting in the gallbladder.
- Draw a circle around the bile duct and label it as the bile duct sphincter. Below this the duct is called the common bile duct.
- Draw the pancreatic duct, from the right to the left side of the page. Draw the pancreatic duct sphincter and sphincter of Oddi on either side of the junction of the pancreatic and common bile duct.

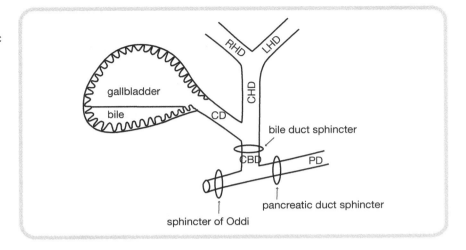

STEP 2

- Draw arrows to represent bile flow. Bile starts in the liver and heads down the left and right hepatic ducts into the common hepatic duct. There is 2-way flow to the gallbladder from there to the CHD. Bile ultimately flows into the second part of the duodenum.

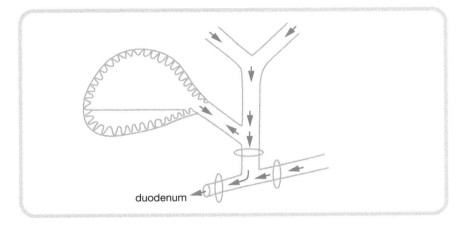

5.1.5 Spleen

To remember key facts about the spleen use the 1, 3, 5, 7, 9, 11 rule:

It is 1 × 3 × 5 inches in size; it is 7 oz in weight; it is positioned between T9 and T11.

(I know that we use metric units in the UK but for the rule to work we need to have it in imperial figures: 7 oz is approximately 200 g!)

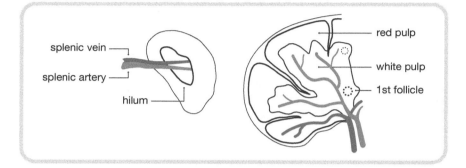

ARTERIAL AND VENOUS SUPPLY

The arterial supply is from the splenic artery. This is the biggest branch of the coeliac artery (also called the coeliac trunk or coeliac axis). It passes through the splenorenal ligament and gives off branches to the pancreas and stomach.

The venous drainage is from the splenic vein. It joins the superior mesenteric vein to form the portal vein.

NERVE SUPPLY

Sympathetic fibres from the coeliac plexus.

COMPONENTS

There are 4 components:

- Supporting tissue – fibroelastic and forms the capsule.
- White pulp – lymphatic nodules arranged around an arteriole.
- Red pulp – comprises connective tissue and many sinuses filled with blood, hence the red colour. The red pulp contains many cells including lymphocytes, red blood cells and macrophages.
- Vascular system.

FUNCTION

This can be remembered using the mnemonic "SHIP":

- **S**torage of red blood cells (8% of circulating RBCs are here).
- **H**aematopoiesis, especially during fetal life and also disease (e.g. chronic myeloid leukaemia/myelosclerosis).
- **I**mmune – antigenic stimulation which leads to the formation of plasma cells and increased lymphopoiesis.
- **P**hagocytosis – removes debris and old red blood cells and microorganisms. The spleen is like a 'filter'. It also initiates the humoral and cellular immune response.

5.1.6   Liver

GROSS ANATOMY

The liver is large, weighing approximately 1.5 kg. It is situated in the right upper quadrant of the peritoneal cavity. It has many functions including synthesis of proteins, hormones, urea and bile, glycogen storage, glucose and fat metabolism, detoxification and clotting factor production.

Blood supply

Blood supply is from the hepatic artery (25%) and hepatic portal vein (75%). Venous drainage is via hepatic veins which open into the inferior vena cava.

Innervation

The liver parenchyma is innervated by the hepatic plexus. This contains sympathetic and parasympathetic nerve fibres from the coeliac plexus and vagus nerve, respectively. The nerve fibres follow the course of the hepatic artery and portal vein.

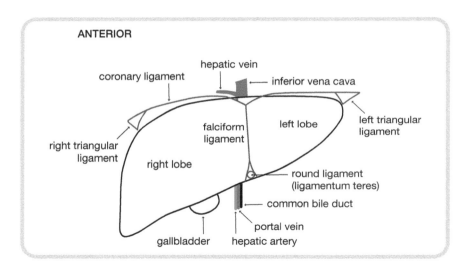

CBD	common bile duct
CHA	common hepatic artery
CL	coronary ligament
IVC	inferior vena cava
LHA	left hepatic artery
PV	portal vein
RHA	right hepatic artery

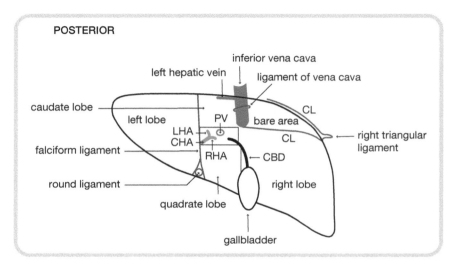

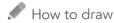 How to draw

Anterior view

STEP ①

- Draw a soft-edged triangle: start by drawing a vertical line up the left side of the page and curve the line to turn 90° and continue it horizontally across the top of the page.
- Join the end of the horizontal line to the bottom end of the vertical line, using curved lines. This completes the outline of the liver.

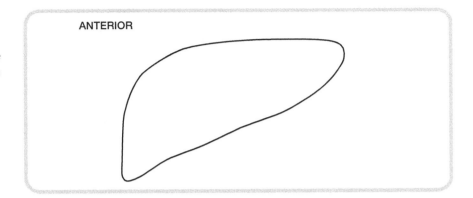

STEP ②

- Above the upper line draw a flattened M shape with a small triangle at each end. This represents the right triangular ligament, the coronary ligament and the left triangular ligament.
- Label the right and left lobe.

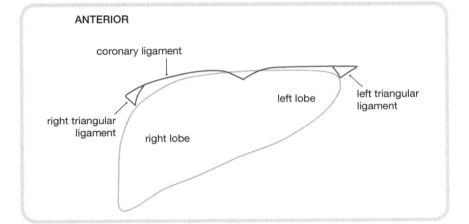

STEP ③

- Draw a line down from the middle of the M, ending in a small triangle. This represents the falciform ligament.
- Draw a circle inside the lower triangle; this is the round ligament (or ligamentum teres – the obliterated umbilical vein). It divides the left lobe into a medial and lateral part underneath (see section on *Posterior view of the liver*).

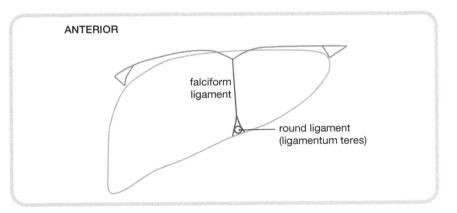

STEP 4

- Draw a semicircle on the lower edge of the right lobe (as shown); this is the gallbladder.
- Above the liver and falciform ligament draw the inferior vena cava and draw the right hepatic vein entering this directly.
- At the lateral edge and inferior to the round ligament draw a black line, a blue line and a red line. These are the common bile duct, portal vein and hepatic artery, respectively.

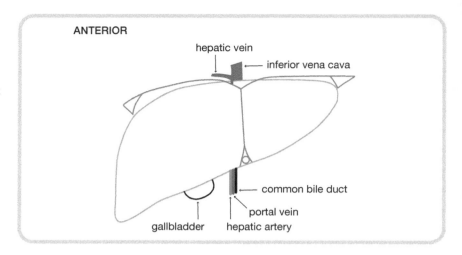

Posterior view

STEP 5

- Draw a soft-edged triangle in a mirror image to the one for the anterior view of the liver.
- This time draw an oval shape about 40% in from the right edge of the liver; this is the gallbladder.

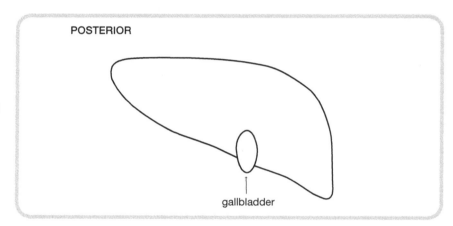

STEP 6

- Draw a vertical grey line about 1/3 in from the left tip; this is the falciform ligament. Draw a triangle at the bottom with a circle in it; this is the round ligament.
- Draw the IVC from about 1/3 up in the middle of the liver, and the left hepatic vein draining into it.
- Draw a grey line horizontally across the middle of the IVC; this is the ligament of the vena cava.
- Draw a grey line horizontally from the IVC to the right side; this is the coronary ligament. Continue it as a curve along the top of the liver. Draw a triangle where these parts meet; this is the right triangular ligament.

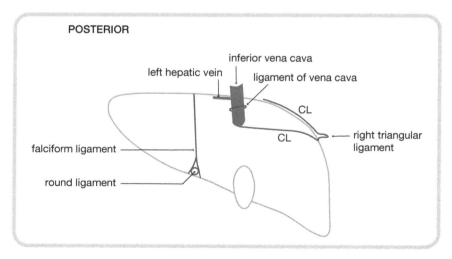

STEP 7

- Label the left lobe on the left side of the page. Label the right lobe on the lower right side, below the CL.
- Label the bare area above the CL.
- From the medial side of the IVC draw a line down to the gallbladder. Then split the middle section into 3. The upper part is the caudate lobe, the lower part is the quadrate lobe and the middle part is where the vessels will be drawn in the next step.

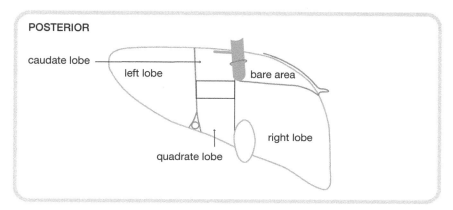

STEP 8

- Draw the CBD from the middle area to the gallbladder.
- Draw a blue circle and label it as the portal vein (PV).
- Draw a red snake's tongue shape; this is the common hepatic artery dividing into the left and right hepatic arteries.

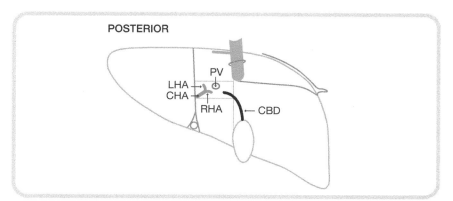

SEGMENTS OF THE LIVER

The liver is divided into 8 functionally independent segments by the Couinaud classification. Each segment has its own blood supply (hepatic artery), venous drainage (branch of the hepatic vein) and common bile duct.

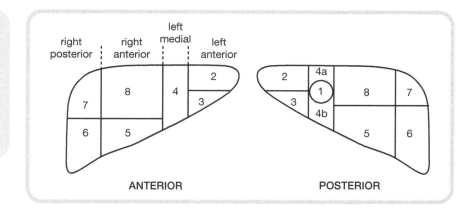

 How to draw

STEP 1

- Draw the outline of the anterior view of the liver.
- Draw a vertical line down the centre of the liver. Divide each side with a further line as shown and label the 4 sections.

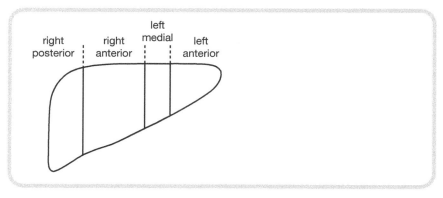

STEP 2

- Draw a horizontal line across the middle of the right half of the liver. Then label the upper 2 segments 7 and 8 and the lower 2 segments 6 and 5 as shown.
- Draw a horizontal line across the left lateral section. Label segment 2 above and 3 below. The left medial section is segment 4.

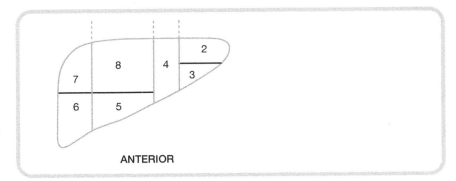

STEP 3

- Draw the posterior view of the liver.
- Draw a vertical line down through the middle of the liver as shown.
- Divide the right side into 4 segments, label 8 and 7 above and 5 and 6 below.

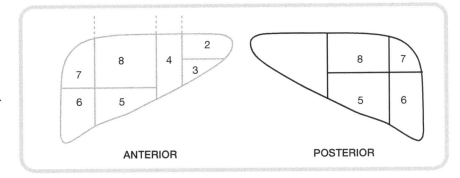

STEP 4

- Draw a vertical line down the middle of the left side of the liver.
- Draw a line horizontally across the left lateral section, label 2 above and 3 below, the same as for the anterior view.

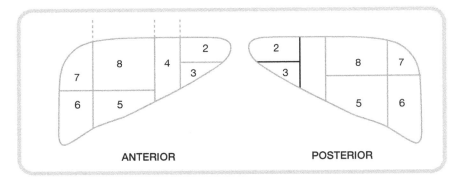

STEP 5

- Draw a circle in the middle of the left medial section. Label this segment 1. Label segment 4a above, and 4b below (I remember this by A for Above, and B for Below).

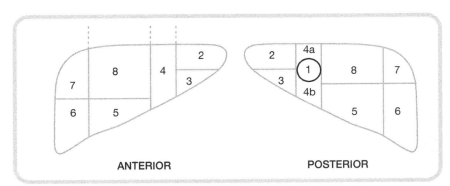

MICROSTRUCTURE OF THE LIVER

- The liver is the second largest organ in the body. It weighs approximately 1.5 kg, and receives 25% of blood flow (approximately 1.5 L/min).
- Blood is supplied by the hepatic artery (25%) and the hepatic portal vein (75%); each supply 50% of oxygen. The hepatic portal vein is responsible for carrying nutrient-rich blood from the GI tract to the liver.
- Venous drainage is via the left, right and middle hepatic veins to the inferior vena cava (IVC).
- The liver is divided into the right and left lobe by the falciform ligament.
- Functionally, the liver is divided into lobules. Blood enters the lobule through the portal vein and hepatic artery. Blood then flows through sinusoids, lined with hepatocytes, to the central hepatic venule.
- The hepatic acinus is the metabolic unit of the liver. Each acinus comprises a diamond shape that runs between the central veins of two lobules. Within the acinus are hepatocytes; the amount of oxygen that the hepatocytes receive is related to distance from the arterioles. There are 3 zones: zone 1 is best oxygenated (it is nearest the arteriole; see image), whereas zone 3 has the least oxygen and hence is at most risk of ischaemia. Because of this the hepatocytes in zone 1 are specialised for oxidative liver functions (gluconeogenesis), and they are at most risk of blood-borne toxins and deposition of haemosiderin in haemochromatosis. Zone 3 hepatocytes carry out glycolysis, lipogenesis and cytochrome P450 drug detoxification. Hence zone 3 cells are at most risk from N-acetyl-p-benzoquinone imine (NAPQI) production in paracetamol overdose.

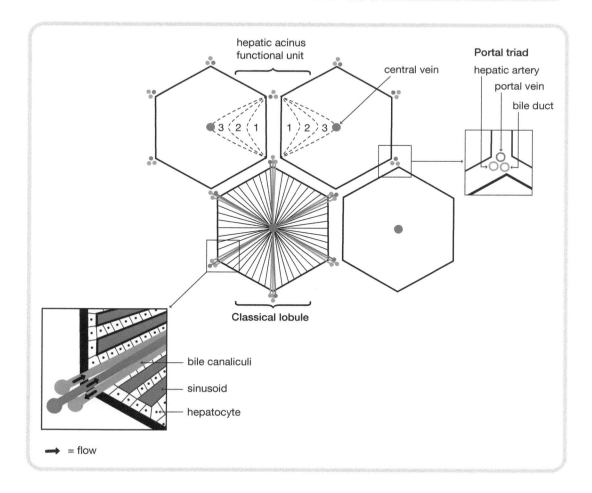

5.1.7 Adrenal gland

The adrenal gland sits on top of the kidney. It is an endocrine gland that produces hormones, as outlined in Table 5.1.

Table 5.1. Hormones produced by the adrenal gland

Adrenal area	Hormone class	Hormones	What they do
Cortex: zona glomerulosa	Mineralocorticoids (corticosteroids)	Aldosterone	Regulation of electrolyte/mineral balance Blood pressure regulation (via blood volume/sodium content in blood)
Cortex: zona fasciculata	Glucocorticoids (corticosteroids)	Cortisol, corticosterone, cortisone	Regulation of glucose metabolism and suppression of immune system
Cortex: zona reticularis	Androgens (precursor to sex hormones)	Dehydroepiandrosterone	Stimulate masculinisation
Adrenal medulla (chromaffin cells)	Catecholamines	Epinephrine and norepinephrine ('stress hormones')	Stimulate sympathetic nervous system

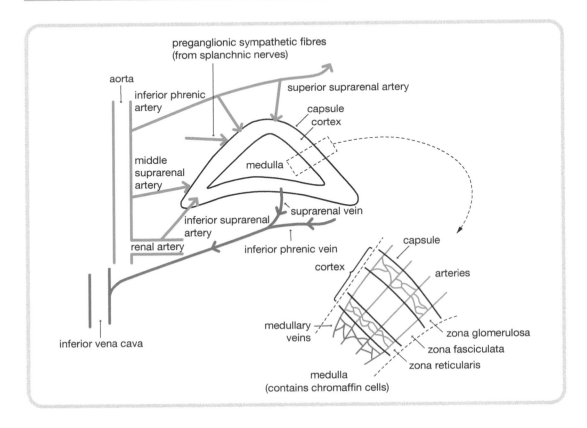

✏️ How to draw

STEP ①

- Draw 2 soft-cornered triangles pointing upwards, one inside the other. This is the adrenal gland.
- Label the capsule on the outside, the cortex in the outer layer and the medulla inside.
- Add an arrow representing the innervation of the adrenal gland, by preganglionic sympathetic fibres from splanchnic nerves.

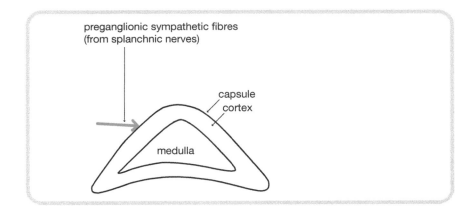

STEP ②

- Now we will zoom in on a section of the gland to draw the layers of the adrenal gland, from the capsule to the medulla, as shown by broken lines.
- Draw 4 lines. The outermost line is the capsule.
- Label the areas between the lines: first 3 form the cortex: zona glomerulosa, zona fasciculata and zona reticularis. (I remember this by GFR, like in the kidneys!) The medulla is the inner layer.

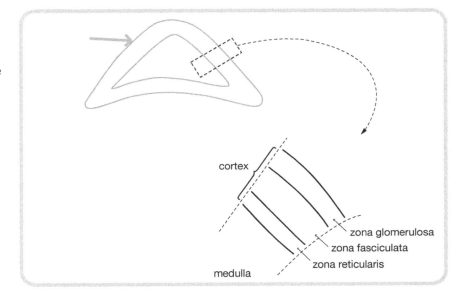

STEP ③

- Add the arteries by first drawing 4 lines perpendicular to the capsule. In the zona glomerulosa and zona reticularis, draw branches to join all 4 together.

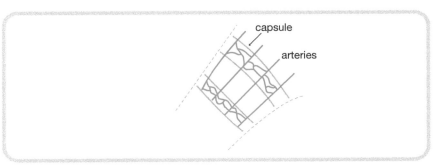

STEP 4

- From the end of the arteries near the medulla draw the medullary veins.
- Add a label to show the medulla also contains chromaffin cells.

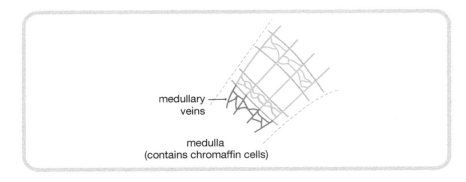

medullary veins

medulla
(contains chromaffin cells)

STEP 5

- We will make this the left adrenal gland. Draw the aorta along the left side of the page. Include the large renal artery branching from it, inferior to the adrenal gland. From here draw an arrow to the lower edge of the adrenal gland; this is the inferior suprarenal artery.
- Draw an arrow directly from the aorta to the nearer edge of the adrenal gland; this is the middle suprarenal artery.
- Draw an arrow from the aorta, superior to the adrenal gland; this is the inferior phrenic artery. Draw 2 arrows from this to the gland; these are the superior suprarenal arteries.

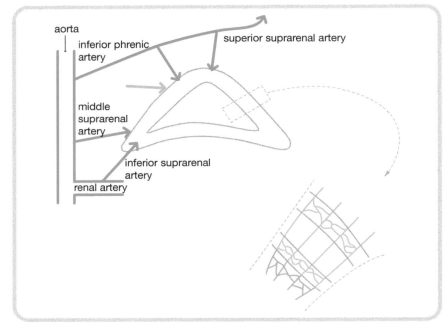

aorta

inferior phrenic artery

superior suprarenal artery

middle suprarenal artery

inferior suprarenal artery

renal artery

STEP 6

- Draw the suprarenal vein, coming out of the bottom of the gland. It joins the inferior phrenic vein and enters the inferior vena cava.

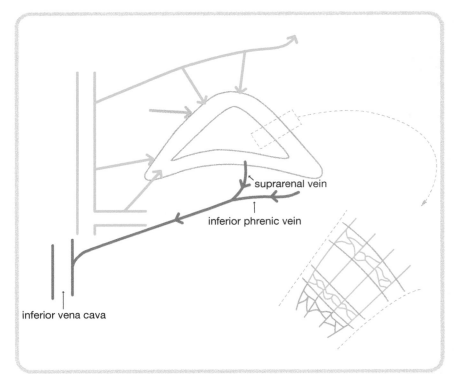

suprarenal vein

inferior phrenic vein

inferior vena cava

5.1.8 Kidney and nephron

In this section, we will draw a section of the kidney and draw a nephron, the functional unit of the kidney. The relationship of the kidney to the urinary tract will be drawn in *Section 5.1.9: Urinary tract*.

KIDNEY

We will draw a coronal section of the kidney.

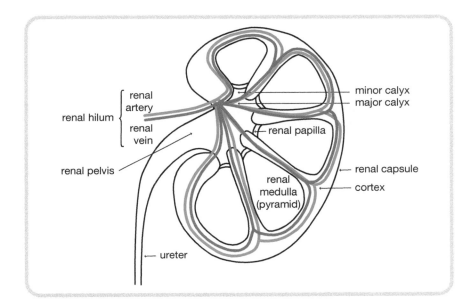

How to draw

STEP 1

- Draw a kidney bean shape. In the middle of the bean, draw 5 flat-topped protrusions joining to form the ureter. This is the renal pelvis. The small area of the protrusion is the minor calyx and the larger part is the major calyx, as labelled.
- Label the renal hilum. The renal hilum is the recessed part of the kidney where blood vessels, nerves and the ureter pass.

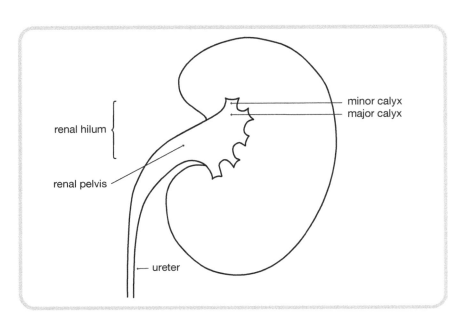

STEP 2

- At the end of each protrusion draw a 'sweetcorn kernel' shape and add a line just above the flat top of each minor calyx. The kernel shape is the renal medulla (meaning 'middle') or pyramid. The area between its base and the renal pelvis is the renal papilla.
- Label the area surrounding the renal medulla as the cortex, and label the outer edge as the renal capsule.
- We have only drawn 5 pyramids but, in reality, there are more in each kidney.

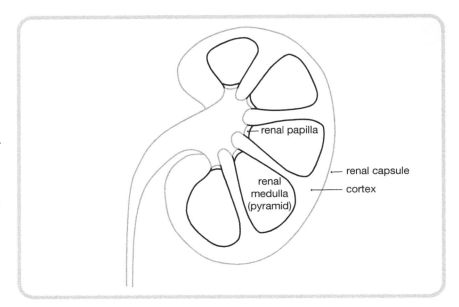

STEP 3

- Draw the renal vein as it exits the kidney, just above the renal pelvis.
- Draw branches around each pyramid.

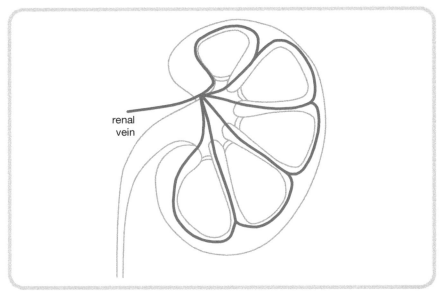

STEP 4

- Just above the renal vein draw the renal artery.
- Again, draw branches around each pyramid.

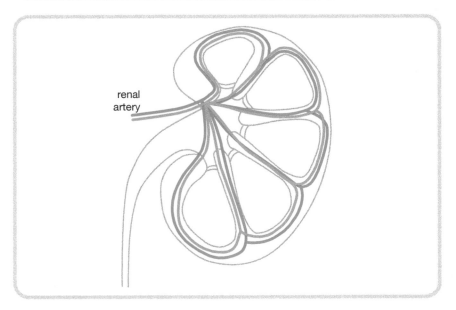

NEPHRON

The kidney is a complicated organ which performs many functions.

- It regulates extracellular fluid volume and electrolyte composition, total body water volume, acid–base balance and blood pressure.
- It produces the active form of vitamin D, renin, erythropoietin and glucose and it excretes waste products.

Most people have 2 kidneys. They are located in the upper abdomen in the retroperitoneal space. They are normally approximately 12 cm in length and 150 g in weight. Each kidney has 2 distinct regions: the outer cortex and the inner medulla.

The basic functional unit of the kidney is called the nephron (see figure). There are about 1.5 million nephrons in each kidney. The glomerulus (a capillary network), Bowman capsule, the proximal tube and the distal convoluted tubule are situated in the cortex. The loop of Henle and collecting duct are in the medulla. The proximal convoluted tubule reabsorbs electrolytes and water lost from the plasma through filtration at the glomerulus. The loop of Henle descends from the renal cortex into the medulla and then returns to the cortex.

The juxtaglomerular apparatus consists of the macula densa (special cells in the wall of the tubule responsible for sensing and responding to tubular composition) and the afferent arteriole granular cells (cells that secrete renin).

The collecting ducts pass through the renal medulla into the renal pelvis.

Blood supply is via the renal artery, a branch from the abdominal aorta. Venous drainage is via the renal vein into the inferior vena cava (IVC).

Kidneys receive 1 L/min blood flow (20% of cardiac output). The cortex receives 90% of this and the medulla receives 10%. The cortex receives 10 × more blood flow than it needs, for oxygenation, whereas the medulla only just receives enough blood for adequate oxygenation. This is because the flow is needed for filtration (the glomerular filtration rate, GFR).

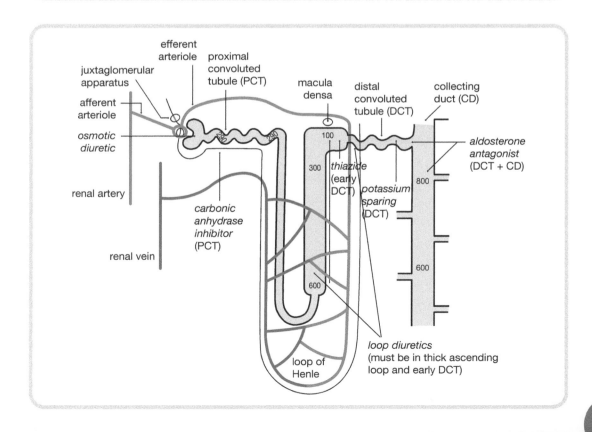

Action of diuretics

Different diuretics act in different parts of the kidney (shown in italic text on the illustration on the previous page).

- **Osmotic diuretic** (mannitol): inhibits reabsorption of water and Na^+, leading to hypertonic hyponatraemia.
- **Carbonic anhydrase inhibitor:** inhibits the enzyme carbonic anhydrase (catalyses hydration of carbon dioxide and dehydration of carbonic acid). This causes renal loss of HCO_3^- ion, which carries Na^+, H_2O and K^+.
- **Loop diuretics:** block $Na^+/K^+/Cl^-$ transporter in the ascending loop of Henle (potassium wasting).
- **Thiazide diuretics:** block Na^+/K^+ transporter (potassium wasting).
- **Potassium-sparing diuretics** (amiloride/spironolactone): block aldosterone receptors in the cortical collecting duct. This decreases Na^+ and water reabsorption and decreases K^+ secretion (potassium sparing).

5.1.9 Urinary tract

URINARY TRACT OVERVIEW (ANTERIOR VIEW)

The male and female urinary tract are the same apart from the area below the bladder. In the male, the urethra is longer and has more than one part, as we will show by drawing the anterior view of the male tract.

Blood supply

Superior vesical branch of the internal iliac artery, plus inferior vesical artery in males and vaginal arteries in females.

Venous drainage

Vesical venous plexus, which empties into the internal iliac veins.

Innervation

- **Sympathetic:** hypogastric nerve (T12–L2) – relaxes the detrusor muscle, with urinary retention.
- **Parasympathetic:** pelvic nerve (S2–S4) – signals lead to detrusor muscle contraction, stimulating micturition.
- **Somatic:** pudendal nerve (S2–S4) – innervates external urethral sphincter, exercising voluntary control over micturition.
- Sensory nerves send signals to the brain to indicate bladder is full.

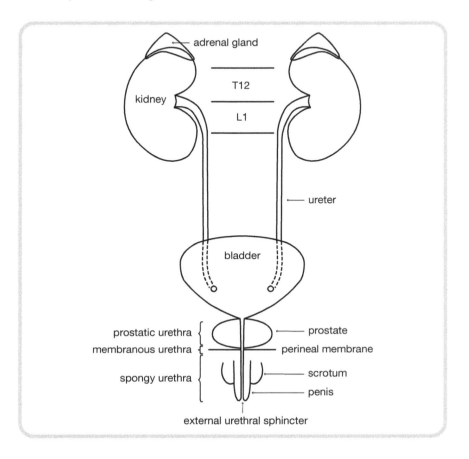

🖉 How to draw

STEP ①

- Draw the level of T12 and L1 in the middle of the top part of the page.
- Either side draw a kidney bean shape, the kidney! Below them draw a 'balloon on a string' shape half-way down the page; this represents the bladder and urethra. Label the opening at the bottom as the external urethral sphincter.
- Draw a tube from the middle of each kidney to the posterior wall of the bladder (use broken lines behind); these are the ureters.
- Draw the adrenal gland on top of the kidneys, looking like a little hat!
- Up to here, male and female tracts are the same.

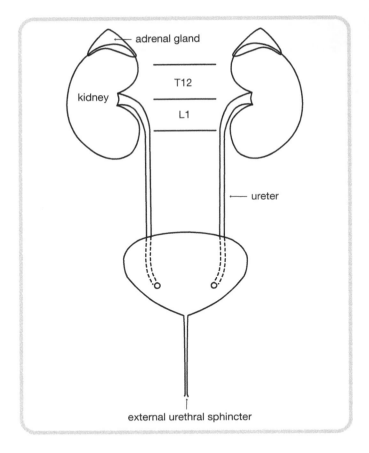

STEP ②

- From here, the images illustrate male anatomy.
- Draw a horizontal oval shape beneath the bladder; this is the prostate gland.
- Beneath this draw a line to represent the perineal membrane.

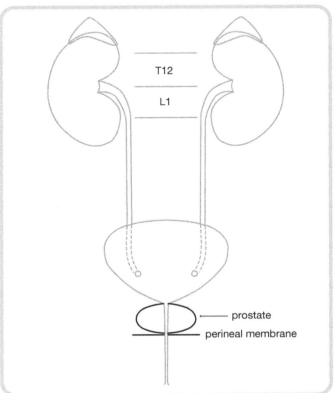

STEP 3

- Draw the scrotum on each side and the penis below this.
- Label the urethra. It is divided into 3 parts: prostatic, membranous and spongy urethra.

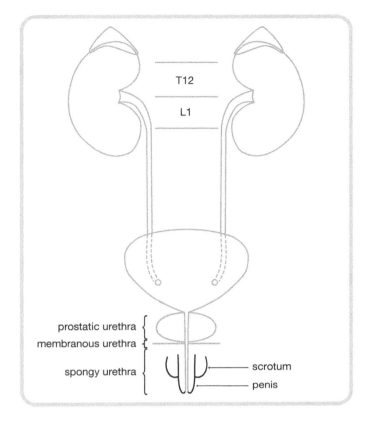

URETER (CROSS-SECTION)

The ureter is 25–30 cm long. It begins at the level of the renal artery and vein and ends in the bladder.

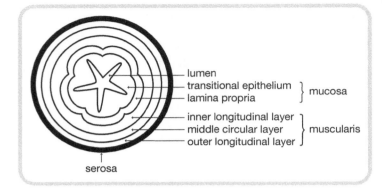

lumen
transitional epithelium ⎱ mucosa
lamina propria

inner longitudinal layer ⎱
middle circular layer ⎰ muscularis
outer longitudinal layer

↑ serosa

 How to draw

STEP 1

- Draw a starfish shape. This is the lumen of the ureter.
- Surround this with a double-line, 5-petal flower shape. Between the star and the flower is transitional epithelium. Between the 1st and 2nd layer of the flower is the lamina propria. These two layers make up the mucosa.

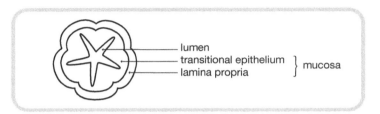

lumen
transitional epithelium ⎱ mucosa
lamina propria

STEP 2

- Draw 3 circles surrounding the flower shape. These are the muscularis: inner longitudinal layer, middle circular and outer longitudinal layers.
- Draw a thickened line around the outer muscular layer; this is the serosa.

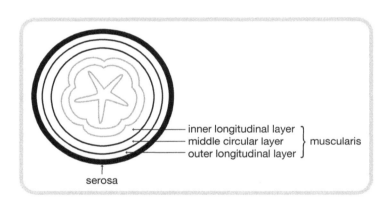

inner longitudinal layer ⎱
middle circular layer ⎰ muscularis
outer longitudinal layer

↑ serosa

SAGITTAL SECTION OF THE URINARY SYSTEM

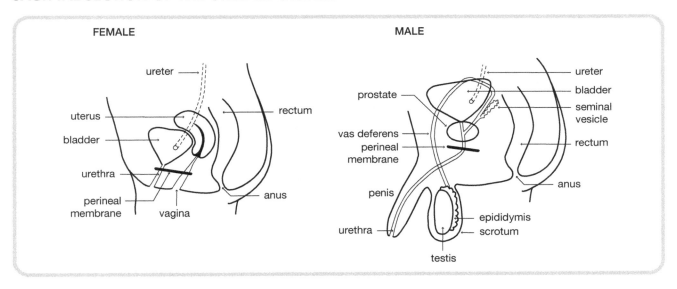

 How to draw

Male urinary system

STEP 1

- Draw the outline of the penis, scrotum and anus as shown.

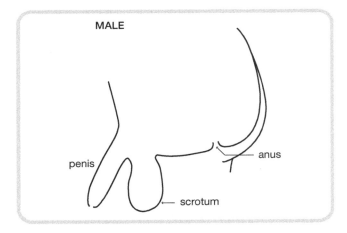

STEP 2

- In the middle, draw an upside-down soft-cornered triangle with an oval below it. These are the bladder and prostate.
- Draw the rectum adjoining the anus.
- Draw a vertical oval in the scrotum, with a bumpy line over its posterior side. These are the testis and epididymis.

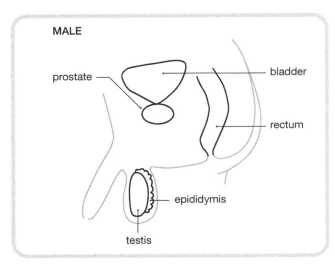

STEP 3

- From the bladder draw a tube to the tip of the penis, with a branch from the middle of the prostate to the 2 o'clock position. The tube to the tip of the penis is the urethra.
- From the 2 o'clock position on the prostate, continue the branch upwards, ready to start the next step.

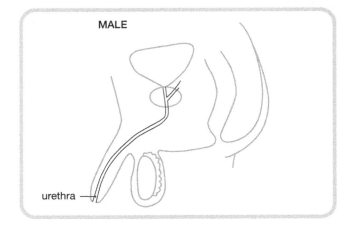

STEP 4

- Joined to this tube, draw a bumpy leaf shape behind the prostate; this is the seminal vesicle. Continue the tube past the seminal vesicle and loop it over the bladder to run down to the epididymis; this is the vas deferens.
- Use a broken line to draw another tube behind the bladder, to represent the position of the ureter.
- Draw a black line beneath the prostate to represent the perineal membrane.

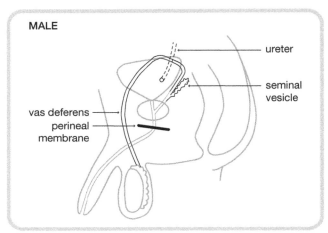

Female urinary system (sagittal section)

STEP 5

- Draw a U-shaped outline sitting on lines representing the front and back of the leg. Leave 3 holes in the lower part of the U, for the urethra, vagina and anus.

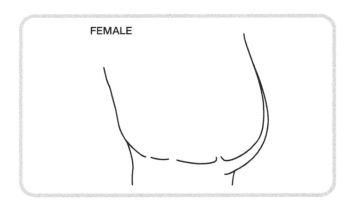

STEP 6

- In the middle draw a triangular 'balloon on a string'; this represents the bladder and urethra.
- Draw a dotted line from behind the bladder upwards; this is the ureter.

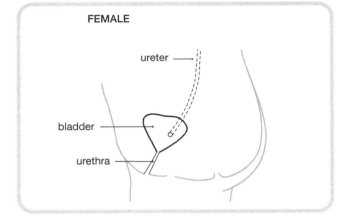

STEP 7

- Draw an upside-down 'aubergine' curved around the back of the bladder; this is the uterus. Add a central curve to represent the uterine cavity.
- Draw the vagina directly below.

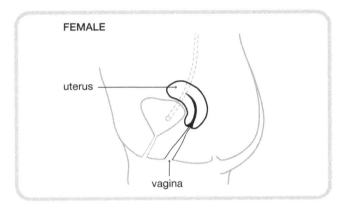

STEP 8

- Draw the rectum above the anus and behind the uterus.
- Draw in the perineal membrane as shown.

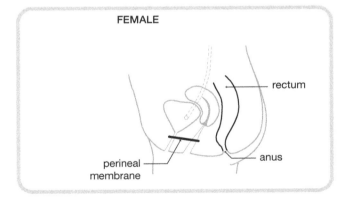

The peritoneum is made up of the parietal peritoneum (lines the inner abdominal wall) and the visceral peritoneum (lines the abdominal viscera). The peritoneal cavity is the space between them; it is divided into the greater sac and lesser sac (see Step 4).

Organs can be described as intraperitoneal or retroperitoneal.

- **Retroperitoneal organs** have peritoneum on their anterior side only. Retroperitoneal organs include adrenal glands, duodenum (2nd and 3rd segments), pancreas, both kidneys and ureters, ascending and descending colon, oesophagus, rectum, aorta and inferior vena cava.
- **Intraperitoneal organs** are contained within the peritoneum and include the stomach, spleen, liver, bulb of the duodenum, jejunum, ileum, sigmoid colon and transverse colon.

There are mnemonics to remember which organs are retroperitoneal – check on line for memory aids!

B	bladder
D	duodenum
GO	greater omentum
J	jejunum
LO	lesser omentum
P	pancreas
R	rectum
S	stomach
TC	transverse colon
TM	transverse mesocolon
U	uterus

SAGITTAL SECTION

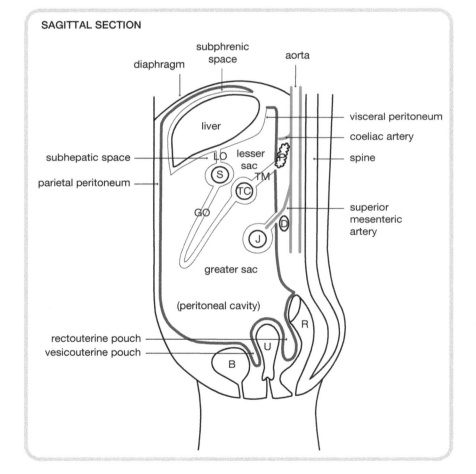

How to draw

STEP 1

- Draw the outline of the abdomen in cross-section, including the bladder, uterus and rectum.
- Draw the outline of the diaphragm and spinal column.
- You don't need to draw the vertebral bodies: the spine is only included in this image to allow you to understand the peritoneum.

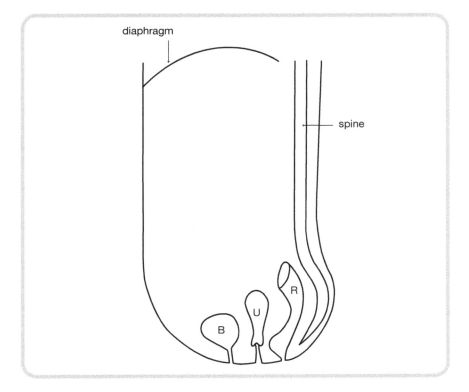

STEP 2

- Draw the liver below the diaphragm.
- Draw the parietal peritoneum as a thick grey line. The line starts below the diaphragm, above the liver. It descends down to form the vesicouterine pouch and the rectouterine pouch as shown. It then ascends anteriorly to the aorta and vertebral column, ending on the other side of the liver – leave 2 gaps in this part of it, as shown.
- Most abdominal contents are within the greater sac (see label and see Step 4 for relations with the lesser sac).

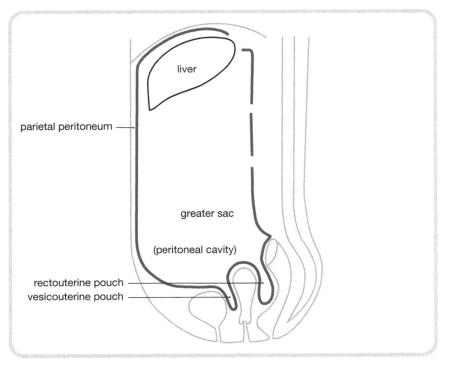

STEP 3

- Draw circles for the stomach, transverse colon and jejunum within the peritoneal cavity.
- Add the pancreas and duodenum as retroperitoneal structures. In this plane the duodenum is retroperitoneal but along its length it is partly intraperitoneal and partly retroperitoneal.
- Draw the visceral peritoneum with a thinner grey line (as shown), starting where it joins the parietal peritoneum above the liver. Show it surrounding certain organs as depicted here.
- Label the lesser sac, subhepatic space, subphrenic space, transverse mesocolon and lesser and greater omentum.

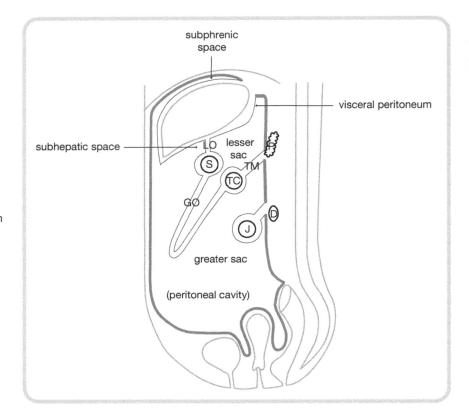

STEP 4

- Draw the aorta, the coeliac artery and the superior mesenteric artery.
- See *Section 5.6: Abdominal aorta* for more detail.

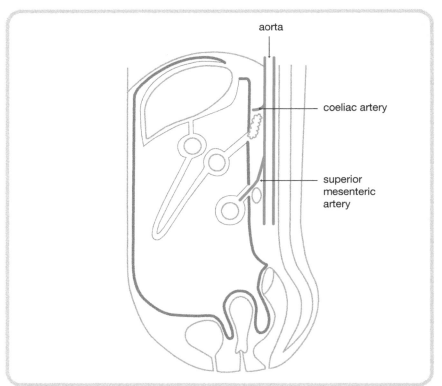

This is a similar diagram to the intercostal nerves. However, the difference is that the three muscles from inner to outer are the:

- transversus abdominis
- internal oblique
- external oblique.

They do not end at the sternum, they end at the rectus muscle.

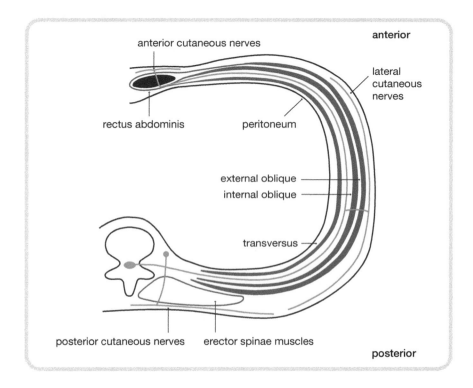

Only the male inguinal canal is depicted, because it is more common to be questioned on it. The inguinal region is complicated so I have just picked out the most important points. The image is transverse in the abdominal part and sagittal in the scrotal part, so you can see how the muscle fascia lies.

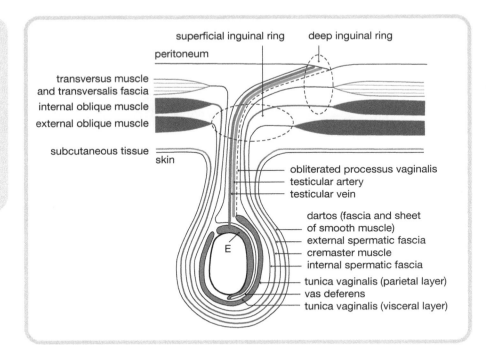

E   epididymis

THE INGUINAL CANAL AND THE SCROTUM

The scrotum is formed by an outpouching through layers of the abdominal wall. The canal carries the ductus deferens, testicular vessels and lymphatics in the male and the round ligament of the uterus in the female.

During its descent the scrotum pushes through the 3 muscular layers of the abdominal wall. The lowest fibres of the internal oblique muscle become the cremaster muscle. External oblique becomes the external spermatic fascia and transversus abdominalis becomes the internal spermatic fascia.

COMMON QUESTIONS

Is the inguinal hernia direct or indirect?

To distinguish between an indirect and direct hernia, put your thumb over the midpoint of the inguinal ligament to block the deep ring.

- If it is an indirect hernia, it will no longer protrude because your thumb prevents it passing through the deep ring.
- If it is a direct hernia, it will still protrude when the patient coughs because it is protruding through a defect in the muscle rather than the deep ring. Direct hernias are more likely to occur medial to the inferior epigastric vessels through Hesselbach's triangle.

Which type of hernia is more common?

The indirect inguinal hernia is more common than the direct hernia, by approximately 5 times. It is 7 times more common in males than females. In males there may be remnants of the processus vaginalis; this is an embryonic developmental outpouching of the peritoneum which normally closes. In some males it remains and allows an indirect hernia to descend into the scrotum.

5.5 Coeliac plexus

This diagram is drawn with the lumbar vertebrae at the bottom of the drawing and can be imagined looking at the patient from the feet towards the head.

The coeliac plexus is also known as the solar plexus. It is the main autonomic nerve supply to intra-abdominal organs. Performing a coeliac plexus nerve block, at L1, can help alleviate chronic pain caused by specific organs, e.g. pancreatitis-related pain.

Sympathetic supply is from the splanchnic nerves, and parasympathetic supply is from the vagus nerves (CN X).

The peritoneum is described in detail in *Section 5.2: Peritoneum*.

C	colon
IVC	inferior vena cava
K	kidney
L	liver
P	pancreas
Sp	spleen

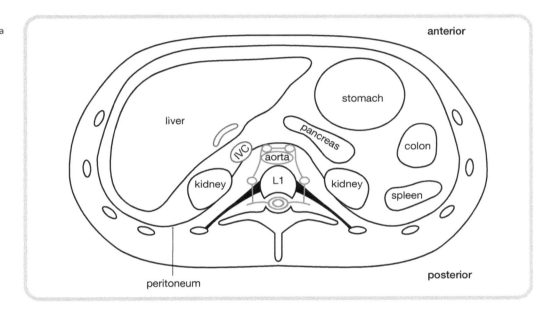

✏️ How to draw

STEP 1

- Draw an oval shape to represent the cross-section of the body.
- Draw one vertebra in the middle, ideally drawn with the main body and spinous processes separately (label it L1).
- Add 5 small ovals around each side to represent the end of the ribs that may be seen in cross-section.

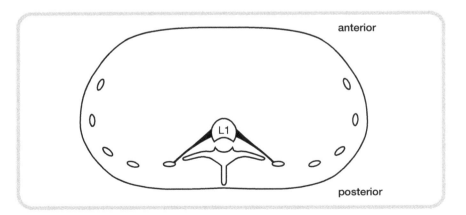

STEP 2

- Draw the peritoneum as one large kidney bean shape (on its side).

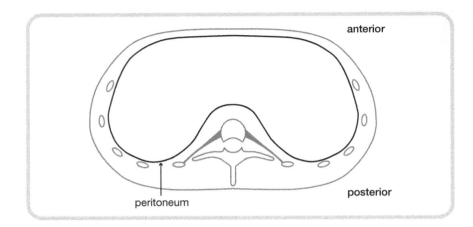

STEP 3

- Add in the organs; 2 kidneys (one either side of the L1 main body), the pancreas (just in front of L1), the stomach (anterior to the pancreas), the spleen and colon (lateral to the stomach) and the liver (the biggest organ in front of the right kidney).

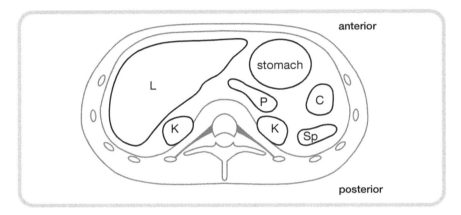

STEP 4

- The aorta lies anteriorly to the L1 main body and posteriorly to the peritoneum. Draw a blue oval to represent the IVC which lies anteriorly to the peritoneum.
- Draw the coeliac plexus as a green structure which encircles the L1 body and aorta. The 2 circles lateral to L1 main body are the sympathetic chain; the 2 anterior to the aorta are the coeliac plexus; the 1 behind the vertebral body is the spinal cord.

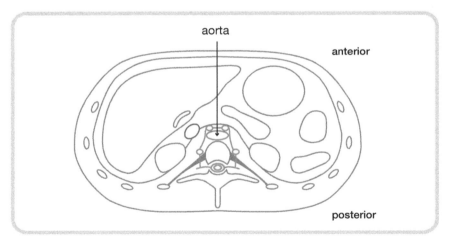

The abdominal aorta is easier to learn on its own because there are many branches and it can get complicated when seen in the same illustration as organs, etc. Here we draw a simplified version.

CHA common hepatic artery
HAP hepatic artery proper
i/c intercostal
IMA inferior mesenteric artery
SMA superior mesenteric artery

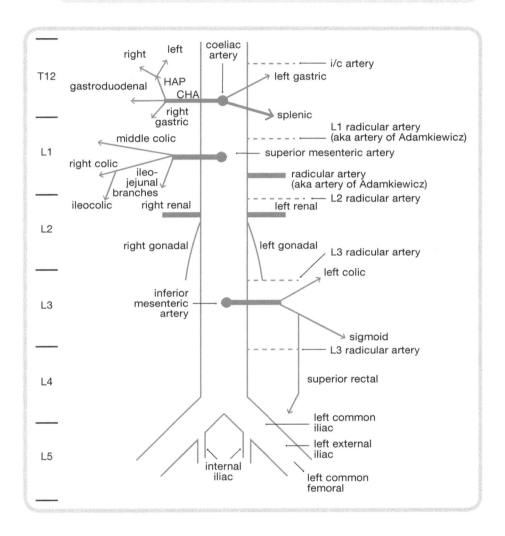

✏ How to draw

STEP 1

- Label the levels from T12 to L5, evenly spaced down the page.
- Draw the aorta. The bifurcation into the two common iliac veins is approximately at the L4 level.
- From the common iliac vessels draw a line downwards on each side; these represent the internal iliac arteries.

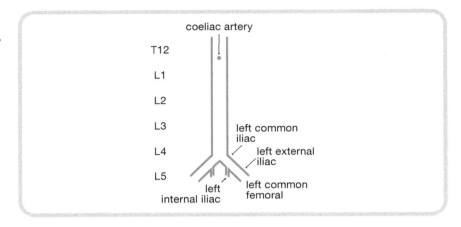

STEP 2

- The coeliac artery branches from the aorta at the T12/L1 level. Draw a horizontal line through the aorta that bifurcates at the left end and splits into 4 on the right side.
- The left side becomes the left gastric and splenic arteries.
- The right side becomes the hepatic (left and right) arteries, the gastroduodenal artery and the right gastric artery.

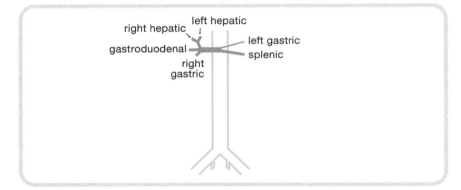

STEP 3

- Just inferior to the coeliac plexus (and to the right side, just for ease) draw the superior mesenteric artery. This divides into the middle colic, right colic, ileocolic and ileojejunal arteries.

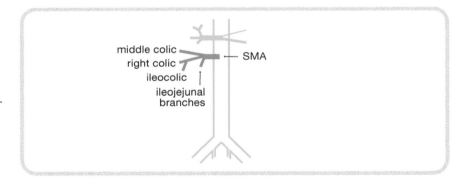

STEP 4

- Between L1/2 level, draw a horizontal line which represents the left and right renal arteries.
- Diagonally downwards from L2 level are the gonadal arteries.

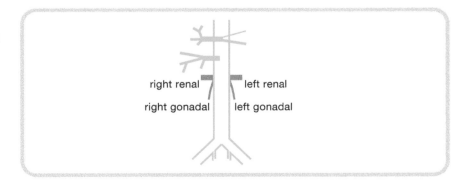

STEP 5

- At approximately L3, draw the inferior mesenteric artery (to the left). This branches into the left colic artery and the sigmoid artery. The superior rectal artery is a continuation of the IMA.

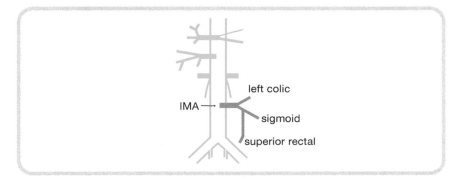

STEP 6

- Finally, draw some dotted lines at each level to represent the intercostal artery and lumbar radicular arteries.

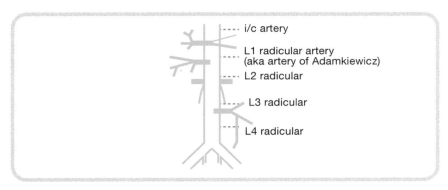

First we will draw the anatomy of the hepatic portal venous system, which returns blood to the inferior vena cava from many abdominal organs. Then we will show this in the context of the venous drainage of other abdominal organs and the major veins draining into the vena cava from the rest of the body.

5.7.1 Hepatic portal venous system

A portal venous system is one when a capillary bed drains into another capillary bed without passing through the heart. The hepatic portal venous system is often simply called the portal venous system and the hepatic portal vein called the portal vein.

In the hepatic portal venous system, capillaries of the gastrointestinal tract and spleen drain into the portal vein. Then the raw nutrients absorbed from the digestive system are processed in the liver before being returned to the rest of the body via the hepatic veins, which drain into the inferior vena cava (IVC).

GB	gallbladder
IMV	inferior mesenteric vein
IVC	inferior vena cava
LCIV	left common iliac vein
LCV	left colic vein
LGEV	left gastroepiploic vein
LGV	left gastric vein
PV	portal vein
RCIV	right common iliac vein
RGEV	right gastroepiploic vein
RGV	right gastric vein
SMV	superior mesenteric vein
SRV	superior rectal vein
SV	sigmoid vein

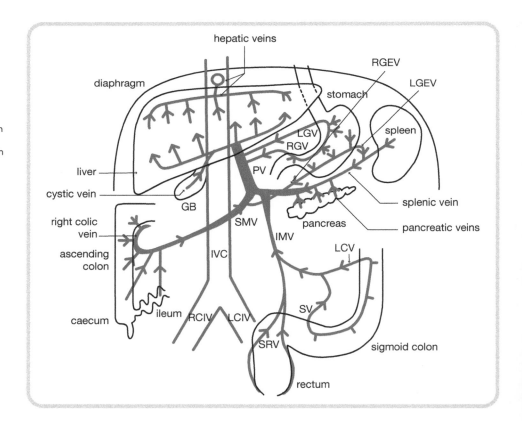

How to draw

STEP 1

- Draw the outline of the liver, gallbladder, oesophagus and stomach, pancreas, spleen, ascending colon and end of ileum and the sigmoid colon and rectum.

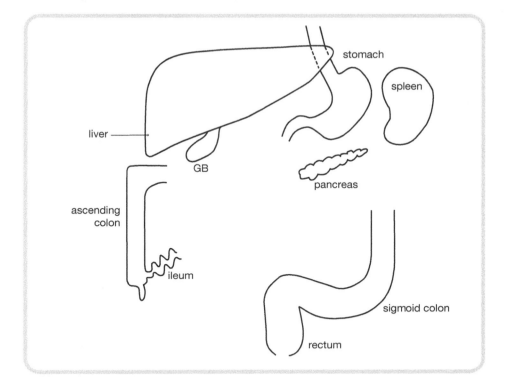

STEP 2

- Draw the diaphragm as a curved dome above the liver, stomach and spleen.
- Draw an upside-down Y shape down the middle of the liver, between the ascending colon and sigmoid colon; this represents the IVC and common iliac veins.

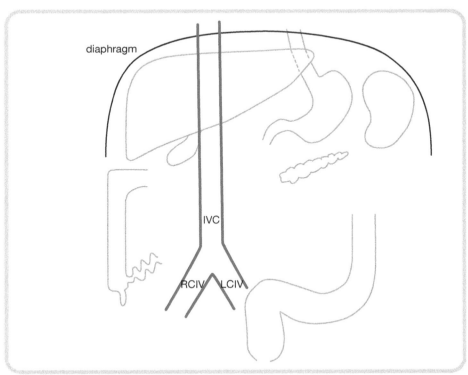

STEP 3

- Draw a tube from the middle of the liver, just medial to the IVC, going down to about the level of the pancreas. This is the portal vein (PV).
- Draw a line fed by the top of the PV with a few arrows pointing upwards; this shows blood flows *to* the liver from the PV.
- Draw a fish-hook shape (the right colic vein) from the top corner of the ascending colon round to form the superior mesenteric vein. This in turn drains into the inferior end of the PV. Draw arrows pointing towards the colic vein from the ascending colon and distal ileum as shown.
- Draw the splenic vein, above the pancreas.
- The splenic vein and superior mesenteric vein drain into the PV directly.

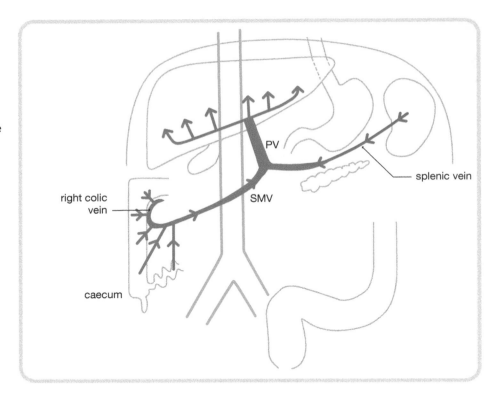

STEP 4

- Draw a loop by the sigmoid colon leading up to the end of the splenic vein. This represents the left colic veins and sigmoid veins. They drain into the inferior mesenteric vein and then the splenic vein.
- Draw 'pincers' around the rectum joining the inferior mesenteric vein; these are the superior rectal veins.
- Draw an arrow from the gallbladder to the veins in the lower half of the liver; this is the cystic vein.

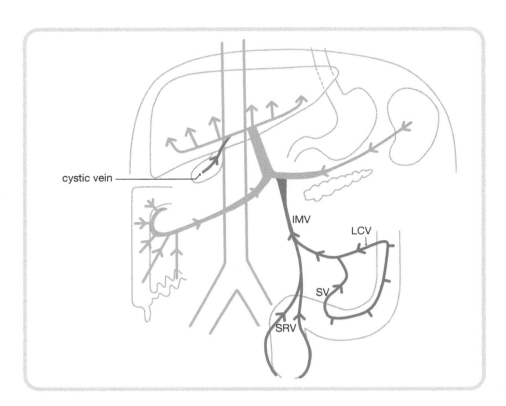

STEP 5

- Draw a loop from the superior mesenteric vein to the lower part of the stomach and then joining the splenic vein. This is initially the right and then the left gastroepiploic vein. It drains blood from the stomach into the splenic and superior mesenteric veins.
- Draw a loop from the PV around the upper part of the stomach; this is the left gastric vein above and the right gastric vein below.
- Draw a few arrows from the pancreas to the splenic vein; these are the pancreatic veins.

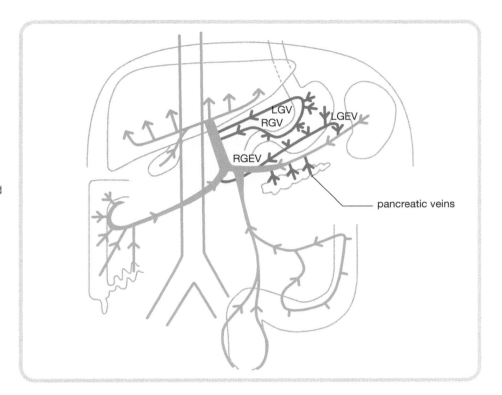

STEP 6

- Draw a line along the superior edge of the liver; this represents the hepatic veins. Add arrows from the top half of the liver draining into them.
- Draw an arrow to a circle drawn in the upper part of the IVC; this represents the right, middle and left hepatic veins draining into the IVC (see *Section 5.7.2: Systemic venous drainage*).
- The hepatic veins drain into the IVC, then the heart.

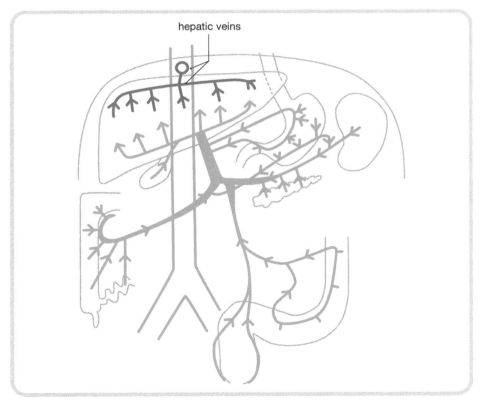

5.7.2 Systemic venous drainage

The superior vena cava (SVC) and inferior vena cava (IVC) are named relative to the right atrium, into which they both drain. This is approximately at the level of the third costal cartilage. The SVC drains everything above the diaphragm and the IVC drains everything below.

This is a complicated diagram, but everything will become clearer as you work through the steps to draw it out.

BCV brachiocephalic vein
CI common iliac vein
EI external iliac vein
EJV external jugular vein
HV hepatic veins
II internal iliac vein
IJV internal jugular vein
IT inferior thyroid vein
IVC inferior vena cava
MT middle thyroid vein
PIV posterior intercostal vein
RA right atrium
SCV subclavian vein
ST superior thyroid vein
SVC superior vena cava

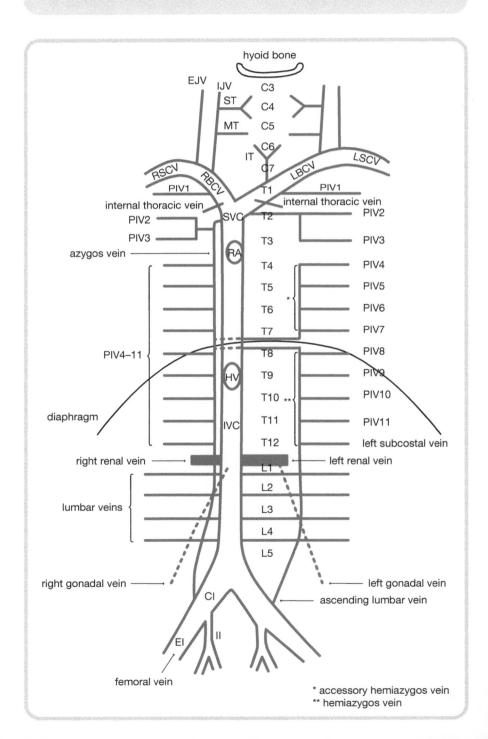

* accessory hemiazygos vein
** hemiazygos vein

How to draw

STEP 1

- Draw from C3 down to L5 in the middle of the paper. Just above C3 draw a flattened U shape, the hyoid bone.
- Draw a dome shape crossing the midline between T7 and T8; this is the diaphragm.

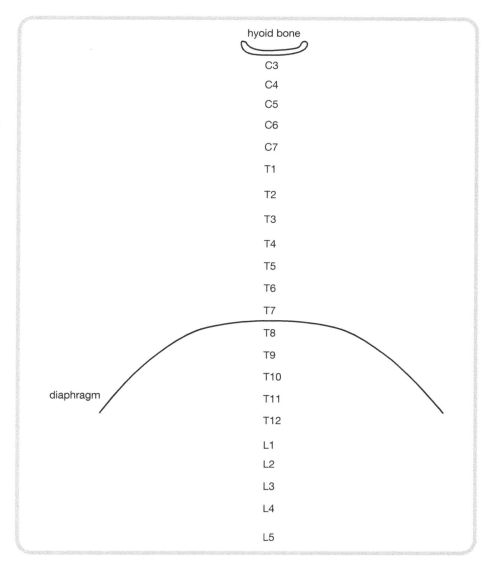

STEP 2

- Draw a tube from T2 to approximately L5 to represent the SVC at the top and the IVC at the bottom.
- At the top of the SVC, draw veins either side forming a bird's wing shape, with the dip meeting the SVC. On each side these represent the subclavian vein draining into the brachiocephalic vein.
- At the lower end of the IVC draw veins in an upside-down V shape, with upside-down Y-shaped vessels draining into them. These represent the femoral vein draining into the external iliac vein, draining into the common iliac vein; the small branch draining in between the external and common iliac veins is the internal iliac vein.
- Draw a circle in the vena cava at approximately T3; this represents the right atrium, into which the SVC and IVC drain.

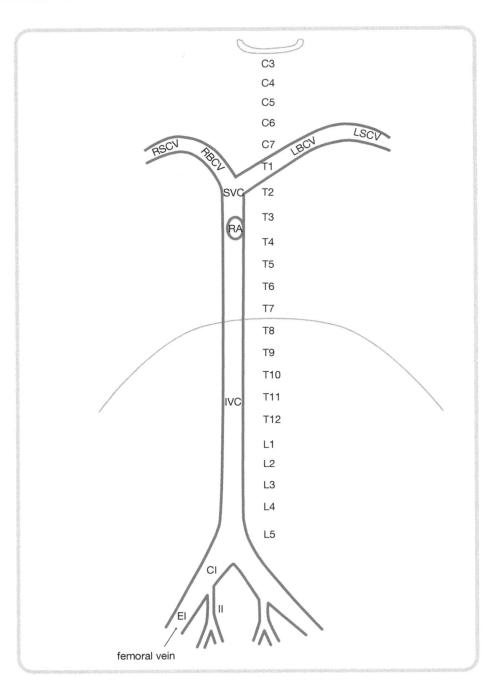

STEP 3

We will now draw the veins of the neck (for more detail see *Section 1.2.4 Venous drainage in the neck*).

- On each side, draw 2 vertical veins draining into the brachiocephalic vein. These are the external jugular veins laterally and the internal jugular veins medially.
- Draw the superior thyroid, middle thyroid and inferior veins as shown on each side (for more detail see the *Thyroid gland* in *Section 1.1.3: Endocrine organs of the head and neck*).

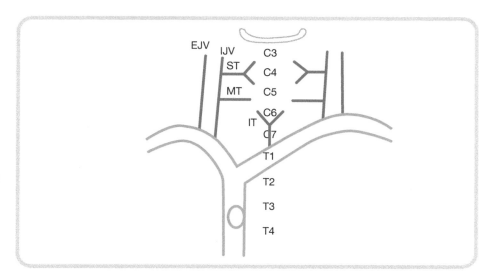

STEP 4

- Draw a horizontal vein exiting from each side of the brachiocephalic vein, approximately in line with T1. These are the 1st posterior intercostal veins (PIVs).
- Just below these 2 veins draw another 2, shorter veins. These are the internal thoracic veins.

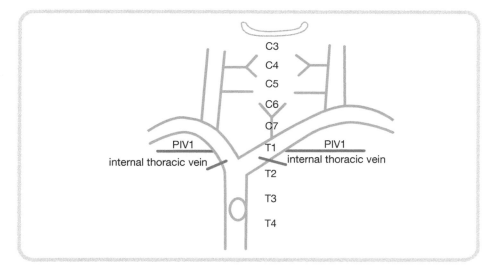

STEP 5

- From the common iliac vein draw a long vein on the left side of the paper, ascending next to the IVC to join the SVC at approximately T2; this is the ascending lumbar vein, which becomes the azygos vein.
- Draw 4 horizontal lines on the left side of the paper, joining the IVC and the ascending lumbar vein at levels L1 to L4; these are the lumbar veins. The first 2 lumbar veins often drain into the ascending lumbar vein and the lower two often drain into the IVC. This can vary between individuals.
- Just above these draw one more vein; this is the right subcostal vein.

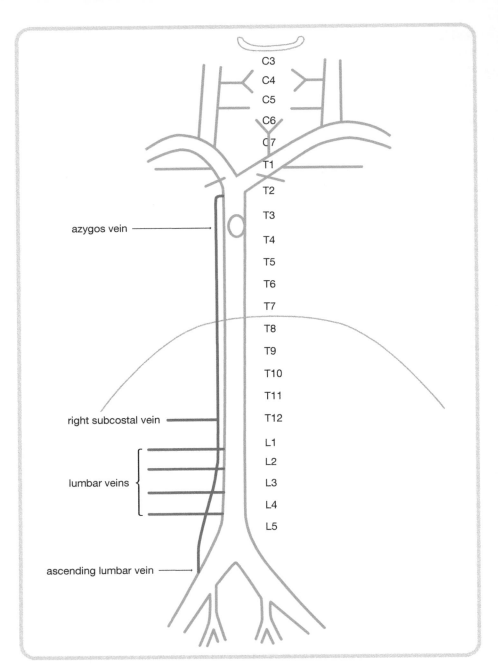

- Draw 8 more horizontal veins from T4 down to T11; these are PIV4 to 11. They drain into the azygos vein.
- Just above this between T2 and T3 draw a short horizontal line and the shape of a tuning fork or 3/4 of a rectangle. These are the PIV2 and 3.
- Below PIV11, draw a vein that drains directly into the IVC. This represents the right renal vein.

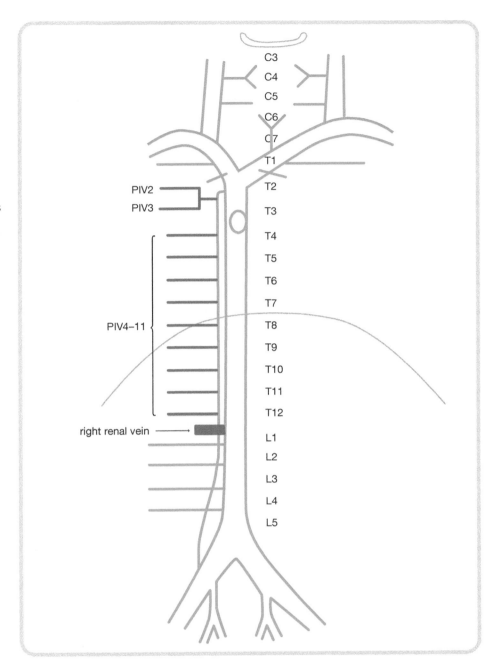

STEP 7

- Draw a horizontal line at T2 on the right side of the paper; this is PIV2. Draw PIV3 below and join it to PIV2.
- Draw a horizontal line at approximately T7 crossing the midline behind the IVC. Extend it upwards to T4 and draw a horizontal line at each level, T4 to T7. These are PIV4–7.
- These PIVs drain into the accessory hemiazygos vein, which in turn drains into the azygos vein.

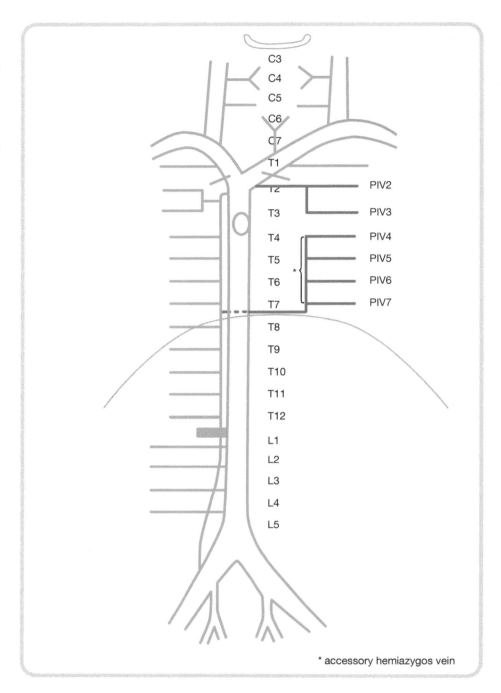

* accessory hemiazygos vein

STEP 8

- Below Step 7, draw a mirror image of it for PIV8–11 and the left subcostal vein.
- These drain into the hemiazygos vein, then the azygos vein.

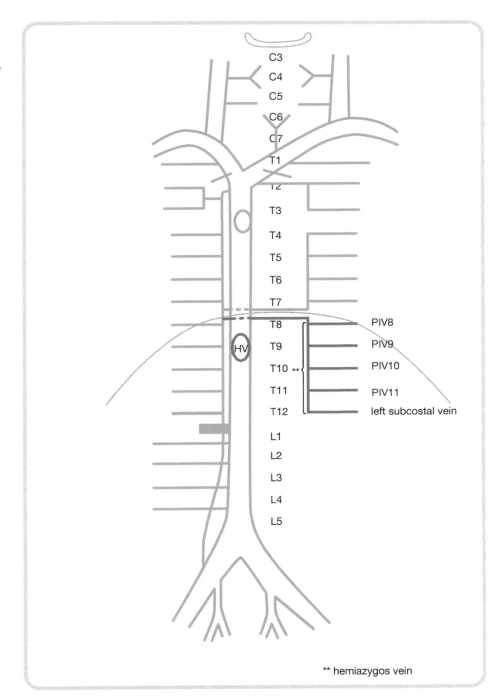

** hemiazygos vein

- Draw a vein opposite the right renal vein to represent the left renal vein.
- Into the left renal vein draw a broken line upwards from below the lumbar veins; this is the left gonadal vein. Still using a broken line, draw the right gonadal vein draining directly into the IVC.
- Draw the left lumbar veins for levels L1 to L4 on the right side of the page.
- Draw a vein joining the common iliac vein to the bottom of the hemiazygos vein; this is the left ascending lumbar vein. Where the ascending lumbar vein crosses the subcostal vein it becomes the azygos vein on the right and the hemiazygos vein on the left.

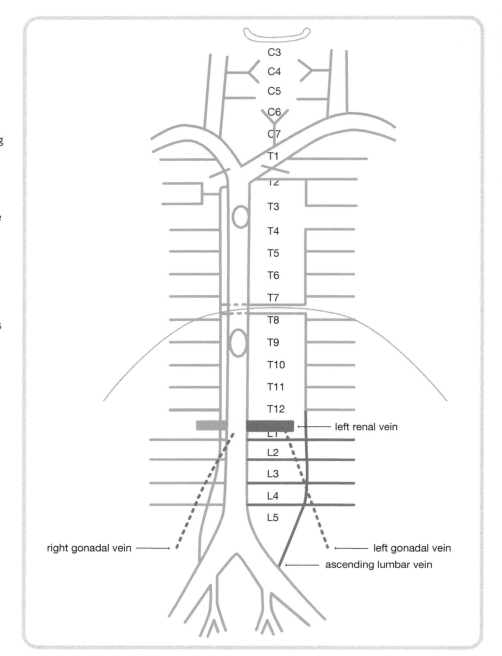

C3
C4
C5
C6
C7
T1
T2
T3
T4
T5
T6
T7
T8
T9
T10
T11
T12
L1
L2
L3
L4
L5

left renal vein

right gonadal vein

left gonadal vein

ascending lumbar vein

- Draw a circle in the middle of the IVC at approximately the level of T9; this represents the hepatic veins.

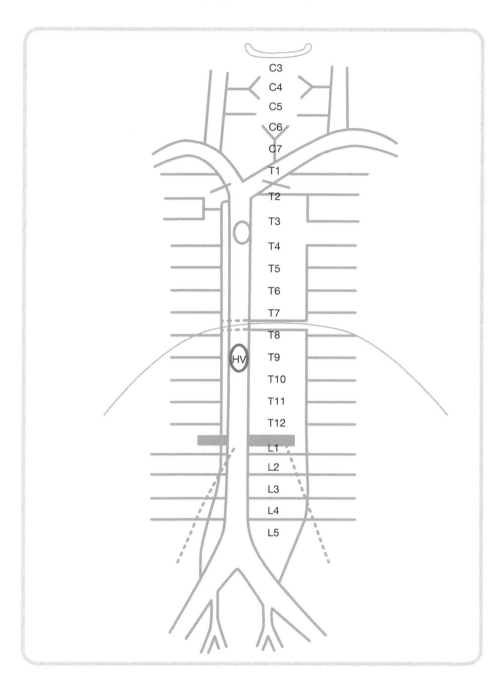

Chapter 6
Pelvis and reproductive systems

06

The pelvis is formed by the sacrum (lower part of the vertebral column) and the paired hip bones. The hip bone connects the vertebral column to the lower limb. It supports the pelvic viscera and contains the intestines, urinary bladder and internal sexual organs. The shape of the pelvis differs in males and females. The images here show the differences.

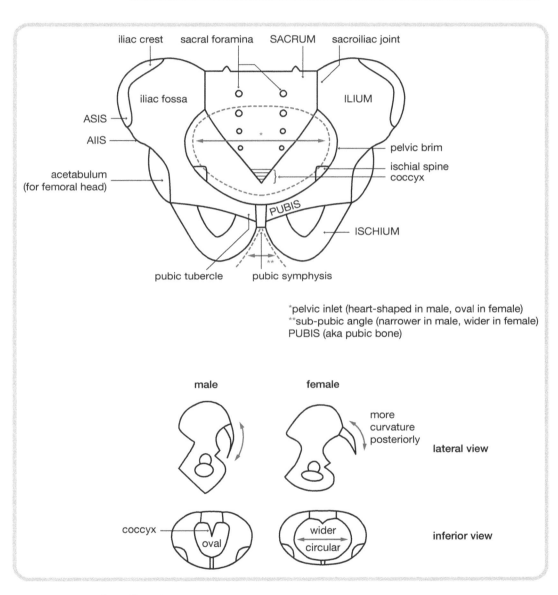

iliac crest   sacral foramina   SACRUM   sacroiliac joint

iliac fossa   ILIUM

ASIS

AIIS

acetabulum
(for femoral head)

pelvic brim

ischial spine
coccyx

PUBIS

ISCHIUM

pubic tubercle   pubic symphysis

*pelvic inlet (heart-shaped in male, oval in female)
**sub-pubic angle (narrower in male, wider in female)
PUBIS (aka pubic bone)

male   female

more
curvature
posteriorly

lateral view

coccyx   wider   inferior view
oval   circular

AIIS   anterior inferior iliac spine
ASIS   anterior superior iliac spine

How to draw

STEP 1

- Draw a pentagon pointing downwards with 2 bumps on top to represent the superior articular facets of S1.
- Draw 4 small circles down each side for the sacral foramina.
- Draw 4 horizontal lines in the bottom of the tail; these are the bones of the coccyx.

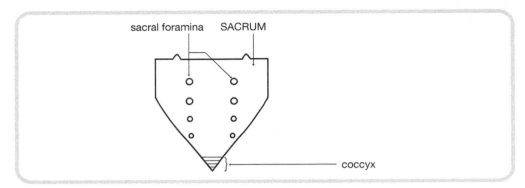

STEP 2

- Draw 2/3 of a circle from the bottom of the vertical side of the sacrum on one side to the same point on the other side; this is the pelvic brim.
- On each side draw a little protrusion at 4 and 8 o'clock; these are the ischial spines (part of the ischium).

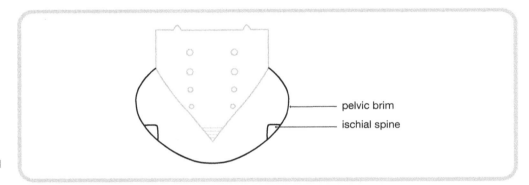

STEP 3

- Draw an outline like butterfly wings from the top of the sacrum as shown on the image.
- Draw a rectangle from the pelvic brim inlet downwards as shown. This is the pubic symphysis.
- Draw a sliver at the top edge of each 'wing'; these represent the iliac crest and the anterior superior iliac spine anteriorly. The superior aspect of the 'wing' is the iliac fossa.
- Label the anterior inferior iliac spine, sacroiliac joint and ilium.

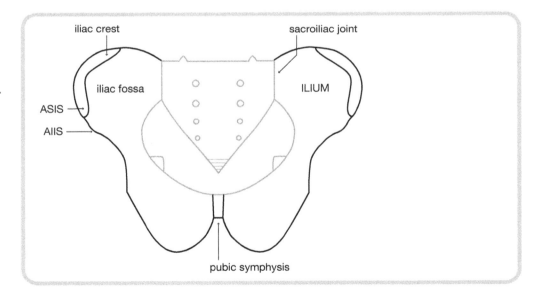

- Draw a straight line from the lower half of the bottom 'wing' on each side to the lower part of the pubic symphysis. The area above this is the pubis (aka pubic bone). The pubic tubercle is on the medial part of the superior ramus of the pubis.
- Draw a semicircle below each of these lines to represent the superior border of the ischium.

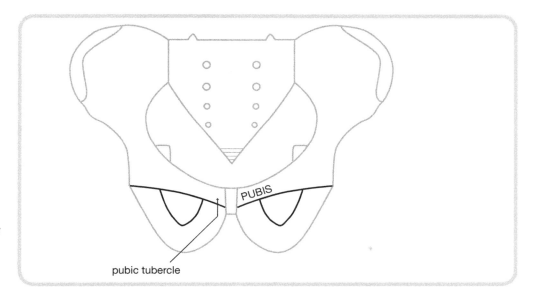

pubic tubercle

- Draw a curve outwards from the anterior inferior iliac spine and back into the corner of the pubic bone; this represents the acetabulum, where the femur articulates.
- Draw a broken purple line around the pubic rim to outline the pelvic inlet. This is wider in females.
- Use broken purple lines to depict the sub-pubic angle anteriorly, below the pubic symphysis. The angle is narrower and V shaped in males, at ≤80°. In females it is more U shaped and normally >90°.

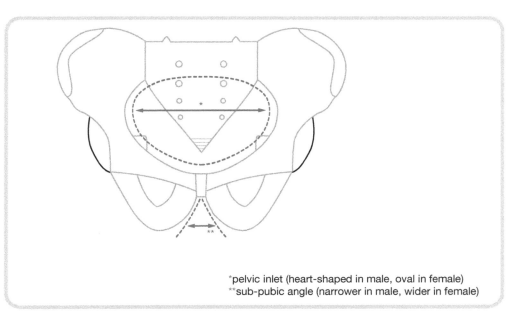

*pelvic inlet (heart-shaped in male, oval in female)
**sub-pubic angle (narrower in male, wider in female)

STEP 6

- Draw lateral and inferior views as shown to learn the difference between the male and female pelvis.

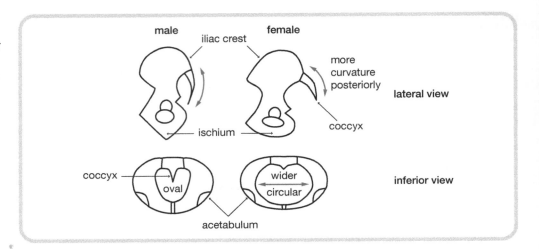

6.2 Perineum

We will consider the perineum of both the male and female in more detail but first we will look at the general areas in the pelvis. The first image we will draw is a schematic view from below.

Table 6.1 describes most of the muscles mentioned in this section. The others are described in *Section 6.3: Muscles of the internal pelvis*.

Table 6.1. Muscles of the perineum and pelvis

Muscle	Action	Blood supply	Innervation
External urethral sphincter	Contraction around urethra, maintains urinary continence	*Female:* internal pudendal artery (internal iliac) *Male:* bulbourethral artery	Pudendal nerve (S2–S4)
Deep transverse perineal muscle	Fixation of perineal body (central tendon of perineum) and support of pelvic floor Squeezes out last drops of urine *Male:* expulsion of semen	Perineal branch of internal pudendal artery	Pudendal nerve (S2–S4)
Superficial transverse perineal muscle	Constricts urethra and maintains urinary continence *Female:* constricts vagina	Perineal branch of internal pudendal artery	Pudendal nerve (S2–S4)
External anal sphincter muscle	Closes anal orifice	Inferior rectal artery and transverse perineal artery	Pudendal nerve (S2–S4), perineal and inferior rectal branches
Bulbospongiosus muscle	*Male:* compresses erectile tissue and the deep dorsal vein of the penis during urination and ejaculation. This aids in emptying the urethra and assists in erection of penis *Female:* constricts the vaginal orifice, and contributes to clitoral erection and contraction of orgasm, assists secretions of greater vestibular gland	Perineal branch of internal pudendal artery	Pudendal nerve (S2–S4), deep branch of perineal nerve
Ischiocavernosus muscle	Compresses the crus in the male to help maintain an erection. It tenses the vagina during an orgasm and helps increase pressure in the clitoris in females	Perineal branch of internal pudendal artery	Pudendal nerve (S2–S4), deep branch of perineal nerve
Coccygeus muscle	Supports pelvic viscera and draws coccyx forwards	Inferior gluteal artery	Ventral rami of lower sacral nerves

6.2.1 Perineal triangles

C   coccyx

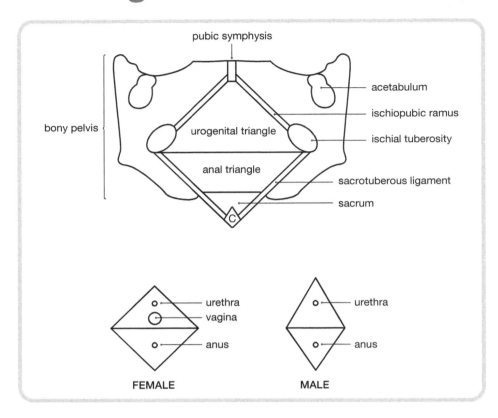

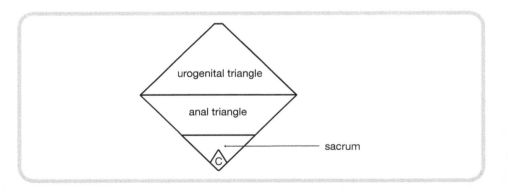

 How to draw

STEP 1

- Draw a blunt-topped diamond in the middle of the page.
- Draw a horizontal line across the middle. The area above this is the urogenital triangle.
- With another horizontal line, divide the lower area into an upper 2/3 and lower 1/3; this is the anal triangle above and the sacrum below.
- Just inside the base of the diamond, draw 2 lines to form a small diamond to represent the coccyx (C).

STEP 2

- At the top of the diamond draw a vertical rectangle; this is the pubic symphysis.
- Draw an oval at 45° on top of each lateral point to represent the ischial tuberosities. On each side, join this to the pubic symphysis to show the ischiopubic rami.
- In the lower half of the large diamond, draw a parallel line on each side; this forms the sacrotuberous ligaments.

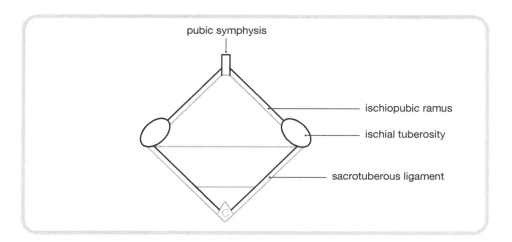

STEP 3

- From the top of the pubic symphysis draw a horizontal line towards the left side of the paper and continue it in curves as far as the leftmost corner, as shown. Take the line vertically down to just below the middle corner of the diamond. Then draw a flattened S-shaped curve to join the sacrotuberous ligament. This is the bony pelvis.
- Draw the acetabulum near the top.
- This step isn't essential to learning shapes but it gives an idea of where the perineum is located.

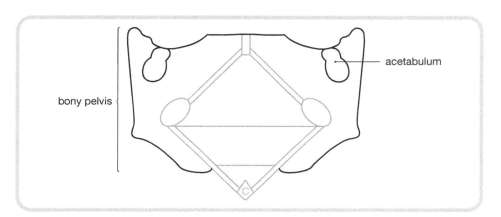

STEP 4

The male and female perineum differ in shape slightly.

- Draw an equal-sided diamond shape on the page. Draw a line horizontally across from one side to the other; this separates the urogenital triangle above from the anal triangle below. These are the wide triangles of the female perineum. Draw circles to show the urethra and vagina in the urogenital triangle and the anus in the anal triangle.
- In the male, draw a narrower diamond (narrower pelvis). Show that only the urethra lies in the urogenital triangle, and draw a circle to represent the anus in the anal triangle.

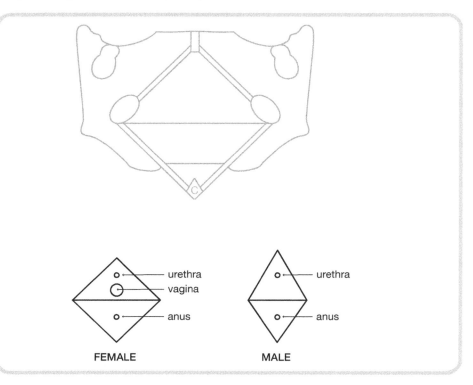

6.2.2 Coronal section of male perineum and pelvic floor

To help you imagine the position of the pelvic diaphragm and the perineal membrane, we will draw a coronal section in the male perineum.

C coccyx
U urethra

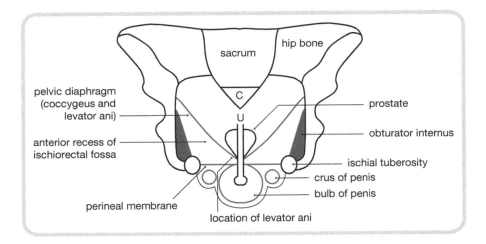

How to draw

STEP 1

- Draw a muscle-brown line across the page with a gap in the middle (for the urethra). This is the perineal membrane.
- Draw a black circle on each end to represent the ischial tuberosities.
- Just above the gap in the middle of the perineal membrane draw a V-shaped muscle with a gap above the same place. This is the pelvic diaphragm.
- The space between the 2 diaphragms is the anterior recess of the ischiorectal fossa.

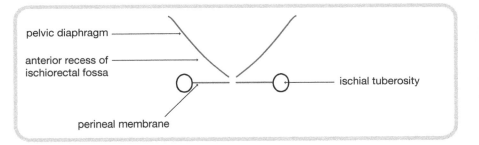

STEP 2

- Draw 2 small circles at the lateral ends and just below the perineal membrane; these are the crura of the penis.
- In the middle and below the perineal membrane draw one bigger circle; this is the bulb of the penis. Draw a small circle in the centre and a tube upwards through the hole in the middle of the perineal membrane and pelvic diaphragm; this is the urethra.
- Draw a circle shape around the urethra in the middle of the 'V' of the pelvic diaphragm; this is the prostate.

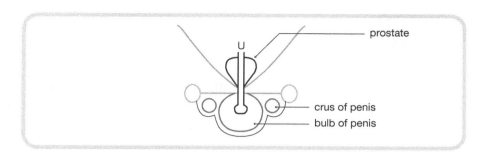

STEP 3

- From the ischial tuberosity draw a line vertically upwards; just medial on each side draw a brown triangular muscle, the obturator internus. The levator ani lies below the prostate and forms the majority of the pelvic diaphragm. (See *Section 6.3: Muscles of the internal pelvis* for details of these muscles.)

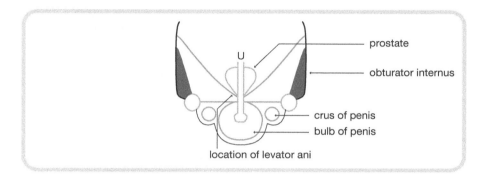

STEP 4

- Draw a cross-section of the pelvis with the sacrum and coccyx, as shown.

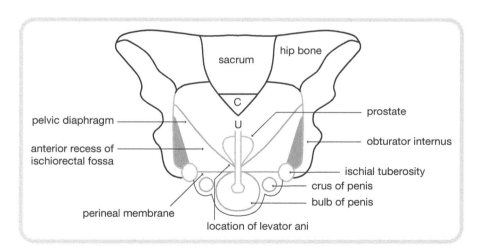

6.2.3 Female perineum

We will now look at the perineum in more detail, starting with the female perinuem.

The pelvic floor or diaphragm consists of the levator ani muscles and the ischiococcygeus muscle. Levator ani is a group of 4 muscles. These are the levator ani, pubococcygeus, iliococcygeus and puborectalis.

The perineal membrane (sometimes called the urogenital diaphragm) lies between the ischiopubic rami. It consists of the external urethral sphincter (sometimes called the urethral sphincter mechanism), the deep transverse perineal muscle and the perineal membrane.

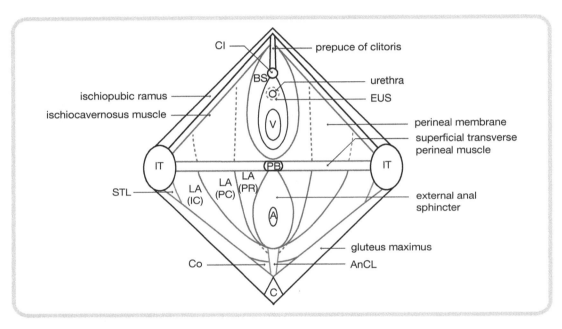

A	anus	**IT**	ischial tuberosity
AnCL	anococcygeal ligament	**LA**	levator ani
BS	bulbospongiosus muscle	**PB**	perineal body
C	coccyx	**PC**	pubococcygeus
CI	clitoris body	**PR**	puborectalis
Co	coccygeus muscle	**STL**	sacrotuberous ligament
EUS	external urethral sphincter	**V**	vagina
IC	iliococcygeus		

How to draw

STEP 1

- Draw a diamond shape, similar to the one you drew in *Section 6.2.1.*
- The ischial tuberosities are at each side with the ischiopubic ramus anteriorly and the gluteus maximus muscle posteriorly. The coccyx is at the base of the perineum.

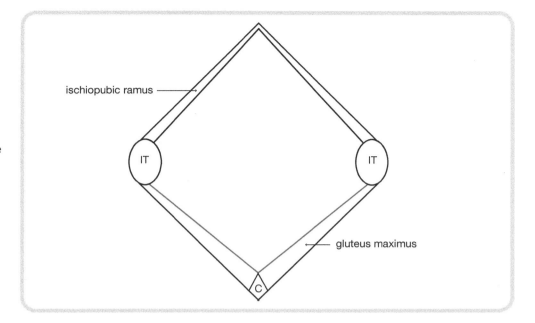

STEP 2

- Draw a brown band across the middle between the 2 ischial tuberosities. This represents the superficial transverse perineal muscles (one on each side); the perineal body lies in its centre.

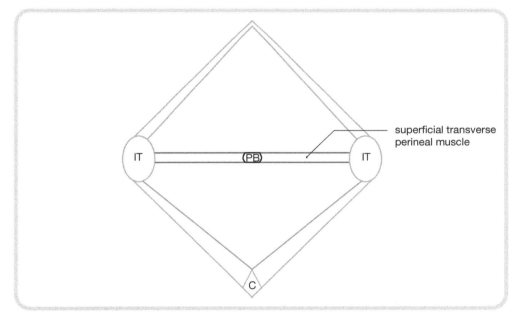

STEP 3

- From 1/3 in on one side of the superficial transverse perineal muscle to the same point on the other, draw a flattened U shape. At its base draw 2 grey lines to join the coccyx; these represent the anococcygeal ligament.
- At each corner below the IT, draw a small grey triangle; this is the sacrotuberous ligament.
- In the middle of the 'U' draw a vertical ellipse. This is the external anal sphincter. In its centre draw a black oval to represent the anus (A).
- Divide the medial levator ani into 2 parts on each side; the medial one is puborectalis, the middle one is pubococcygeus and the outer one is iliococcygeus.

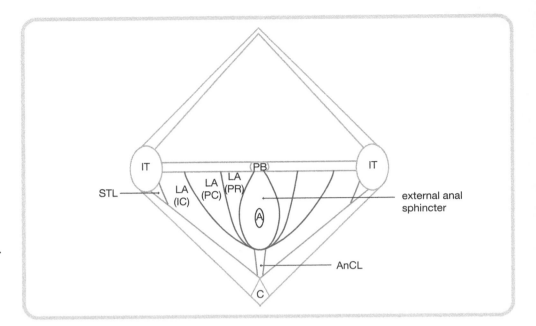

STEP 4

- From the top of the middle of the diamond draw 2 lines about 1/4 of the way down to the superficial transverse perineal muscle. These represent the prepuce of the clitoris.
- Below this draw a small circle, the body of the clitoris. Then below this draw a slim oval with a small circle in its upper half and a larger oval below that and inside the oval. These are the urethra and vagina (V), respectively.

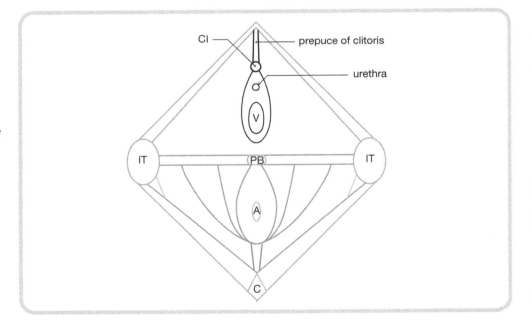

STEP 5

- Draw a brown line around the vagina and urethra to join the top of the diamond. This represents the outer border of the bulbospongiosus muscle, which overlies the bulb of the vestibule.
- Draw a brown line parallel to the ischiopubic ramus; this is the ischiocavernosus muscle.
- Label the area between bulbospongiosus and ischiocavernosus as the perineal membrane.

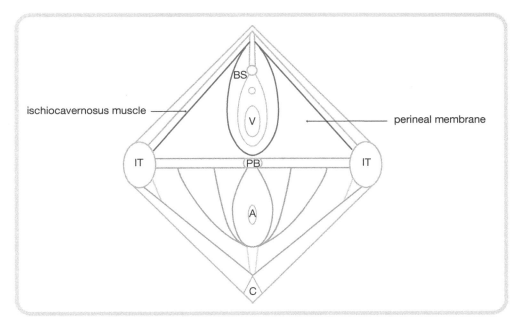

STEP 6

- Draw a short brown line across the base of each posterior triangle; this is the coccygeus muscle (deep to gluteus maximus, drawn here so you can imagine where it is!).
- Draw broken lines continuing from the LA muscles posteriorly (straight up the page) to show that they continue anteriorly, deep to the perineal membrane.

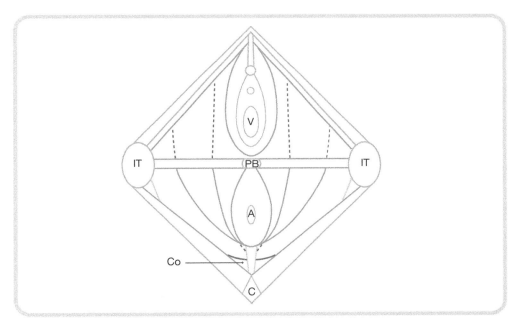

STEP 7

- Draw a broken line around the urethra in brown, to represent the external urethral sphincter.

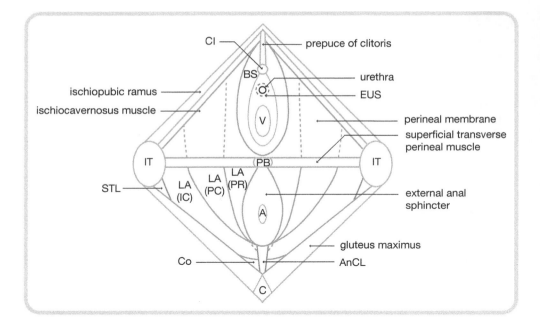

6.2.4 Male perineum

Now we will look at the male perineum.

BS bulbospongiosus
IT ischial tuberosity

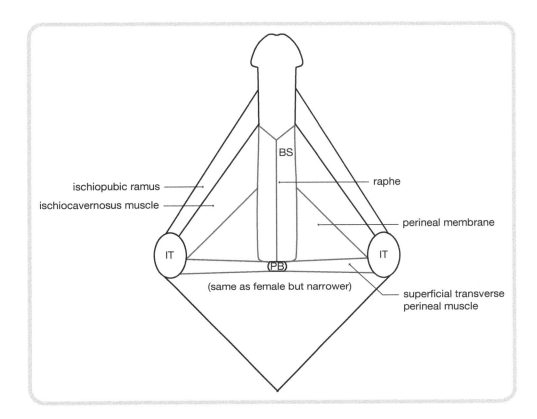

ischiopubic ramus

ischiocavernosus muscle

BS

raphe

perineal membrane

IT

IT

(PB)

(same as female but narrower)

superficial transverse perineal muscle

 How to draw

STEP ❶

- Draw a narrow diamond with a gap at the top (so the body of the penis can be drawn here later).
- At each lateral part draw an oval which represents the ischial tuberosities.

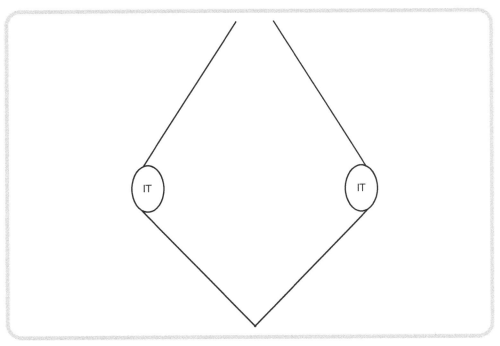

IT

IT

STEP 2

- Draw a band from one IT to the other. Draw a black circle in the middle to represent the perineal body (PB). Each side of this is one of the superficial transverse perineal muscles.
- The posterior part of the male perineum is the same as the female so the details are not drawn here. Overall it is a narrower shape.

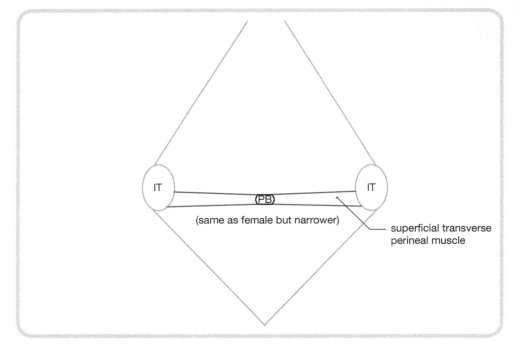

STEP 3

- In brown pen, from the perineal body draw a narrow U shape with a line down the middle and a 'V' at the top. This is the bulbospongiosus muscle. The line down the middle is the raphe.
- Above this draw the shaft and head of the penis.

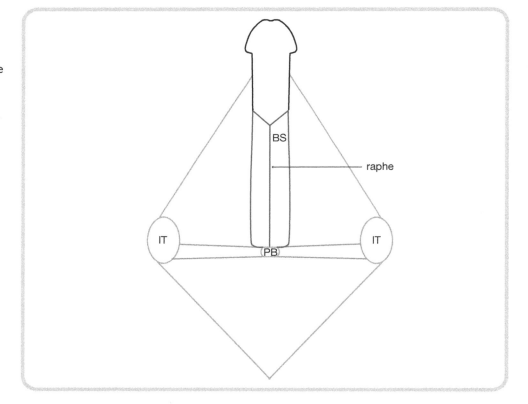

STEP ④

- Draw lines parallel to the top of the diamond on each side; these are the ischiopubic rami (same as in female).

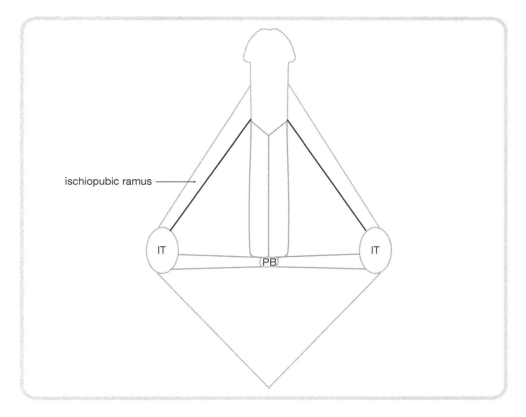

STEP ⑤

- Draw a line from the middle of bulbospongiosus to the ischial tuberosity. The muscle above this line is the ischiocavernosus muscle which lies over the crus of the penis. The part below the ischiocavernosus is the perineal membrane.

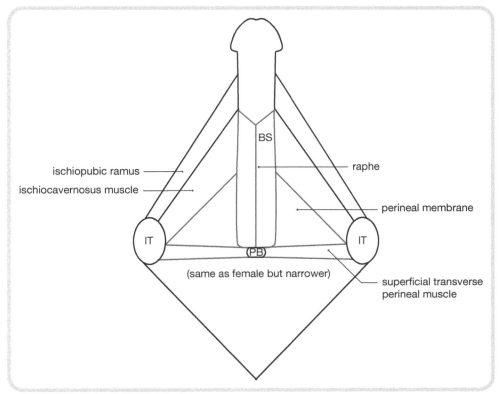

In this section we will draw the muscles of the pelvic floor (levator ani) and the muscles attached to the inside of the pelvis.

To learn where they lie we will draw a sagittal section of the pelvis. Imagine the pelvis cut in half and you are looking from the middle towards the outside of the person.

Steps 1 to 6 describe the deep and intermediate muscles, and their actions and innervation.

The muscles forming levator ani are described from Step 7 onwards. They are the 3 components of the levator ani:

- puborectalis
- pubococcygeus
- iliococcygeus.

Action: puborectalis and pubococcygeus both work to lift the pelvic and perineal structures (preventing prolapse in females). They also reinforce the anal sphincter. Iliococcygeus assists puborectalis in achieving anorectal and urinary continence. Levator ani contracts with abdominal muscles to increase intra-abdominal pressure.

Innervation: branches of the sacral plexus (mainly S3 and S4, with some contribution from S2).

Blood supply: inferior gluteal artery.

DEEP MUSCLES

sacrum
ASIS
arcuate line
piriformis
coccyx
SSL
STL
obturator canal
obturator foramen (aperture in bone)
ischial spine
pubic symphysis
ischial tuberosity

INTERMEDIATE MUSCLES

obturator internus
ischiopubic ramus

SUPERFICIAL MUSCLES

iliococcygeus
obturator internus
PC
PR
tendinous arch of levator ani
rectum
vagina
PC
urethra
perineal membrane

ASIS	anterior superior iliac spine
PC	pubococcygeus
PR	puborectalis (superficial to PC)
SSL	sacrospinous ligament
STL	sacrotuberous ligament

DEEP MUSCLES

 How to draw

STEP 1

- Start by drawing a 'tail' or claw shape on the right side of the page, with a line across its tip. This represents the coccyx (at the tip), the sacrum and the base of the lumbar spine.
- Draw a soft wave shape from the top of the sacrum to just above the level of the coccyx. This represents the iliac crest and anterior superior iliac spine (ASIS).
- Draw the arcuate line as shown.
- At the lowest part of the line, draw an oval to represent the pubic symphysis anteriorly. From here draw an S shape to join the sacrum just above the coccyx; interrupt the 'S' with a little protrusion behind the pubic symphysis to represent the ischial spine.
- Label the lowest part as the ischial tuberosity.
- Draw an oval behind the pubic symphysis; this is the obturator foramen.

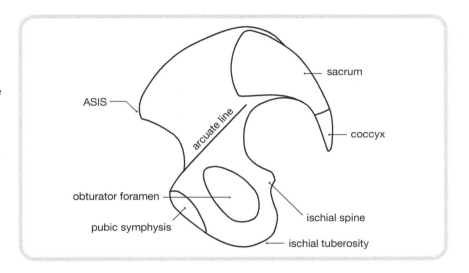

STEP 2

- Draw a grey line in the top of the obturator foramen; the part above this line is the obturator canal.
- The part below is a fascial layer called the obturator fascia or membrane.

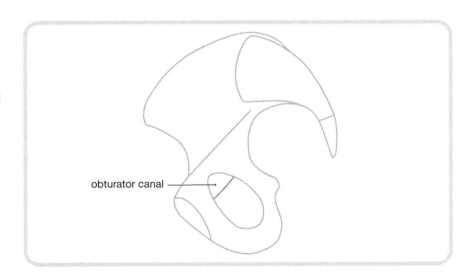

STEP 3

- Draw the piriformis muscle from its origin on the sacrum and disappearing behind the ischium (to insert onto the greater trochanter).
- **Action**: externally rotate the thigh.
- **Innervation**: nerve to piriformis (mainly S1 and S2, with some contributions from L5).
- **Blood supply**: mainly by the superior gluteal artery, some from the internal pudendal artery and sometimes the inferior gluteal artery. In the pelvis the main supply is from the lateral sacral artery.

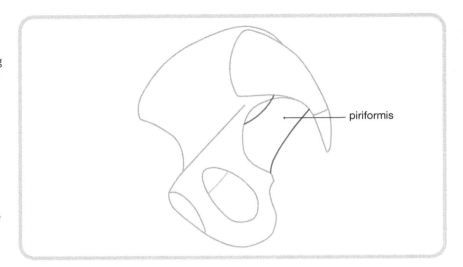

STEP 4

- Draw a grey line from the ischial spine to the coccyx; this is the sacrospinous ligament.
- Draw a 2nd grey line, from the ischial tuberosity to midway down the anterior side of the sacrum; this is the sacrotuberous ligament. It is a fan-shaped ligament present on both sides.

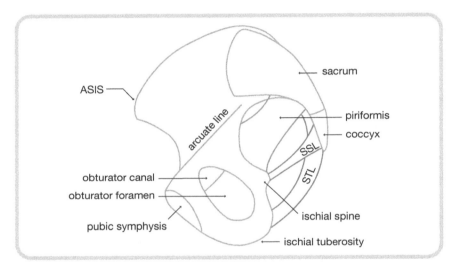

INTERMEDIATE MUSCLES

STEP 5

- Start with the basic drawing from Step 4 of the deep muscles but without labels and with an empty obturator foramen.

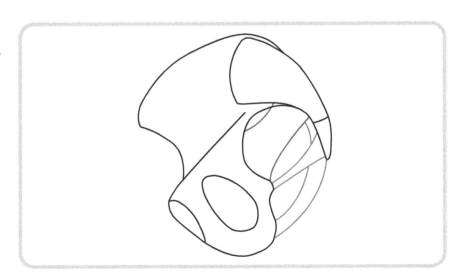

STEP 6

- From the obturator foramen draw the obturator internus; its origin is the ischiopubic ramus and obturator membrane. It inserts into the greater trochanter (not shown).
- It lies on the posterior side of the obturator foramen between the superior and inferior gemelli muscles (these are not shown).
- **Action**: slightly varies depending on whether the hip is extended or flexed. In an extended hip the obturator internus abducts and laterally rotates the thigh. If the hip is flexed it abducts the thigh at the hip.
- **Innervation**: nerve to obturator internus (directly from the sacral plexus, L5–S2).
- **Blood supply**: inferior gluteal artery.

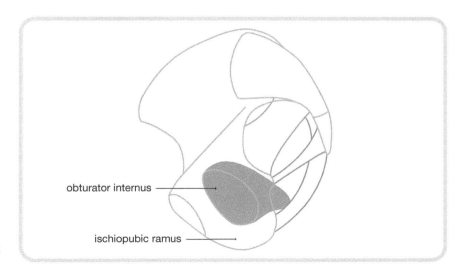

SUPERFICIAL MUSCLES

STEP 7

- Start again from Step 5.
- Draw a thick grey line through the middle of the obturator foramen; this is the tendinous arch of levator ani. Show the portion of obturator internus that lies above the arch; we will not draw its lower half because the superficial muscles we are going to draw next would lie over it and make the image confusing. However, it is useful to have this visual reminder that obturator internus lies deep to them.

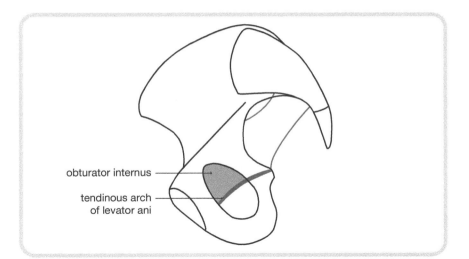

STEP 8

- Below the tendinous arch, draw the pubococcygeus muscle, part of the levator ani. This arises from the pubic bone and inserts into the coccyx, as suggested by the name!
- Start by drawing a brown line downwards from the anterior end of the tendinous arch at the inner edge of the obturator foramen.
- Then draw 2 lines to join this to the coccyx.

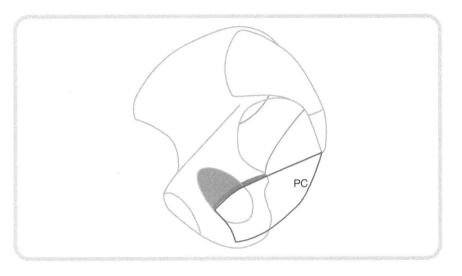

STEP 9

- Just above the pubococcygeus draw the iliococcygeus. This arises from the inner side of the ilium and inserts into the coccyx, also indicated by the name!

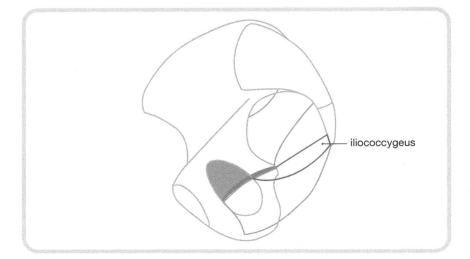

iliococcygeus

STEP 10

- Draw a 3rd muscle in the middle of PC. This is the puborectalis (PR). It is a sling-like muscle around the rectum. It arises from the pubic symphysis and inserts into the midline sling posterior to the rectum.
- PR is not visible from the inside of the pelvis because it sits superficial to PC. It is drawn here so you can see where it lies in relation to PC.

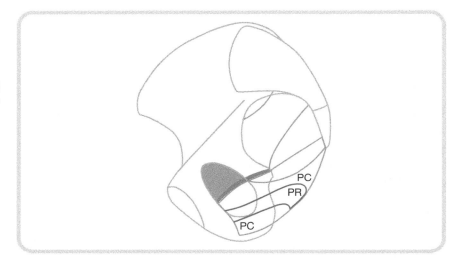

PC
PR
PC

STEP 11

- To help you visualise how the urogenital organs fit into this image, draw a urethra, vagina and rectum.
- Below the pubococcygeus, draw a line between the urethra, vagina and rectum; this is the perineal membrane.

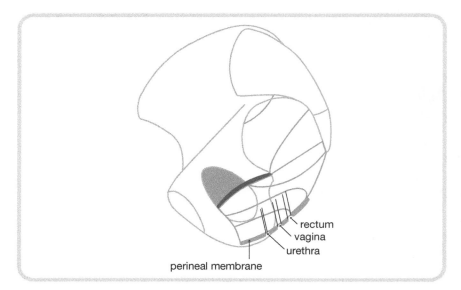

rectum
vagina
urethra
perineal membrane

6.4 Male reproductive system

As well as the drawings shown here, see also *Section 5.1.9: Urinary tract* and *Section 5.4: Inguinal canal* for drawings of the testis, epididymis, vas deferens and seminal vesicle.

6.4.1 Cross-section of the penis

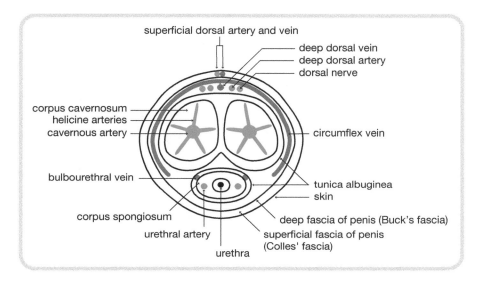

How to draw

STEP 1

- Draw one circle just inside another.
- Label the outer circle as the skin, the inner circle as the deep fascia of the penis (Buck's fascia) and the gap between as the superficial fascia of the penis (aka Colles' fascia).

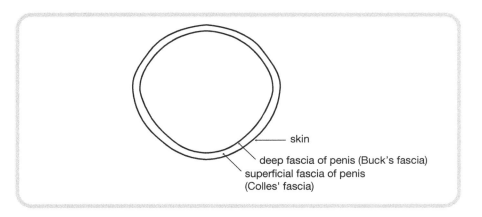

STEP 2

- Draw 2 oval shapes, one just inside the other in the lower 1/3 of the inner circle. The outer oval is the tunica albuginea.
- Draw a 'goggles' shape with 2 'lenses' (circles) in the upper 2/3 of the inner circle. The outer layer of this is also the tunica albuginea.

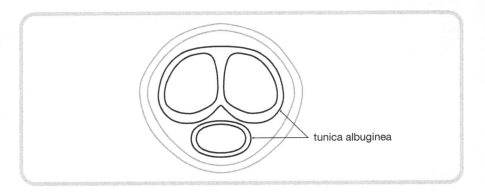

tunica albuginea

STEP 3

- In the middle of the oval draw a small circle to represent the urethra.
- Draw a red dot on either side of the urethra to represent the urethral arteries.
- Label the area surrounding these as the corpus spongiosum muscle.

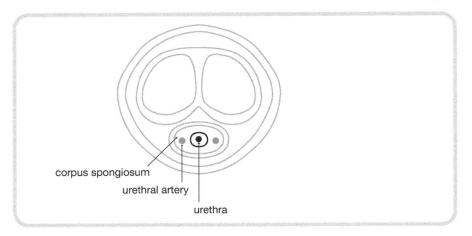

corpus spongiosum

urethral artery

urethra

STEP 4

The next image looks like a little face with very blood-shot eyes to me!

- Draw a red dot in the middle of each circle and then draw 'spokes' from here to the edge of the circle. These are the helicine arteries. The central dot is the cavernous artery. The area surrounding these is the corpus cavernosum.
- Draw 2 blue dots just above the arteries of the bulb of the penis; these are the bulbourethral veins.

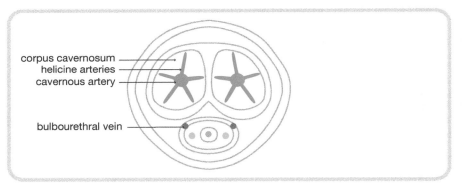

corpus cavernosum
helicine arteries
cavernous artery

bulbourethral vein

STEP 5

- Between the deep fascia at the top of the image and the tunica albuginea draw a line of dots using colour in the order green, red, blue, red and green, leaving a slim band of space between them and the deep fascia of penis. These are the dorsal nerves, arteries and vein.

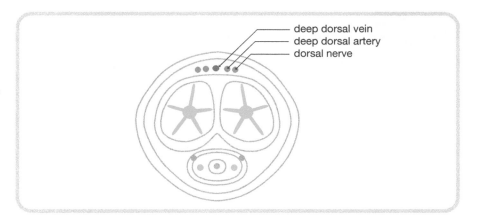

deep dorsal vein
deep dorsal artery
dorsal nerve

STEP 6

- Just above these vessels draw an artery and vein in the superficial fascia; these are the superficial dorsal artery and vein.

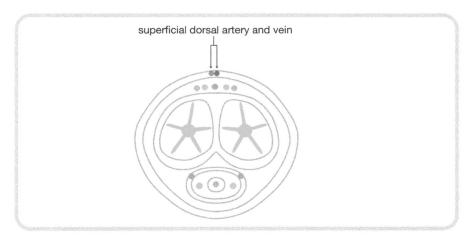

superficial dorsal artery and vein

STEP 7

- Draw a blue semicircle from approximately 8 o'clock to 4 o'clock, under the deep fascia of penis. This is the circumflex vein, which arises from the deep dorsal vein.

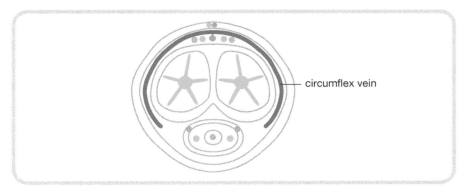

circumflex vein

6.4.2 Midline sagittal section of the male reproductive system

Because this image is in the mid-sagittal plane, it does not show the testis, epididymis, vas deferens and seminal vesicles. There are 2 of each of these, situated either side of the midline as shown in relation to the male urinary system in *Section 5.1.9: Urinary tract*. For internal anatomy of the testis, see *Section 5.4: Inguinal canal*.

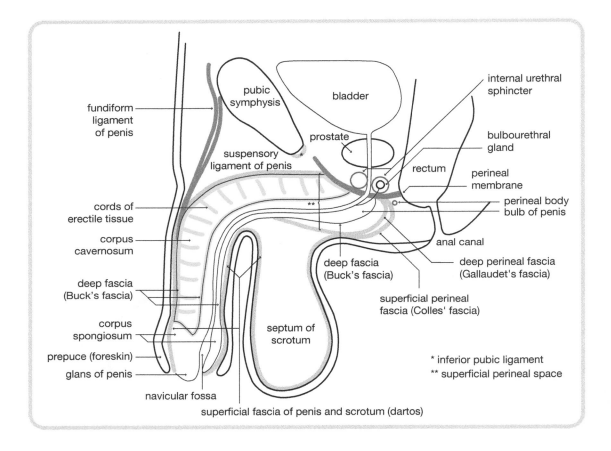

* inferior pubic ligament
** superficial perineal space

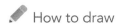 How to draw

STEP 1

- Draw a double and almost straight line down the left side of the page. End it with a slightly curved shape for the head of the penis.
- Label the prepuce (foreskin) at the head of the penis.
- Just behind this, draw a second double line from the posterior side of the head of the penis up to about 40% of the height of the first set of lines and then back down, drawing a sac shape for the scrotum. The centre of the scrotum is the septum. From here continue horizontally to the anus.
- Draw the rectum and anal canal as shown.

STEP 2

- Draw a worm-like shape in the anterior part of the penis, with a right-angle curve above the scrotum as shown. This represents the corpus cavernosum. The lines across it represent the cords of erectile tissue.
- Behind the corpus cavernosum draw a curved line to just in front of the rectum, and leave a small gap in it as shown, for the urethra. This is the perineal membrane.
- Draw a small brown circle just below the posterior end of the ligament, label the perineal body (or central tendon of the perineum). This is a fibromuscular mass in the midline of the perineum at the junction between the urogenital triangle and the anal triangle.

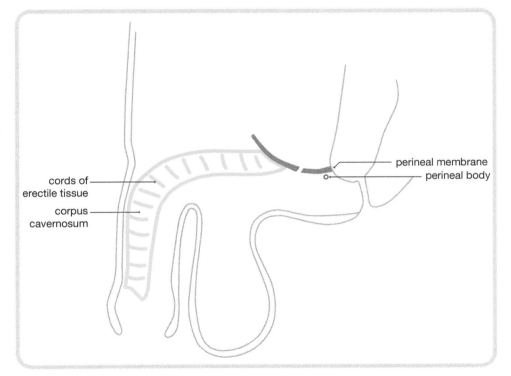

STEP 3

- Posterior to the abdominal wall draw a grey line down to the anterior edge of the corpus cavernosum. This represents the fundiform ligament of the penis; it is made of two bundles that pass downward from the abdominal wall to the penis, here each bundle widens and forms a sling-like shape under the corpus cavernosum and corpus spongiosum (not shown).
- Behind here draw a slanted oval shape in black pen; this is the pubic symphysis where the left and right pelvic bones join. At its posteroinferior end draw a grey line; this represents the inferior arcuate ligament.

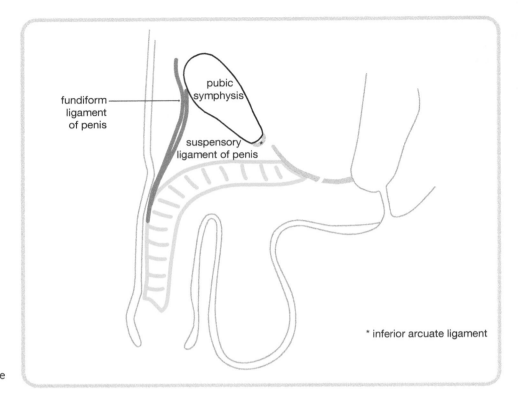

- Just below the pubic symphysis, label the triangle-shaped area as the suspensory ligament of the penis.

STEP 4

- Draw a grey line from the lower anterior edge of the corpus cavernosum just behind the anterior foreskin, along the top of the corpus cavernosum to the transverse perineal ligament.
- Draw a second grey line starting just anterior to the posterior edge of the head of penis and continuing all the way around the edge of the penis and scrotum to join the posterior half of the transverse perineal ligament; this is the superficial fascia of penis and scrotum anteriorly and superficial perineal fascia (Colles' fascia) posteriorly.
- Draw a thin black line under the superficial fascia and above the corpus cavernosum. This represents the deep fascia (Buck's fascia).

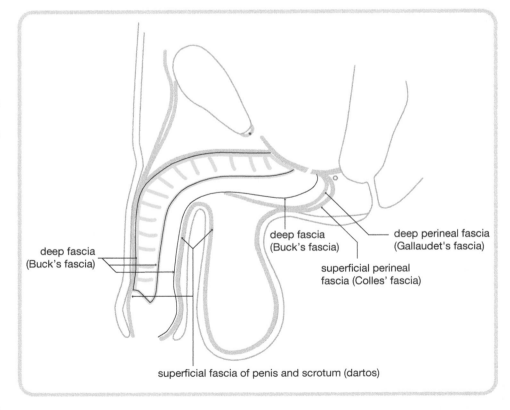

- Draw a second thin dark grey line on the anterior side of the superficial fascia on the underside of the penis. Instead of following the superficial fascia into the scrotum, continue the line to join the transverse perineal ligament.
- Draw a short grey line from Buck's fascia to the transverse perineal ligament; this lies on top of the superficial fascia and deep to Buck's fascia. This represents the deep perineal fascia (Gallaudet's fascia).

STEP 5

- From the hole in the transverse perineal ligament draw the urethra running to the end of the penis. Draw a wider section just before the tip; this is the navicular fossa.
- Label the glans of penis in front and behind the fossa. Draw a line from the urethral opening to the inferior end of the superficial fascia of the penis.
- Label the corpus spongiosum.

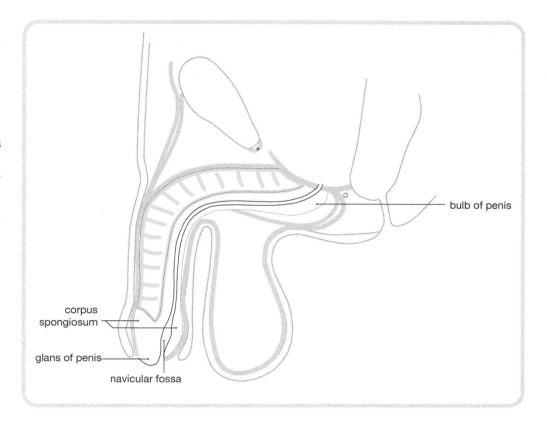

STEP 6

- Draw the urethra and bladder between the pubic symphysis and rectum.
- Draw the prostate around the urethra above the transverse perineal ligament.
- Draw 2 brown circles either side of the urethra above the ligament; these represent the internal urethral sphincter. The bulbourethral gland lies in here; draw it as a small circle and draw a curve to represent its duct to the urethra below.
- Label the superficial perineal space as shown.

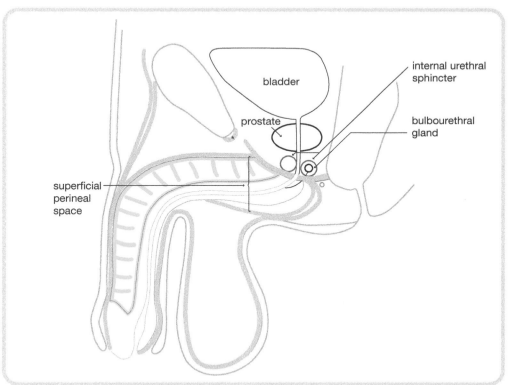

6.4.3 Nerve supply of male reproductive system

A simplified line diagram is shown here to help you understand the nerve supply and its origins for the reproductive system and pelvis.

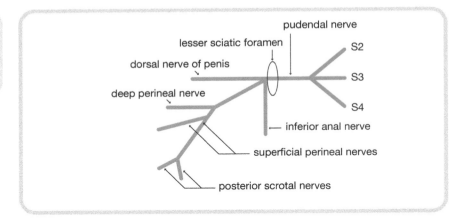

How to draw

STEP 1

- Draw the nerve roots S2, S3 and S4 joining together to form the pudendal nerve.
- Draw a black oval around the nerve, to represent the lesser sciatic foramen.

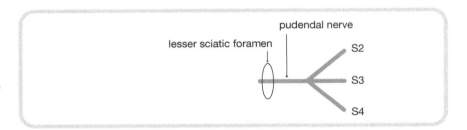

STEP 2

- Continue the pudendal nerve further across the page, where it becomes the dorsal nerve of the penis.
- Draw a branch off the pudendal nerve going downwards; this is the inferior anal nerve.
- Draw another branch in the direction of 8 o'clock; this is the deep perineal nerve.

STEP 3

- Draw a number of superficial branches from the deep perineal nerve.
- Some of these become the posterior scrotal nerves; label these.

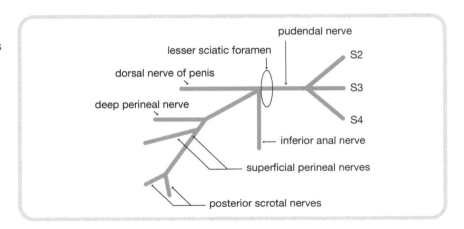

6.5 Female reproductive system

6.5.1 Mid-sagittal section of the female reproductive system

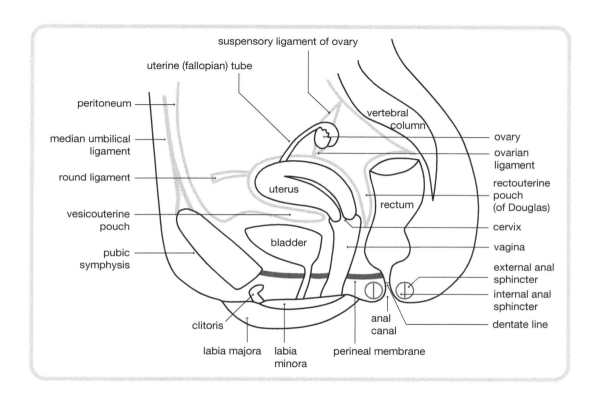

✏️ How to draw

STEP 1

- On the right side of the page draw a tail shape to represent the vertebral column.
- Draw the outline of the back and the anal canal and rectum.

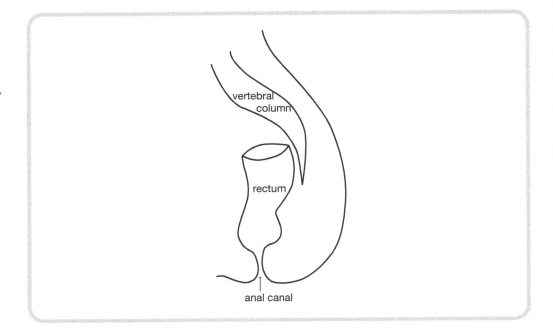

STEP 2

- Draw the anterior abdominal wall and follow the line round to meet the anus. Draw a black shape anteriorly to represent the pubic symphysis.
- From the top of the pubic bone draw a narrow, vertical triangle in grey. This is the medial umbilical ligament.
- Just in front of the rectum, draw the outline of the vagina.
- Above this, draw the uterus and cervix as shown (ensure there is some space between these and the rectum – see Step 3).
- Just in front of the vagina draw the urethra and bladder (ensure there is space above it, below the uterus – see Step 3).

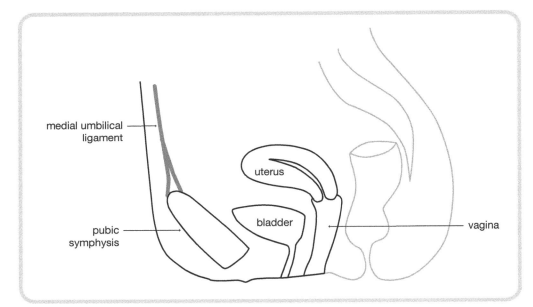

STEP 3

- Start drawing a grey line just posterior to the median umbilical ligament to about 1/4 of the way down the pubic symphysis then horizontally into the space between the bladder and uterus (forming the vesico-uterine pouch).
- Continue with a curve around the uterus as shown, and then continue past the rectum.
- Finish the line by continuing up the anterior side of the spine.
- The grey line represents the peritoneum.
- The region between the uterus and rectum is the rectouterine pouch (pouch of Douglas).

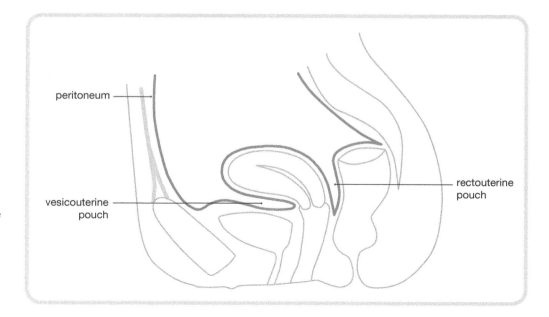

peritoneum

vesicouterine pouch

rectouterine pouch

STEP 4

- Draw 2 half ellipses below the bladder and vagina on the underside of the image. These are the labia minora and labia majora.
- Just above the anterior end of the labia minora draw a cashew-nut shaped clitoris.

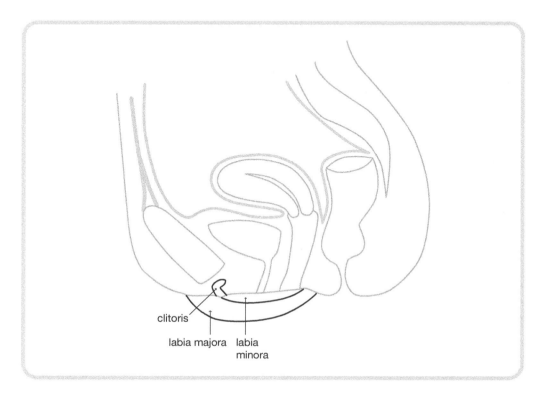

clitoris

labia majora   labia minora

STEP 5

- From the top of the uterus draw the uterine (fallopian) tube 'holding' the ovary.
- The ovaries and uterine tube lie lateral to the uterus (see *Section 6.5.3: Uterus, fallopian tubes, ovaries and uterine ligaments*). That would be difficult to depict so we will draw one, as shown, and you can imagine where they lie.

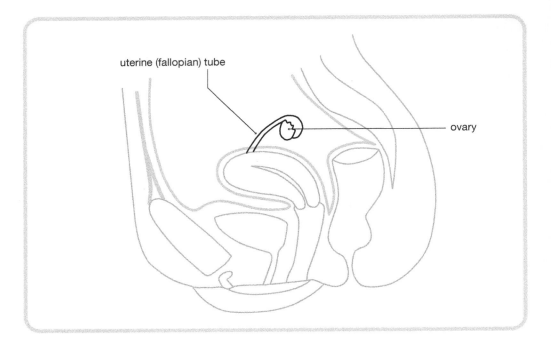

STEP 6

- Draw 2 brown circles, 1 just in front and 1 behind the anus. Draw a line down the middle of each. The inner half is the internal anal sphincter and the outer part is the external anal sphincter.
- Draw a small black line between the inner boundaries of the internal anal sphincter. This is the dentate line; above this point you would feel stretch but no pain and below it you would feel sharp well-localised pain.
- Draw a grey line from the pubic bone anteriorly to the rectum; this represents the perineal membrane.
- Draw a grey horizontal rectangle just anterior to the uterus; this is the round ligament.
- Draw a small grey triangle above the uterus joining the ovary; this is the ovarian ligament.
- Draw a 2nd grey triangle above the ovary joining the peritoneum; this is the suspensory ligament of the ovary.

6.5.2 Inferior external view of the female reproductive system

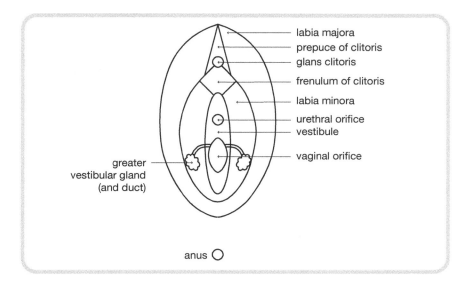

How to draw

STEP 1

- Draw a vertical leaf shape; this is the vestibule. The vestibule is the cavity that lies between the labia minora. It contains the urethral orifice, vaginal orifice and the openings of the two greater vestibular (Bartholin's) glands.
- Draw the anus behind it.

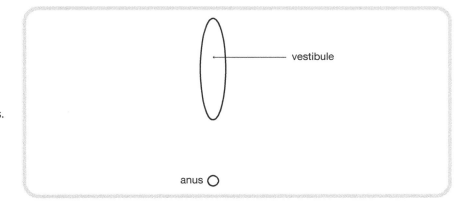

STEP 2

- Draw a small circle in the top half, the urethral orifice, and a larger oval below, the vaginal orifice.

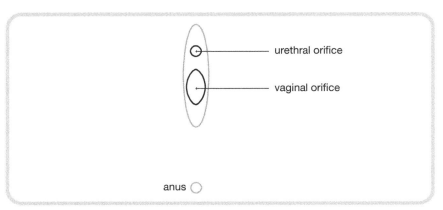

STEP 3

- Draw a larger leaf shape around the vestibule. Draw 2 short diagonal lines from the top of the vestibule to this new line. Below these 2 new lines are the labia minora. The area above is the frenulum of the clitoris.
- At the top of the drawing draw a circle; this is the glans clitoris.

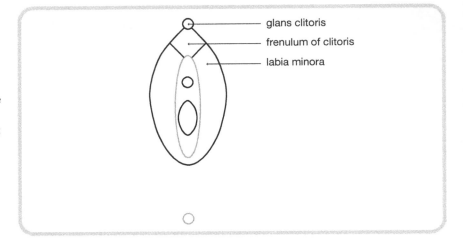

glans clitoris

frenulum of clitoris

labia minora

STEP 4

- Draw an ellipse around this image; this shows the labia majora.
- Draw a triangle shape above the clitoral glans; this is the prepuce of the clitoris.

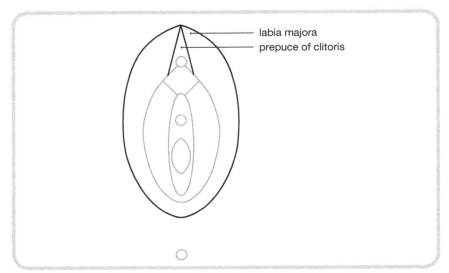

labia majora

prepuce of clitoris

STEP 5

- On both sides of the vaginal orifice, draw a little tube and gland; these represent the greater vestibular glands (aka Bartholin's glands).

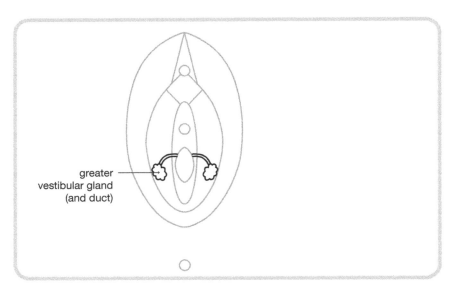

greater vestibular gland (and duct)

6.5.3 Uterus, fallopian tubes, ovaries and uterine ligaments

On the left side of the image we will draw the interior of the uterus and uterine (fallopian) tube in more detail, and on the right we will draw the uterine ligaments.

BL	broad ligament
MM	mesometrium
MS	mesosalpinx
O	ovary
OL	ovarian ligament
SL	suspensory ligament of ovary

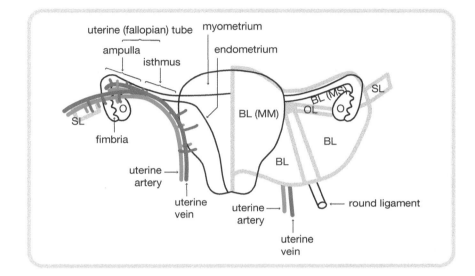

How to draw

STEP 1

- Draw a 'sheep's head' with 'horns', and add an oval on the end of the 'horns'. These are the uterus, uterine (fallopian) tubes and ovaries.
- On the left side of the page, label the parts of the uterine tube.
- Label the myometrium and endometrium inside the uterus.

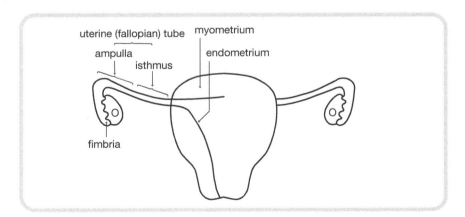

STEP ②

- On the right side of the page, draw 2 short grey lines from the ovary to the uterus; these represent the ovarian ligament.
- Draw a grey rectangle emerging from behind the fimbria laterally; this is the suspensory ligament of the ovary.
- Draw a grey line enclosing the uterus and fallopian tube in a wing shape. This is the broad ligament. The part over the uterus is mesometrium and the part between the ovary and the ovarian ligament is the mesosalpinx.
- Draw a long thin grey rectangle from the uterine end of the fallopian tube towards 5 o'clock. Underneath this is the round ligament: draw this protruding below.
- Draw the uterine artery and vein medial to the round ligament.

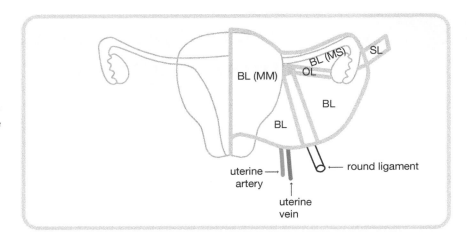

STEP ③

- On the left side of the page draw the uterine artery and vein curving around the edge of the uterus, along the lower edge of the fallopian tube and above the ovary.
- These supply the ovary, fallopian tube and uterus: add small branches to show this.

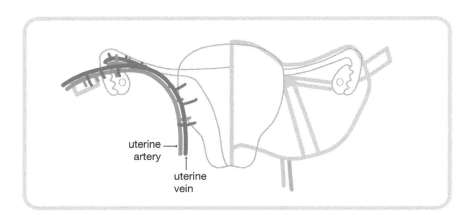

6.6 Breast

The breast (or mammary gland) is located between the 2nd and 6th intercostal cartilages (or ribs) and is superficial to the pectoralis muscles (located within the superficial fascia). In women they are made of fatty tissue and glandular tissue which is organised into lobes. There are 15–20 lobes which are comprised of lobules, each containing 10–100 alveoli that are approximately 0.12mm in diameter. It is the alveoli that are the site of milk production.

Men and women develop breasts from the same embryological tissue but production of oestrogen and growth hormones initiates breast development in females.

6.6.1 Sagittal section, midline of breast

i/c   intercostal

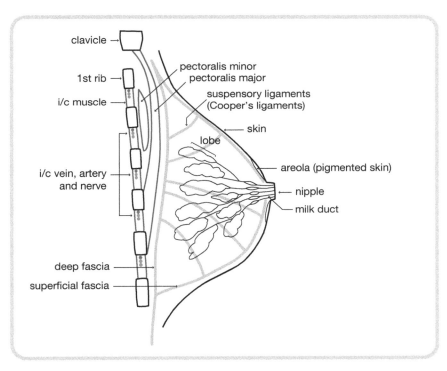

How to draw

STEP 1

- Draw a small square on the left side of the page; this represents a cross-section through the clavicle.
- Draw 6 small rectangles in a row downwards; these are the 1st 6 ribs.

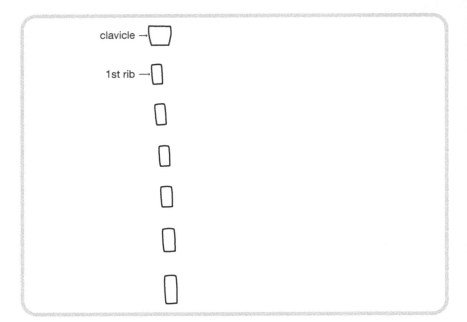

STEP 2

- Draw 2 brown lines joining each rib to the next one down. These are the intercostal muscles.
- Draw a blue, red and green dot just below each rib, to represent the intercostal vein, artery and nerve.

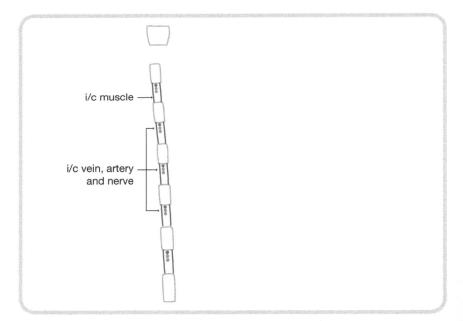

STEP 3

- Draw the outline of a breast, including the nipple.
- Just in front of ribs 1 and 2 draw a small elliptical muscle. This is the pectoralis minor, which arises from the 3rd to 5th ribs by the costochondral junction and inserts into the coracoid process of the scapula (not shown).
- From the clavicle to approximately the 5th rib, draw a curved muscle. This is the pectoralis major. It arises from the clavicular head, medial half of the clavicle, the sternocostal head, the upper 6 costal cartilages, and the aponeurosis of the external oblique muscle. It inserts into the bicipital groove of the humerus.
- See *Section 4.10: Muscles of the thorax* for action, innervation and blood supply of the pectoralis muscles.

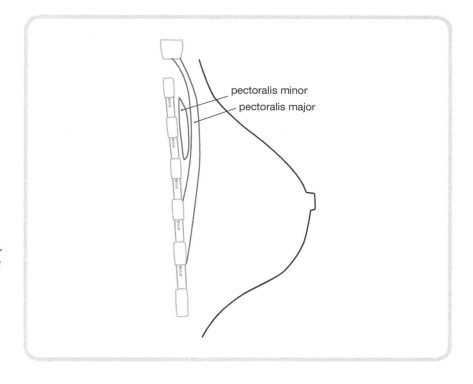

STEP 4

- Draw a line in grey just under the skin of the breast, from the clavicle down to the 6th rib. Leave a gap where the nipple lies. This is the superficial fascia.
- Draw a grey line downwards from the clavicle, parallel to pectoralis major, to meet the superficial fascia. This is the deep fascia.
- Draw a few lines from the deep fascia to the superficial fascia. These represent the suspensory ligaments (Cooper's ligaments).

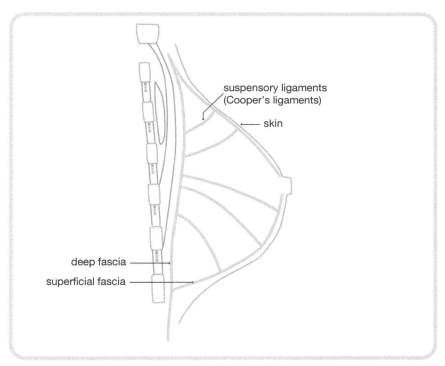

STEP 5

- Draw about 5 black lines from the end of the nipple to just inside the breast. These are milk ducts (each breast normally has 5–18 ducts, but sometimes only 5–12 eject at the nipple).
- Continue the ducts inwards, into groups of 'clouds'; these represent the lobes of the breast.
- Draw 2 short black lines from the edge of the nipple, between skin and fascia, upwards and downwards; these show the areola (pigmented skin).

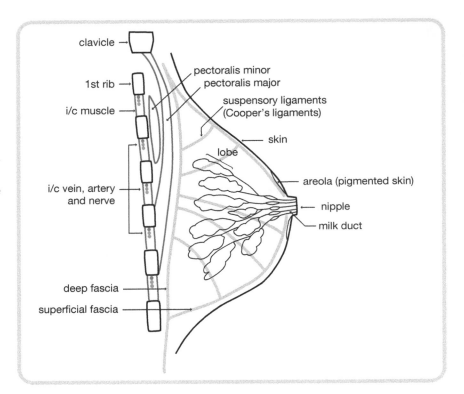

6.6.2 Blood supply to the breast

A anterior cutaneous branches of the intercostal nerves
L lateral cutaneous branches of the intercostal nerves
LMV lateral mammary vein
LTV lateral thoracic vein
SVC superior vena cava

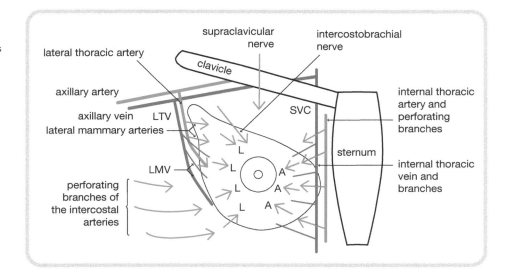

How to draw

STEP ①

- Draw a slim rectangle sloping downwards from the left side of the page to the centre. This is the clavicle.
- At its medial end draw a vertical rectangle-like shape to represent the sternum.
- Under the clavicle draw the outline of the tissue of the right breast, a tilted teardrop shape. This is also known as the axillary tail or axillary process.
- In its centre, draw a smaller circle inside a larger circle; this is the nipple and areola, respectively.

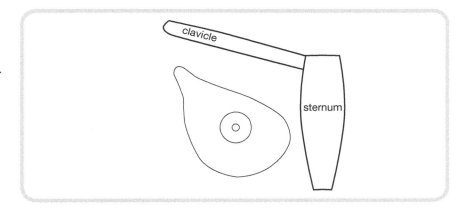

STEP ②

- Draw an artery down the lateral edge of the sternum with arrows pointing towards the breast. These are the internal thoracic artery and perforating branches.
- From just below the lateral 1/3 of the clavicle, draw the axillary artery going towards the arm, and from here draw the lateral thoracic artery descending down the lateral side of the breast, with lateral mammary branches as shown.
- Draw a few red arrows from the left to approximately 7, 8 and 9 o'clock; these

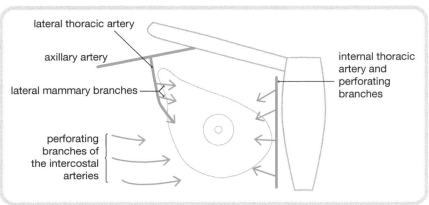

represent the perforating branches of the intercostal arteries (aka posterior intercostal arteries).

STEP 3

- Draw a vein medial to the internal thoracic artery, with branches from the breast; this represents the internal thoracic vein and branches.
- Just below the axillary artery, draw the axillary vein. Alongside the lateral thoracic artery draw the lateral thoracic vein; draw a few branches to represent the lateral mammary veins.
- Draw in the superior vena cava behind the sternum and clavicle; the axillary vein and the internal thoracic vein both drain into here.

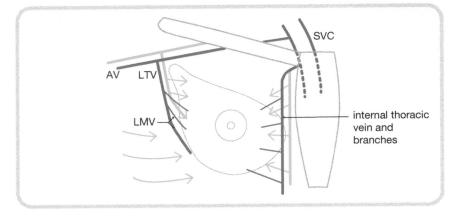

STEP 4

- Draw a green arrow down from above the clavicle to the upper part of the breast; this represents the supraclavicular nerve.
- Draw an arrow from below the lateral clavicle toward approximately 5 o'clock; this is the intercostobrachial nerve.
- Draw a few green arrows on the left side of the page towards the centre of the breast, to represent the lateral cutaneous branches of the intercostal nerves. Draw similar green arrows on the medial side of the breast towards the centre of the breast; these are the anterior cutaneous branches of the intercostal nerves.

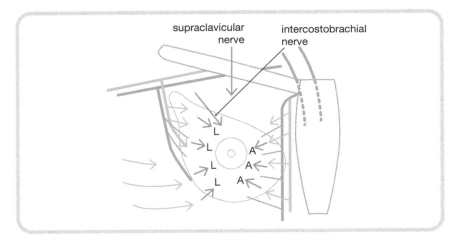

Chapter 7
Upper limb

07

7.1 Blood vessels

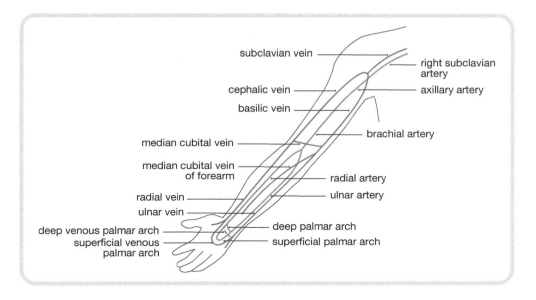

ARTERIES

- The arteries can be seen as one line from the axilla to the cubital fossa (CF), and it then forms a loop from the CF to the hand.
- The subclavian artery becomes the axillary artery which becomes the brachial artery.
- This then divides in the CF to become the radial artery (laterally, near the thumb) and the ulnar artery (medially and near the little finger).
- They join in 2 loops in the hand, the deep palmar arch and the superficial palmar arch.

VEINS

- The venous system has a superficial part and a deep part. The superficial veins include the superficial venous palmar arch, the median cubital vein, the cephalic vein, and the basilic vein. The deep part comprises the deep venous palmar arch, many perforating veins, radial vein, and the ulnar veins which drain into the brachial vein (not shown).
- This is not an exact replica of venous drainage because I have simplified the anatomy for ease of learning.
- The veins drain from the hand towards the axilla.
- The basilic vein starts in the medial side of the wrist and runs superficially along the medial side of the arm to drain into the brachial vein.
- The cephalic vein runs from the anatomical snuff box along the lateral side of the arm.
- The venous drainage of the arm ends in the subclavian vein.
- To help remember which vein is on which side of the arm, put your arm out with your thumb pointing up: the basilic vein is at the bottom (base) and the cephalic vein is nearer the head (cephalad).

7.2 Brachial plexus

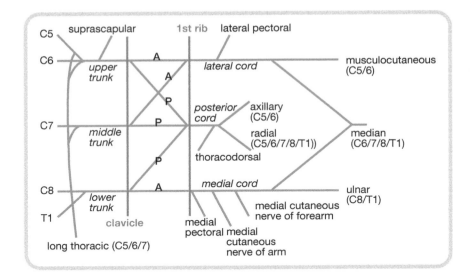

A	anterior
CNA	cutaneous nerve of arm
CNF	cutaneous nerve of forearm
LT	lower trunk
MT	middle trunk
P	posterior
UT	upper trunk

🖊 How to draw

STEP ①

- Draw 3 lines horizontally.
- The middle line should be approximately 2/3 the length of the outside lines.

STEP ②

- Add in the landmarks: the clavicle and 1st rib. These should be perpendicular lines at approximately 1/3 and 2/3 along the middle line.

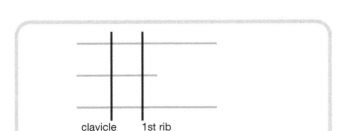

STEP ③

- Add the roots and label: C5, C6, C7, C8 and T1.
- Add in the long thoracic nerve; this usually comes off near the roots of C5, C6 and C7.
- Label the upper, middle and lower trunks.

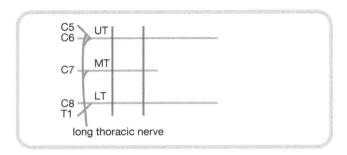

STEP 4

- Draw in the divisions – these usually occur between the clavicle and first rib. Each trunk has an anterior (A) and posterior (P) division.
- Draw them in by drawing an arrowhead from the outer two lines to meet in the posterior cord and then cross the top half of the arrow.
- The posterior division of each trunk joins to form the posterior cord.
- The anterior divisions of the upper and middle trunk join to form the lateral cord and the anterior division of the lower trunk forms the medial cord.

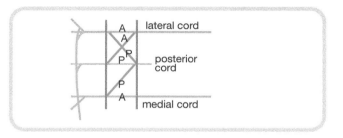

STEP 5

- Draw a second arrowhead joining the lateral and medial cord. These form the median nerve.

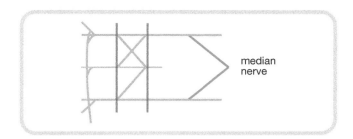

STEP 6

- Draw a 'snake's tongue'; this is the posterior cord dividing to form the axillary nerve (upper) and the radial nerve (lower).
- Label the musculocutaneous (M/C) nerve and the ulnar nerve.

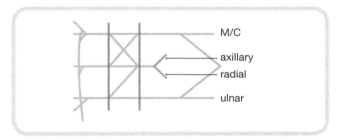

STEP 7

- Add in one branch from the lateral cord – this is the lateral pectoral nerve.
- Add in three branches from the medial cord – these are the medial cutaneous nerve of the forearm, the medial cutaneous nerve of the arm and the medial pectoral nerve.

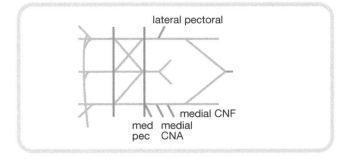

STEP 8

- Add in one branch from the posterior cord – this is the thoracodorsal nerve (reminder: dorsal and posterior both mean behind/back).
- Add in one branch from the upper trunk – this is the suprascapular nerve (this can be missed in a supraclavicular block; it usually supplies the lateral skin of the shoulder and so can lead to pain in shoulder surgery if missed).

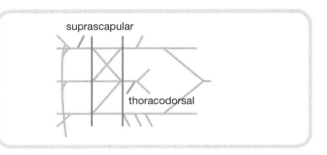

7.3 | Axilla

BB biceps brachii muscle
BR brachialis muscle
CB coracobrachialis muscle
M/C musculocutaneous nerve

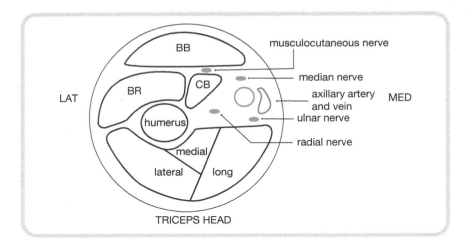

There are few good simplistic versions of the axilla. I found it difficult to represent the anatomy exactly. This diagram of the right axilla shows a view from distal to proximal. It should help you label any diagram of the axilla, but it is not an exact anatomical replica.

How to draw

STEP 1

- Draw a large circle to represent the cross-section of the axilla with a small circle in the middle just lateral to the centre – this represents the humerus.

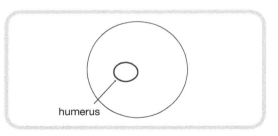

STEP 2

- Draw a semicircular shape, split into 3, below the humerus. This represents the triceps muscle.
- There are 3 heads: the lateral head (left), the medial head (middle) and the long head (right).

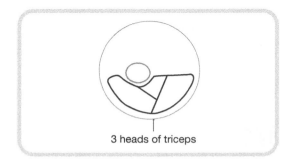

STEP ③

Draw 3 shapes as shown above the humerus:
- the brachialis muscle
- the biceps brachii muscle
- the coracobrachialis muscle.

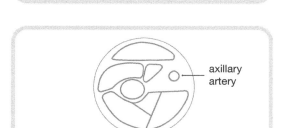

STEP ④

- Draw a red circle medial to the humerus – this represents the axillary artery.

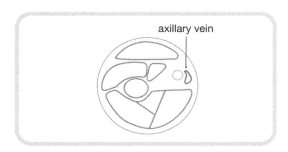

STEP ⑤

- Draw a blue shape lateral to the axillary artery – this represents the axillary vein.

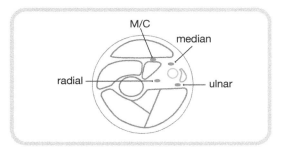

STEP ⑥

- Draw 4 green dots, 3 encircling the axillary artery at approximately 12 o'clock (median nerve), 5 o'clock (ulnar nerve) and 8 o'clock (radial nerve), and 1 between the biceps brachii and coracobrachialis muscles, the musculocutaneous nerve.

> To help remember this image, think of it as 'the triangle'. Using different shapes for different areas will help to differentiate them in your mind as you draw this image of the right cubital fossa.

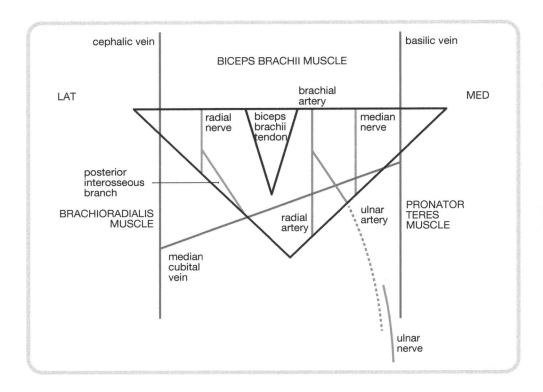

 How to draw

STEP 1

- Draw an isosceles triangle pointing downwards. Label the borders: biceps brachii muscle above, pronator teres medially and brachioradialis laterally.
- Draw a smaller triangle just lateral to the centre to represent the biceps brachii tendon.

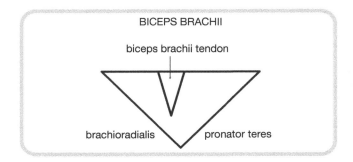

STEP 2

- Draw the brachial artery as a straight line down just medial to the biceps brachii tendon.
- This divides into the ulnar artery medially and the radial artery laterally. The ulnar artery passes under the pronator teres where it joins the ulnar nerve.

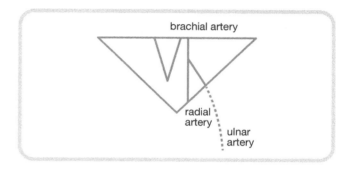

STEP 3

- Add in the ulnar nerve part-way down by the dotted ulnar artery.
- Add in the median nerve medial to the brachial artery.
- Add in the radial nerve lateral to the biceps brachii tendon; draw in the posterior interosseous branch. (This is important because a radial nerve block that is too low can miss this branch and hence the patient can experience wrist pain during surgery.)

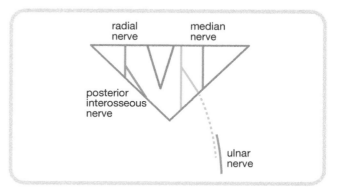

STEP 4

- Add in the veins. Draw an H shape with a diagonal crossbar from lower to higher, lateral to medial.
- Label these: cephalic, basilic and median cubital veins.

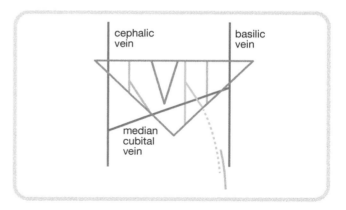

TIP!

Put your arm out with your thumb pointing upwards. The basilic vein is on the 'base' of the arm and the cephalic vein is nearer the head.

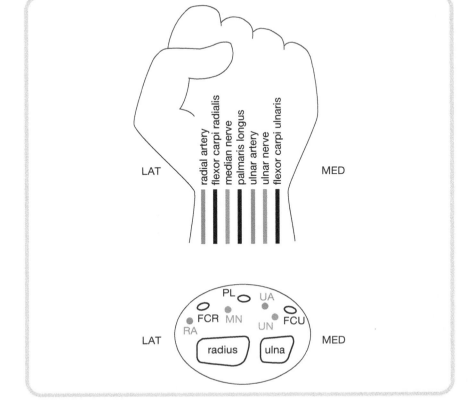

FCR	flexor carpi radialis tendon
FCU	flexor carpi ulnaris tendon
MN	median nerve
PL	palmaris longus
R	radius
RA	radial artery
U	ulna
UA	ulnar artery
UN	ulnar nerve

It's important to know the basic anatomy of the wrist so that when you perform procedures, you know what vital structures you may damage. To help remember it, think of it as the '7 lines' of the wrist. This drawing shows you the cross-section of the wrist in your left arm, as you look down the arm.

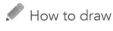 How to draw

 STEP **1**

- Draw a hand shape.

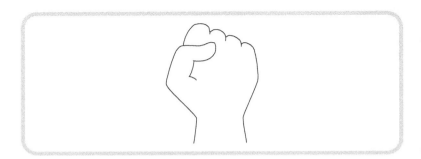

STEP 2

- Draw 7 lines in the following order: red, black, green, black, red, green and black. The lines represent the tendons (black), nerves (green) and arteries (red).
- From lateral to medial these are: the radial artery, flexor carpi radialis (FCR), the median nerve, palmaris longus, ulnar artery, ulnar nerve and flexor carpi ulnaris (FCU).
- Nerves are often 'protected' by tendons and so you can see that the median nerve lies between and below 2 tendons and the ulnar nerve lies just below FCU.
- The radial artery can be easily found by feeling for FCR and palpating just laterally.

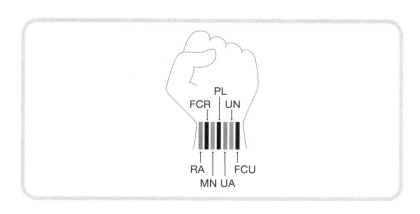

 How to draw the cross-section

STEP 1

- Draw an oval shape with 2 squares in it to represent the radius and ulna.

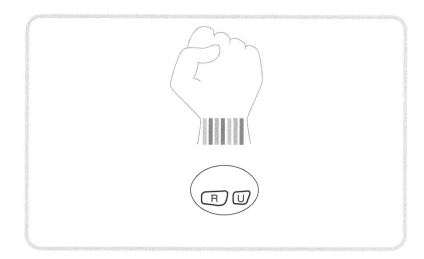

STEP 2

- Draw 7 coloured dots/circles that correspond to the picture above. Note that nerves are deep compared with the tendons.

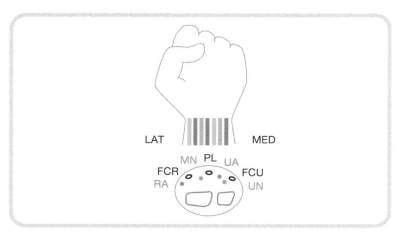

Bones of the upper limb

All the bones drawn here relate to the right side of the body.

7.6.1 Scapula and clavicle

SCAPULA

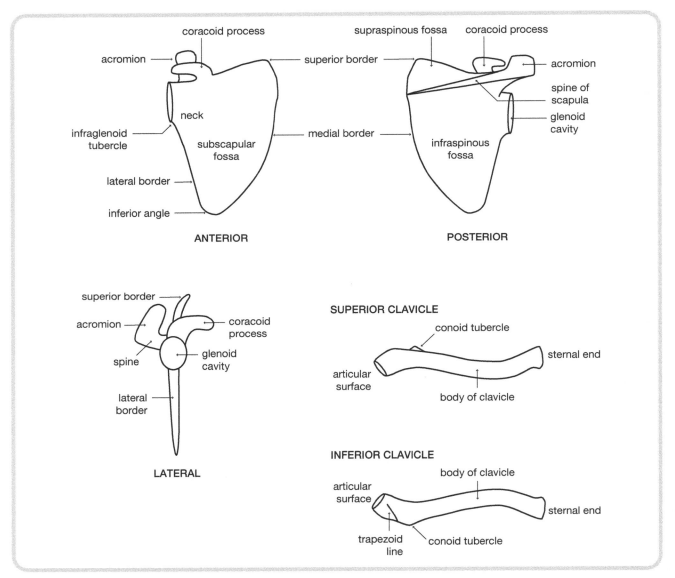

ANTERIOR

POSTERIOR

LATERAL

Anterior view

 How to draw

- Draw a triangular shape with 2 protrusions at the top, the coracoid process anteriorly and the acromion posteriorly, as shown.
- Draw the top of the lateral border as a convex shape to show the glenoid cavity for the humeral head.
- On the anterior side the large flattish area is the subscapular fossa. This is where the subscapularis muscle attaches.

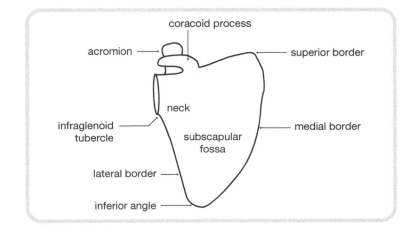

Posterior view

 How to draw

- Begin by drawing a mirror image of the anterior view in pencil, then add detail. For now, leave out the acromion and coracoid process.
- Starting at the medial border, draw a long thin triangle that broadens as it runs at an upward angle; this is the spine of the scapula, projecting out of the page. At its lateral end, complete it with an outline mirroring the anterior view of the acromion.
- Now add the mirror image of the coracoid process beyond (anterior to) the acromion.
- Label the supraspinous fossa above the spine and the infraspinous fossa below. These are where supraspinatus and infraspinatus muscles sit, respectively.

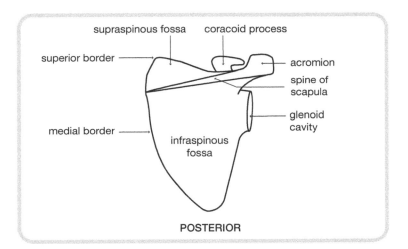

Lateral view

 How to draw

- Draw the glenoid cavity as an oval with the long lateral border of the scapula tapering below it.
- Add the acromion and coracoid process: they look like 2 blades on a fan.
- Show that the superior border can be seen in a lateral view.

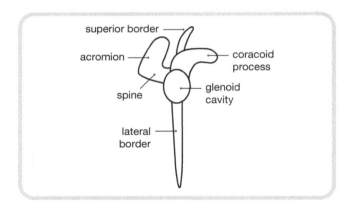

CLAVICLE

Superior view

 How to draw

- Draw a back-to-front 'S' shape horizontally across the page, with flattened ends as shown. The end on the right side of the page is the medial end and articulates with the sternum (sternoclavicular joint).
- Draw a thin line at the lateral end, just in from the border of the bone on the left side of the page; this delineates the articular surface where the clavicle and the acromion of the scapula meet in the acromioclavicular joint.
- About 1/3 of the way in from the lateral end, draw a small protrusion; this is the small part of the conoid tubercle seen from above.

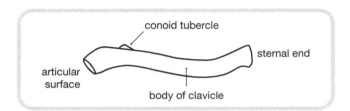

Inferior view

 How to draw

- Draw a mirror image of the superior view. Show the conoid tubercle (also called coracoid tubercle). The tubercle is an attachment point for the conoid ligament, which is the part of the coracoclavicular ligament that attaches the clavicle to the coracoid process of the scapula.
- Draw a line from here towards the lateral end; this is the trapezoid line.

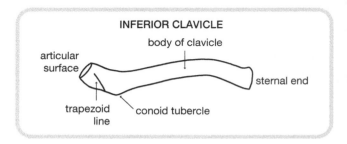

7.6.2 Humerus

The humerus is the long bone in the arm between the elbow and the shoulder joint. At the shoulder, the humeral head sits in the glenoid fossa of the scapula, forming the glenohumeral joint.

At the elbow the capitulum of the humerus articulates with the radius, and the trochlea with the ulna.

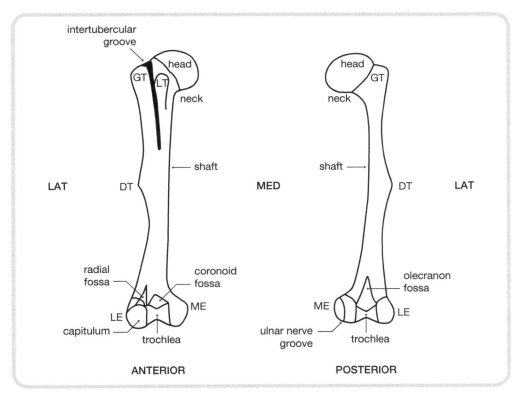

DT   deltoid tuberosity
GT   greater tuberosity
LE   lateral epicondyle
LT   lesser tuberosity
ME   medial epicondyle

Anterior view

✏️ How to draw

STEP ①

Start by drawing the outline of the humerus as a fairly straight bone with a rounded head on a narrow neck.

- In the middle of the shaft on the lateral side, draw a slight protrusion. This is the deltoid tuberosity; unsurprisingly, it is where the deltoid muscle attaches.
- Show bulges in the outline at the distal end; these are the medial epicondyle and lateral epicondyle (the smaller of the two).
- Label the head, neck and shaft

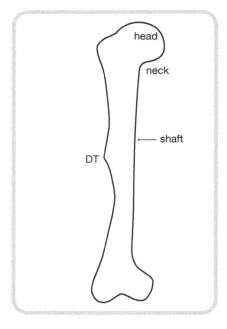

STEP ②

- Draw a very narrow, long V shape; this is the intertubercular groove, which separates the 2 tuberosities.
- At the top, label the greater tuberosity (or tubercle).
- On the medial side of the groove, draw a hairpin shape; this is the lesser tuberosity.

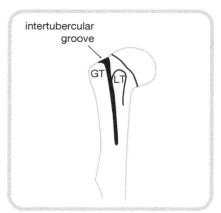

STEP ③

- Create a circle on the lateral side at the distal end; this is the capitulum.
- Medial to the capitulum draw a straight-edged 'bow tie', in the middle of the bone's width; this is the trochlea, the articular surface of the humerus in its pivot joint with the ulna.
- Draw the coronoid fossa as a diamond shape above the trochlea.
- Draw the radial fossa as a triangle just above the capitulum.
- Finish by drawing a line above the capitulum to the outer edge; this shows where the lateral epicondyle lies.

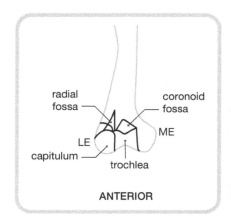

Posterior view

 How to draw

STEP 1

- Draw the mirror image of *Anterior view* Step 1, showing a posterior view of the humerus.
- Label the head, neck, shaft, greater tuberosity and deltoid tuberosity, and medial and lateral epicondyles.

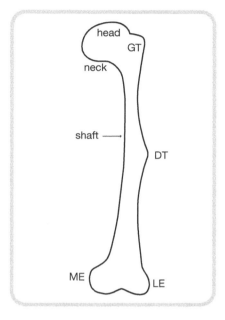

STEP 2

- Draw a line at the proximal end to show the boundary between the head and neck of the humerus.

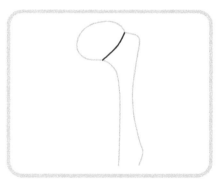

STEP 3

- Draw a straight-edged 'bow tie' in the middle to represent the posterior portion of the trochlea.
- On each side draw a curve up and out from the trochlea, to delineate the medial and lateral epicondyles.
- On the medial side draw a line down the middle; this represents the ulnar nerve groove.
- Above the trochlea draw a diamond shape; this is the olecranon fossa.

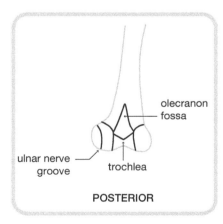

7.6.3	# Radius and ulna

In the anatomical position, with the palms facing forward:

- The radius lies on the lateral side and supports the thumb side of the forearm.
- The ulna lies on the medial side and supports the little finger side of the forearm.

NOTE: the bone is called the ulna, without the 'r' of the ulnar nerve, artery and vein. The radius is small proximally and wide distally; the ulna is the opposite.

The radius articulates with the capitulum of the humerus superiorly and the carpal bones at the hand end. The ulna articulates with the trochlea of the humerus and the carpal bones at the hand.

The radius and ulna also articulate with each other. Proximally the radial head forms a joint with the radial notch on the ulna. Distally the head of the ulna forms a joint with the ulnar notch of the radius.

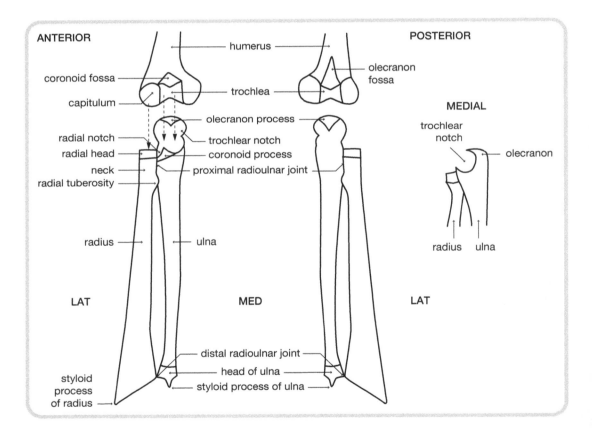

ANTERIOR VIEW

 How to draw

STEP ①

- Draw a long trapezoid shape, with its lower edge having a downward slant from the middle to the left side of the page and with a bump on the medial side near the top of the bone just below its neck. This is the radius.
- Label the lower corner as the styloid process of radius.
- Label the bump as the radial tuberosity.
- Draw a horizontal line in a little way in from the top; the area above is the radial head and the area below is the radial neck.

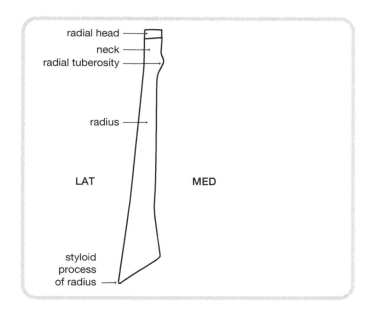

STEP ②

- Draw a shape a bit like a butterfly for the head of the ulna, as shown.
- Join the top of both 'wings' with a curved line. The area below this line is the olecranon process. The 'butterfly' is the trochlear notch (see the later *Medial view*, which shows how this is concave).
- The ulnar area in contact with the radial head is the radial notch, at the proximal radioulnar joint.

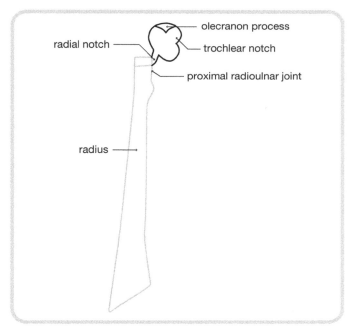

STEP 3

- Draw a line joining the bottom of the 'wings'; the area above this is the coronoid process.
- Draw a narrowing trapezoid shape to the same length as the medial side of the bottom of the radius. On the medial side of its lower edge, draw a protrusion; this is the styloid process of ulna.
- Draw a line across the ulna at the distal end; the area below this is the head of the ulna. The area where the ulna and radius touch distally is the distal radioulnar joint.

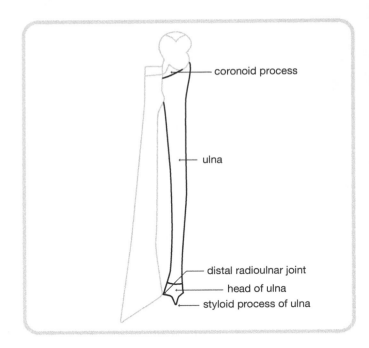

STEP 4

- Draw the distal end of the humerus above the radius and ulna, as shown.
- Draw the 'bow-tie'-shaped trochlea in the middle with the coronoid fossa as a triangle above it. Draw a circle shape on the lateral side; this is the capitulum.
- Draw 3 dashed arrows to show where the radius and ulna articulate with the humerus: from the capitulum to the radial head and from the trochlea to the 'wings' of the trochlear notch of the ulna.

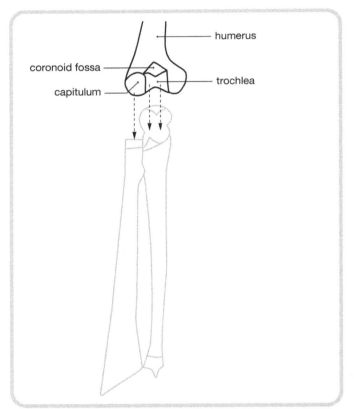

POSTERIOR VIEW

 How to draw

STEP 1

- Draw a mirror image of the radius in *Anterior view* Step 1 as shown, omitting the radial tuberosity.

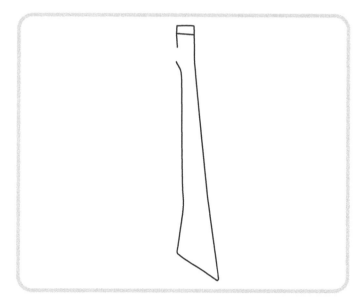

STEP 2

- Draw a mirror image of the ulna as shown. It obscures the radial tuberosity in this view.
- At the proximal end, draw a small triangle; this represents the posterior area of the olecranon (the trochlear notch can only be seen from the anterior side).

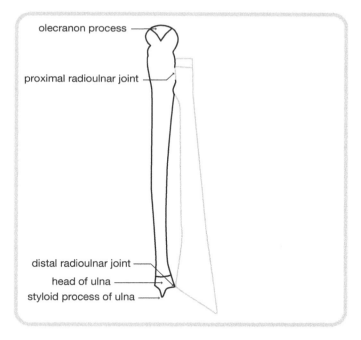

olecranon process

proximal radioulnar joint

distal radioulnar joint

head of ulna

styloid process of ulna

STEP 3

- Draw the distal end of the posterior humerus above the radius and ulna.
- On this, draw a 'bow-tie' for the trochlea, with a triangle above for the olecranon fossa.

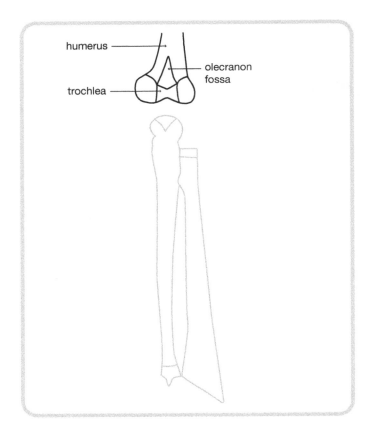

MEDIAL VIEW

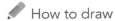 How to draw

- Draw a straight line up the right side of the paper.
- At the top of the line turn 90° and draw a short line across. From here draw a semicircle, from 1 to 7 o'clock, and then turn sharply and continue down the page.
- The concave semicircle is the trochlear notch. The humerus sits here. The upper part is the olecranon process.
- Draw the radial head sitting lateral to and just below the trochlear notch.

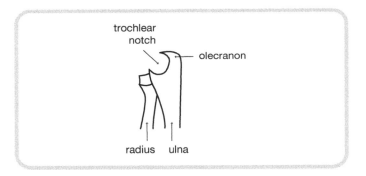

7.6.4 Bones of the hand

The wrist joint (also known as the radiocarpal joint) is a synovial joint and marks the area of transition between the forearm and the hand. The distal end of the radius above articulates with the scaphoid, lunate and triquetral bones below.

The hand is made up of 5 metacarpal bones and 14 phalanges. Each finger is made up of 3 phalanges; the thumb is made up of 2. These 19 bones collectively form 14 separate joints.

C	capitate
H	hamate
Ln	lunate
P	pisiform
Sc	scaphoid
Td	trapezoid
Tq	triquetral
Tr	trapezium

R	radius
U	ulna

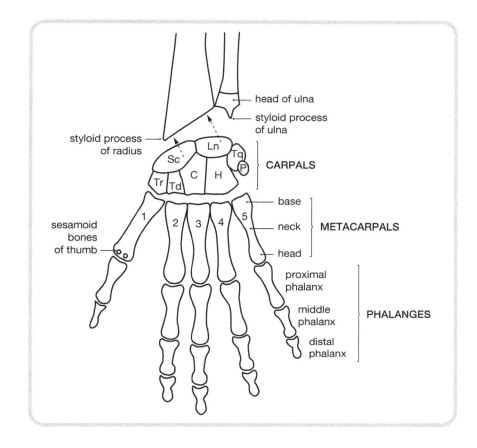

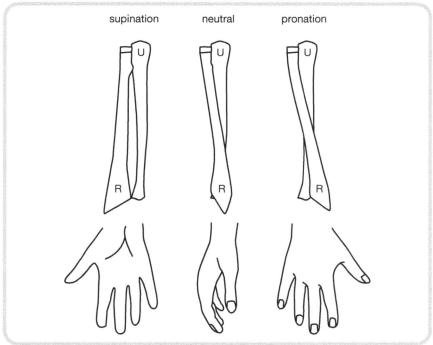

CARPALS: ANTERIOR VIEW

 How to draw

STEP 1

- Copy and label the distal end of the anterior view from *Section 7.6.3: Radius and ulna*.
- Draw 4 horizontal oval shapes in a slightly curved line just below the radius and ulna.
- From lateral to medial these are the scaphoid, lunate, triquetral and pisiform bones.

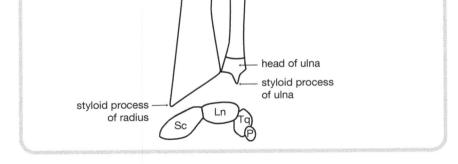

STEP 2

- Draw a 2nd line of bones, with different shapes as follows.
- Draw a pentagon on the lateral side for the trapezium, followed by a trapezoid shape for the trapezoid, then a pentagonal shape for the capitate and a similar shape for the hamate bone.

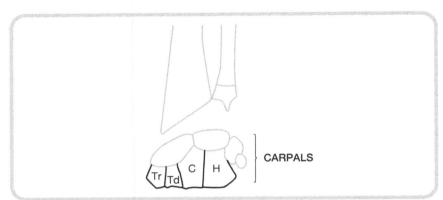

STEP 3

- Draw 2 dashed arrows: 1 from the scaphoid to the lateral part of the distal radius and 1 from the lunate to the medial part of the distal radius. These show where the bones articulate.

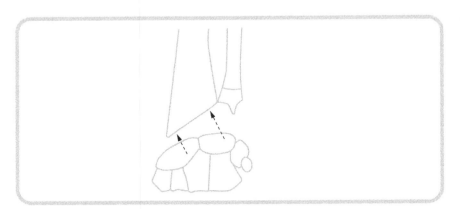

STEP 4

- Draw 5 metacarpals starting from the radial side, the thumb. On the 1st metacarpal draw 2 small circles, the sesamoid bones.
- Label the base, neck and head of the metacarpals.

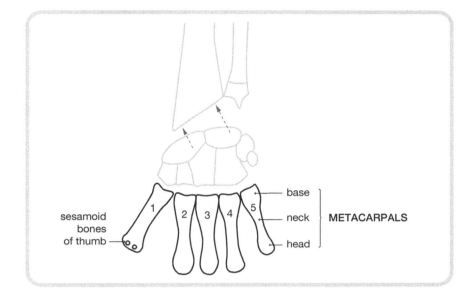

STEP 5

- At the distal end of the 2nd to 5th digits, draw 3 phalanges: proximal, middle and distal.
- At the distal end of the thumb draw only 2 phalanges, distal and proximal.

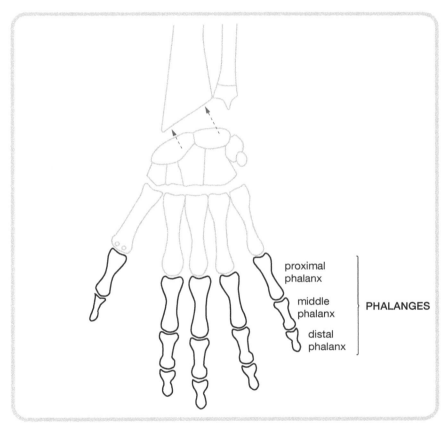

7.7 Muscles of the upper limb

Muscles of the upper limb are summarised at the end of this section in Table 7.2; this gives their innervation, blood supply and actions. In the images, tendons are distinguished from their muscles by switching from the muscle brown colour to grey where a muscle belly ends and its long tendon starts.

Note the table lists muscles by area. However, each drawing includes muscles seen in a specific view, which is sometimes different from the table. For example, brachioradialis and supinator are in the posterior compartment of the forearm arm in the table. But brachioradialis has its origin in the arm and supinator inserts onto the anterior radius, so they first appear in drawings of the arm and anterior forearm, respectively, as well as the posterior forearm drawing.

7.7.1 Muscles of the upper arm

For more details of the muscles on the scapula, see *Section 2.7.8: Superficial muscles of the back and muscles of the lumbar region*. Blood supply and innervation are shown separately later on in this section to avoid overcomplicating these images.

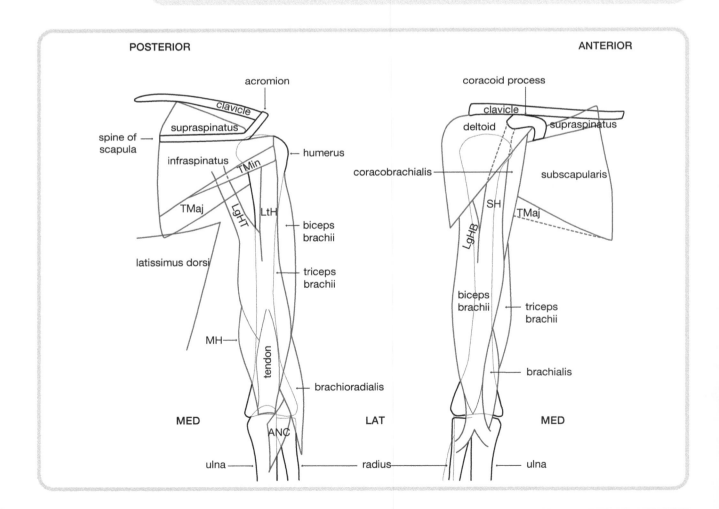

Aa	axillary artery	LtH	lateral head of triceps brachii	SH	short head of biceps brachii
ACa	anterior circumflex artery	MH	medial head of triceps brachii	SubSa	subscapular artery
ANC	anconeus			SupSa	suprascapular artery
Ba	brachial artery	PBa	profunda brachii artery	TMaj	teres major
LgH	long head (B, biceps; T, triceps)	PCa	posterior circumflex artery	TMin	teres minor

POSTERIOR VIEW

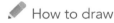 How to draw

STEP 1

- Draw a horizontal 'hockey stick' across the page to represent the spine of the scapula and the acromion.
- In pencil draw a rough outline for the humerus and the upper ends of the ulna and radius.
- From the end of the acromion draw a curved line backwards, above and past the supraspinatus; this is the clavicle.
- On the superior edge of the scapula draw a brown horizontal triangle; this is the **supraspinatus**. It originates from the supraspinous fossa and inserts onto the superior facet on the greater tuberosity of the humerus.

STEP 2

- Below the spine of scapula draw a brown triangle; this is **infraspinatus**. It originates from the infraspinous fossa and inserts onto the middle facet on the greater tuberosity of the humerus, inferior to the supraspinatus.
- Below this draw 2 smaller triangles: the **teres minor**, which originates from the lateral border of the scapula and inserts onto the humeral head below the infraspinatus, and **teres major**, which originates from the inferior angle of the scapula and inserts onto the humerus below and medial to the infraspinatus and teres minor.
- Go over the outlines of the glenoid tubercle and the shaft of the humerus in black, as shown.

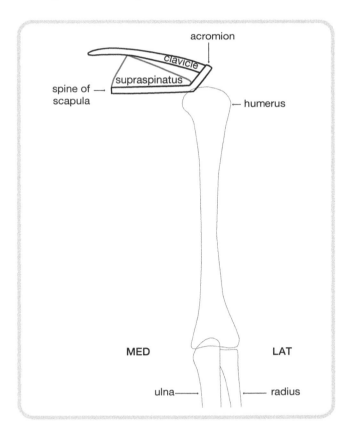

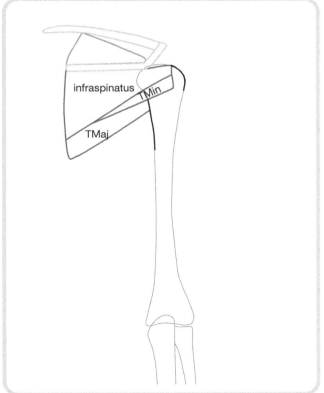

STEP 3

- **Triceps brachii** has 3 proximal heads (see Box 7.1): long, lateral and medial.
- From just below the insertion of teres minor on the humeral head draw a thin rectangle down almost half the length of the humerus; this is the triceps' lateral head.
- Draw the long head similarly: it arises from the infraglenoid tubercle of the scapula and passes anterior to the teres minor and posterior to the teres major.
- Draw the medial head emerging from behind the main muscle belly medially (most of it lies beyond the long and lateral heads).
- Join the heads to form the main muscle belly, converging as a tendon that inserts onto the olecranon process of the ulna.
- Draw a triangle below teres major to show **latissimus dorsi**. This originates from the spinous processes of T7–T12, thoracolumbar fascia, iliac crest and the inferior 3 or 4 ribs. It inserts onto the intertubercular groove of the humerus (not shown).

STEP 4

- Along the lateral edge of triceps brachii draw a slim line. This is **biceps brachii**. Its short head originates on the coracoid process and the long head on the supraglenoid tubercle. The heads combine and insert onto the radial tuberosity on the radius.
- Draw a triangular shape below the lateral lower end of triceps brachii. This is **brachioradialis**, which arises from the lateral supracondylar ridge of the humerus and inserts onto the styloid process of the distal radius.
- Draw **anconeus**, which arises from the lateral epicondyle of the humerus (obscured by brachioradialis here). Show its insertion on the lateral surface of the olecranon process of the ulna (the insertion on the posterior, proximal part of the ulna is not visible below the muscle).
- Now ink in the outlines of the proximal humerus and the ulna and radius in the regions where they aren't hidden by muscle.

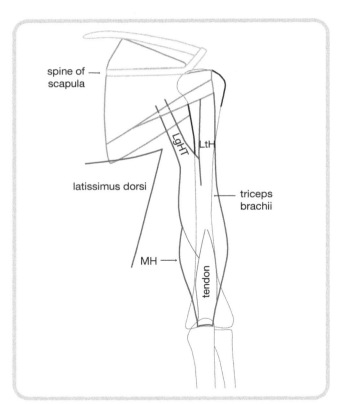

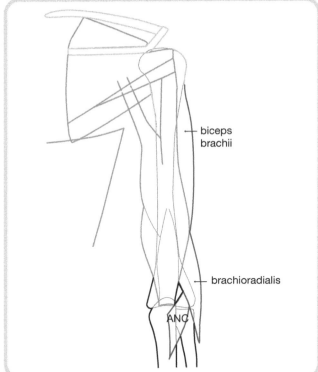

ANTERIOR VIEW

 How to draw

STEP 1

- Draw a horizontal rectangle for the clavicle. Below and inferior to the lateral 1/3 of the clavicle, draw the coracoid process. Pencil in a mirror image of the humerus, radius and ulna bones from *Posterior view* Step 1.
- Medial to the coracoid process and inferior to the clavicle draw the **supraspinatus** over the area that would be the supraspinous part of the scapula.
- Below this draw the triangular **subscapularis**, which originates on the subscapular fossa; its insertion onto the lesser tubercle of the humerus is omitted here because later steps will show this.

STEP 2

- Draw the **deltoid** as a right-angled triangle below the clavicle and ending behind the coracoid.
- The muscle is named after the shape of the Greek letter *delta*. Its origins are on the anterior upper border of the lateral 1/3 of the clavicle, the acromion and the spine of the scapula. It inserts onto the deltoid tuberosity of the humerus.

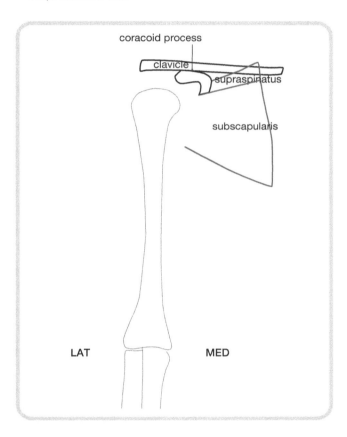

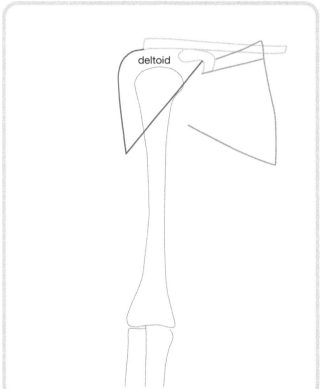

STEP 3

- Draw the short head of the **biceps brachii** as a dotted line underneath the deltoid, originating from the coracoid process.
- Draw the long head appearing from below the deltoid muscle; it arises from the supraglenoid tubercle of the scapula.
- Join the 2 heads to form the main muscle belly; continue it downwards and then divide it to insert onto the medial side of the radius (radial tuberosity) and the bicipital aponeurosis anterior to the ulna.
- Ink in the distal end of the humerus (both medial and lateral epicondyles) and the proximal end of the radius and ulna.

Box 7.1: Tips to help you remember

- For biceps the **Long** head is **Lateral**
- Biceps has 2 heads (*bi* = 2)
- Triceps has 3 heads (*tri* = 3)

STEP 4

- Draw a 'lens' just medial to the lower part of biceps brachii. This is **brachialis**, a short fat muscle that originates below deltoid's insertion point on the humerus and inserts onto the coronoid process of the ulna. It lies deep to biceps brachii and makes up the floor of the cubital fossa.
- Draw a small triangular muscle medial to the short head of the biceps. This is **coracobrachialis**, a fairly small muscle that arises from the coracoid process of the scapula and inserts onto the anteromedial edge of the humerus.
- Draw part of **triceps brachii** medial to and showing from behind brachialis and coracobrachialis. The origins of its 3 heads are: lateral on the upper half of the posterior side of the humerus (above the radial groove), medial on the posterior side of the humerus (below the radial groove) and long on the infraglenoid tubercle of scapula. The muscle bellies join and insert onto the olecranon process of the ulna.
- Draw **teres major** as a broken line under subscapularis.

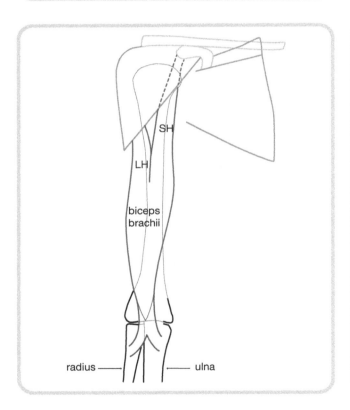

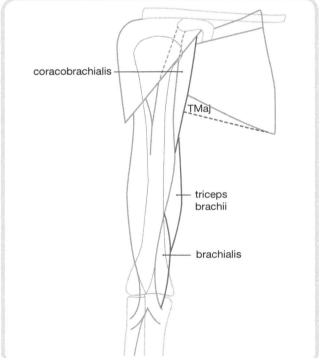

NERVES AND ARTERIES SUPPLYING THE UPPER ARM

STEP ①

- Draw the axillary nerve supplying the teres minor on the posterior view and the deltoid on the anterior view.
- On the posterior view show the subscapular nerve innervating the teres major, and on the anterior view show it innervating the subscapularis.

Then add the rest of the posterior nerves as follows.

- Draw the posterior cutaneous nerve to the triceps.
- Draw the radial nerve coming down the middle of the posterior of the arm, giving branches to the triceps muscle, brachioradialis and anconeus muscles.
- Draw the suprascapular nerve branching to supply the supraspinatus and infraspinatus.

Finally, add the rest of the anterior nerves as follows.

- Draw the musculocutaneous nerve emerging from the coracobrachialis and giving branches to the biceps brachii and brachialis.

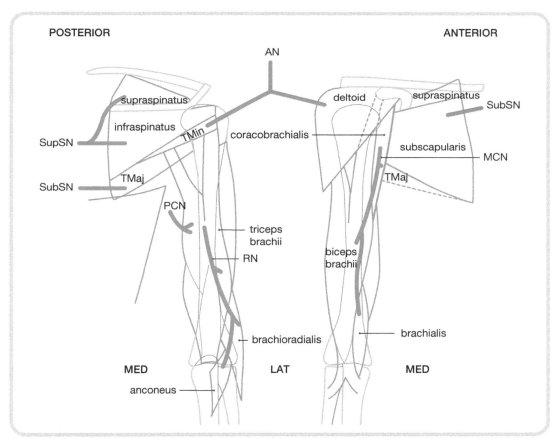

| AN | axillary nerve (C5–6) | PCN | posterior cutaneous | SubSN | subscapular nerve |
| MCN | musculocutaneous nerve (C5–7) | RN | nerve radial nerve (C5–8/T1) | SupSN | suprascapular nerve |

STEP 2

- On the posterior view, draw the profunda brachii artery, which branches off the brachial artery to supply the posterior compartment of the arm.
- On the anterior view, draw a long artery from above the clavicle down the full length of the arm; this is called the axillary artery in the axillary region and becomes the brachial artery, the major artery of the arm.
- Show the suprascapular artery supplying the supraspinatus muscle.
- Add branches from the brachial artery: laterally, the anterior and posterior circumflex arteries which form a loop around the humerus; medially, the subscapular artery supplying the subscapularis and teres major. The circumflex artery is called posterior on the posterior side and anterior on the anterior side.

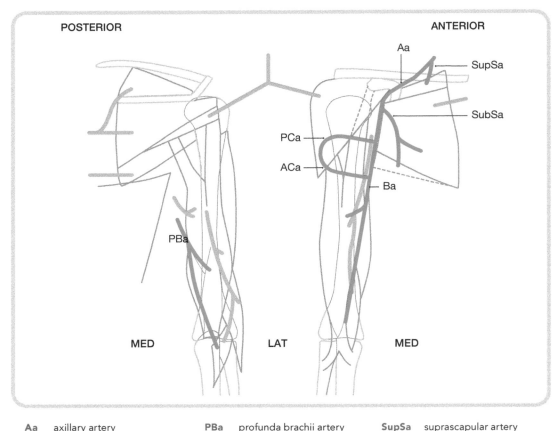

Aa	axillary artery	**PBa**	profunda brachii artery	**SupSa**	suprascapular artery
ACa	anterior circumflex artery	**PCa**	posterior circumflex artery		
Ba	brachial artery	**SubSa**	subscapular artery		

Note: Profunda means deep. Hence the profunda brachii artery is also known as the deep brachial artery.

7.7.2 Muscles of the anterior compartment of the forearm

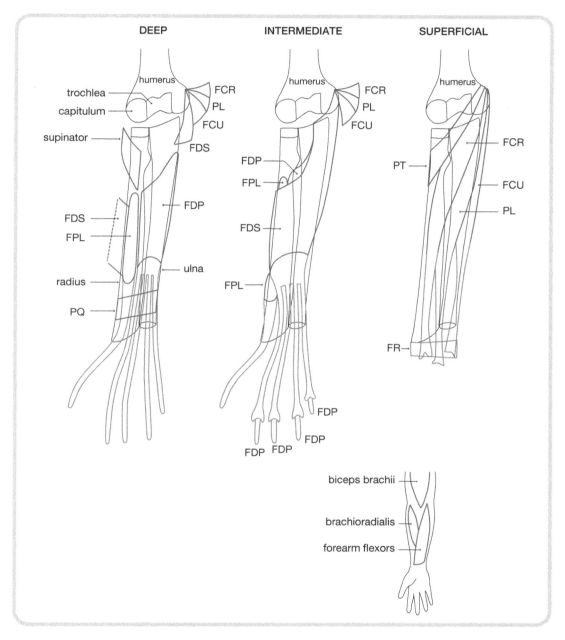

FCR	flexor carpi radialis	**FDS**	flexor digitorum superficialis	**PL**	palmaris longus
FCU	flexor carpi ulnaris	**FPL**	flexor pollicis longus	**PQ**	pronator quadratus
FDP	flexor digitorum profundus	**FR**	flexor retinaculum	**PT**	pronator teres

Muscles of the anterior compartment of the forearm are flexors. The inset in the image helps you see the forearm flexors as a group, and the biceps brachii and brachioradialis on the anterior side of your lower arm.

DEEP FLEXORS OF THE FOREARM

 How to draw

- Draw the outline of the distal humerus, including the trochlea, capitulum, radius and ulna as shown (see *Section 7.6.3: Radius and ulna* and *7.6.4: Bones of the hand*).
- Draw **supinator** coming from the posterior side around to the front; it arises from the lateral epicondyle of the humerus and the supinator crest of the ulna. Give it a triangular shape near the radial head as shown. It inserts onto the lateral edge of the upper half of the radius.
- Attached to the medial epicondyle, draw 4 retracted and cut muscles: the **flexor carpi radialis, palmaris longus, flexor carpi ulnaris** and **flexor digitorum superficialis**. This is the common flexor tendon, the upper attachment point for superficial muscles of the forearm. These muscles are more superficial than the supinator: their full lengths are shown in *Intermediate flexors of the forearm* and *Superficial flexors of the forearm* (see later).

- Draw a rectangle crossing the distal radius and ulna. This is the **pronator quadratus**. It is not a flexor but is shown here because it lies deep to the flexors.
- Draw **flexor digitorum profundus** (FDP) covering the ulna from a level just below supinator on the lateral side and just above on the medial side. It arises from the anterior and medial part of the ulna and is an extrinsic muscle of the hand (see Box 7.2).
- Continue FDP down the forearm where it divides into 4 tendons. Each tendon inserts onto the distal phalanx of 1 of the 4 fingers (not the thumb).
- Draw a line to separate the muscle belly above from the tendons below.

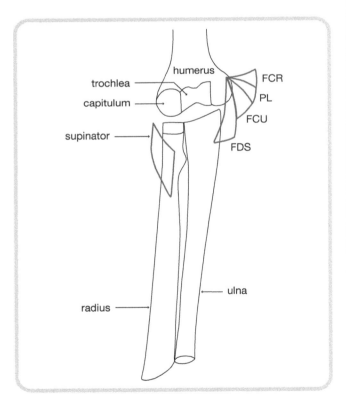

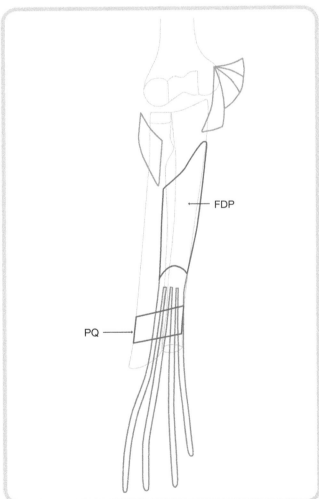

- Lateral to FDP draw a slim muscle that originates on the anterior side of the radius and interosseous membrane and then forms a long tendon that inserts onto the distal phalanx of the thumb. This is the **flexor pollicis longus** (FPL).

- Draw the radial part of the origin of the **flexor digitorum superficialis** (FDS) next to FPL. FDS also arises from the medial epicondyle and the coronoid process of the ulna, and its body lies more superficially and is shown in *Intermediate flexors of the forearm* Step 2 (see later).

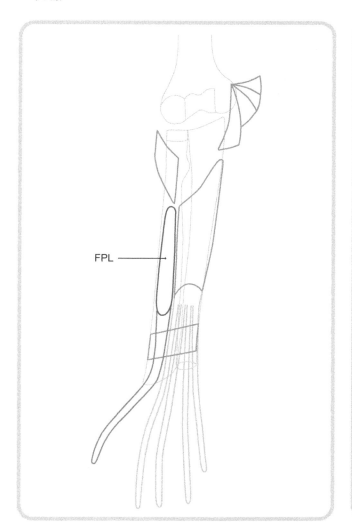

FPL

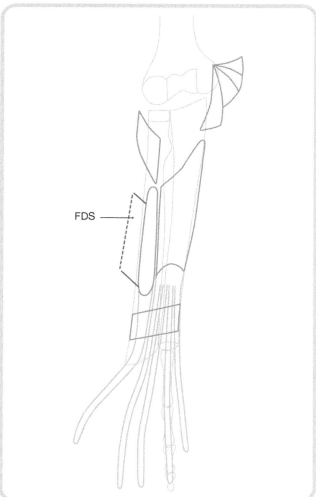

FDS

Box 7.2: Extrinsic muscles of the hand

- Muscles that originate outside the hand but insert onto structures within the hand and produce movements of the hand and digits.
- Two solely originate from the humerus: flexor carpi radialis and palmaris longus.
- The rest originate from the humerus and forearm, and they include all the forearm flexors and extensors listed in Table 7.2, as well as abductor pollicis longus.

INTERMEDIATE FLEXORS OF THE FOREARM

 How to draw

STEP 1

- Copy the image from *Deep flexors of the forearm* Step 1 (see earlier), with the following changes.
- Omit supinator from the radius.
- Omit the flexor digitorum superficialis.

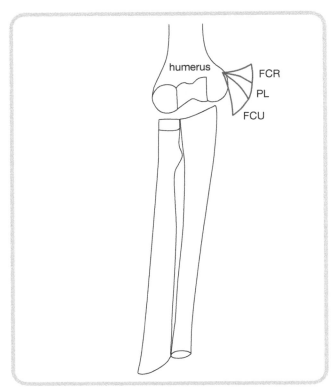

STEP 2

We will now draw the **flexor digitorum superficialis** (FDS).

- Start at the medial epicondyle and the radius (the origin at the coronoid process of the ulna is not shown), extend the body of the muscle down and divide it into the 4 tendons that insert onto the middle phalanges on the 4 fingers.
- At the end of each tendon, draw a small 'snake's tongue'. This shows the tendon's insertions either side of each middle phalanx.
- Draw a little 'bud' protruding from each 'snake's tongue'. This is flexor digitorum profundus (FDP) emerging from underneath FDS and inserting onto the distal phalanx (see *Deep flexors of the forearm* Step 2, above).

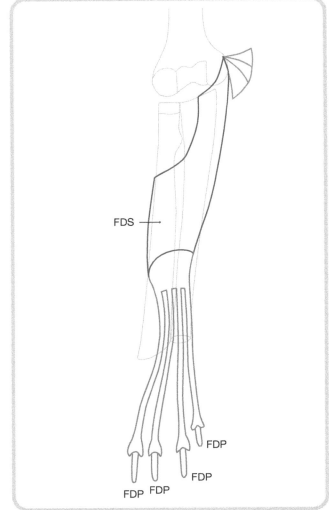

STEP 3

- Draw the proximal part of FDP that is visible behind FDS.
- Draw in the proximal end of **flexor pollicis longus** (FPL) arising from just above FDS.
- Draw **flexor pollicis longus** (FPL) emerging from beneath FDS and inserting onto the distal phalanx of the thumb as seen above in *Deep flexors* Step 4.

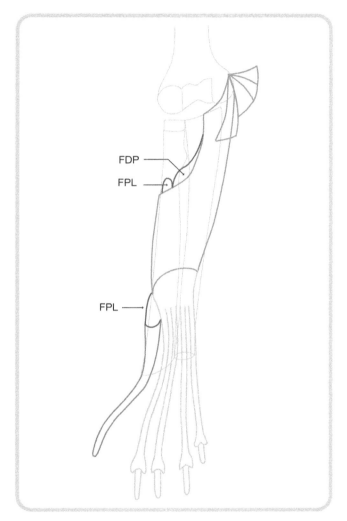

SUPERFICIAL FLEXORS OF THE FOREARM

 How to draw

STEP 1

- Copy the humerus, radius and ulna from *Deep flexors of the forearm* Step 1.
- Add **pronator teres** as a long thin triangle with its origin at the medial epicondyle and inserting onto the lateral edge of the radius. It also has an origin on the coronoid process of the ulna (not shown).

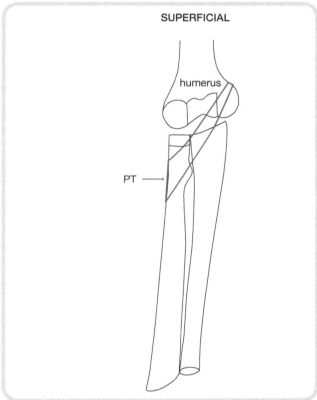

SUPERFICIAL

humerus

PT

STEP 2

- Draw the **flexor carpi radialis** (FCR), arising from the common flexor tendon at the medial epicondyle of the humerus and inserting onto the base of the 2nd and 3rd metacarpal bones.
- NOTE: 'carpi' means 'of the wrist' so flexor carpi radialis means flexor of the wrist on the radial side; it's all in the name!

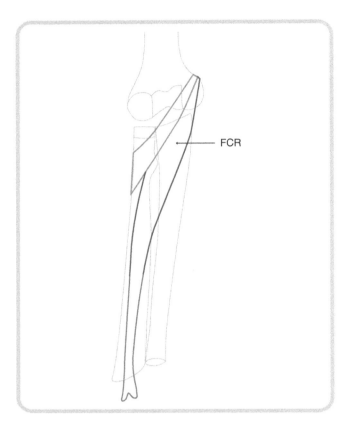

STEP 3

- Draw **palmaris longus** (PL), originating from the common flexor tendon at the medial epicondyle. It inserts onto the palmar aponeurosis and flexor retinaculum of the hand.
- Draw **flexor carpi ulnaris** (FCU) lateral to PL, arising from the common flexor tendon at the medial epicondyle and (not shown) the olecranon of ulna. It inserts onto the pisiform, part of the hamate and the 5th metacarpal bone.
- Draw a rectangle at the distal end of the palmaris longus tendon and FCU tendon. This represents the flexor retinaculum (FR) (see Box 7.3).

NOTE: PL is present in approximately 85% of the population. If you put your thumb and little finger together and flex your wrist slightly, you will see its tendon between FCR and FCU.

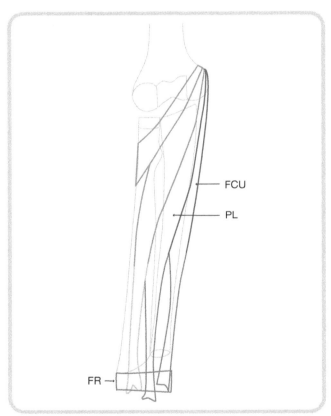

Box 7.3: The flexor retinaculum (FR)

- A fibrous band that forms a 'tunnel' for tendons to pass under.
- Attached to carpal bones on each side: scaphoid and trapezium laterally and pisiform and hamate medially.
- Partially attached to tendons of PL and FCU.

The median nerve and tendons of FCR, FPL, FDS and FDP pass under the FR. If there is swelling or inflammation within the carpal tunnel then median nerve entrapment can occur, commonly referred to as carpal tunnel syndrome. Symptoms include tingling and muscle weakness in the flexors of the hand.

7.7.3 Muscles of the posterior compartment of the forearm

Muscles of the posterior compartment of the forearm are extensors.

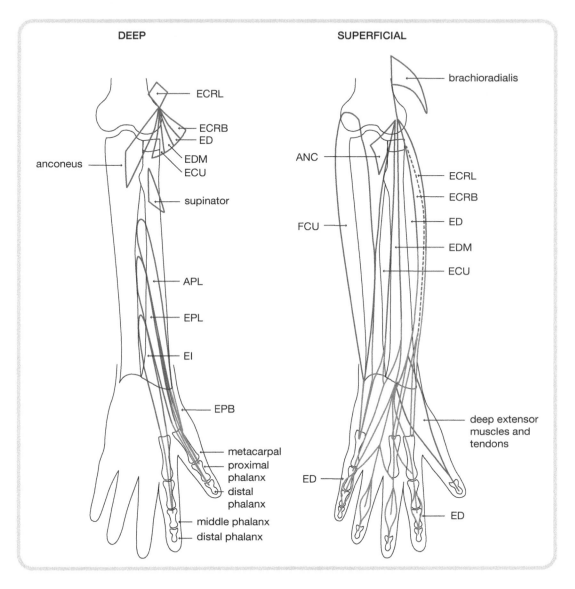

ANC	anconeus
APL	abductor pollicis longus
ECRB	extensor carpi radialis brevis
ECRL	extensor carpi radialis longus
ECU	extensor carpi ulnaris
ED	extensor digitorum
EDM	extensor digiti minimi
EI	extensor indicis
EPB	extensor pollicis brevis
EPL	extensor pollicis longus
FCU	flexor carpi ulnaris

DEEP EXTENSORS OF THE FOREARM

 How to draw

STEP 1

- Draw the mirror image of Step 1 from *Section 7.7.2: Muscles of the anterior compartment of the forearm*, to show the bones in posterior view.
- Add the outline of the hand.
- Draw in the metacarpal, proximal phalanx and distal phalanx of the thumb.
- Add the metacarpal, proximal, middle and distal phalanx of the first finger.

STEP 2

Now we will draw the **extensor indicis**, a narrow muscle from the ulna to the middle phalanx.

- Draw a line representing its origin at the posterior distal 1/3 of the ulna and from the interosseous membrane.
- Draw a long thin triangle for the muscle body, tapering it to a single line representing the tendon.
- Show the tendon inserting onto the middle phalanx of the index finger.

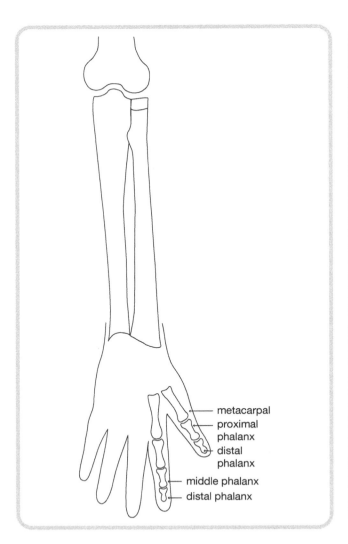

metacarpal
proximal phalanx
distal phalanx
middle phalanx
distal phalanx

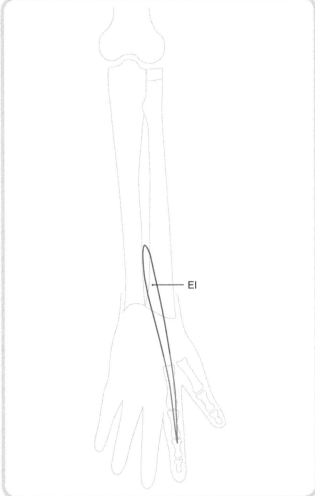

EI

STEP 3

- Draw **extensor pollicis longus** (EPL) as a similar shape to extensor indicis but originating above, from the middle 1/3 of the posterior ulna and interosseous membrane.
- Show it inserting onto the distal phalanx of the thumb.

STEP 4

- Draw the origin of **abductor pollicis longus** (APL) above EPL on the ulna, below the level of the insertion of the anconeus on the radius (see Step 5).
- Draw the rest of the muscle as a long thin triangle, as for EPL and extensor indicis. Show it inserting into the lateral side of the base of the 1st metacarpal. It also inserts onto the trapezium and the belly of the abductor pollicis brevis.
- From behind and below APL, draw a sliver of **EPB** following the same direction as APL and inserting onto the proximal end of the proximal phalanx of the thumb.

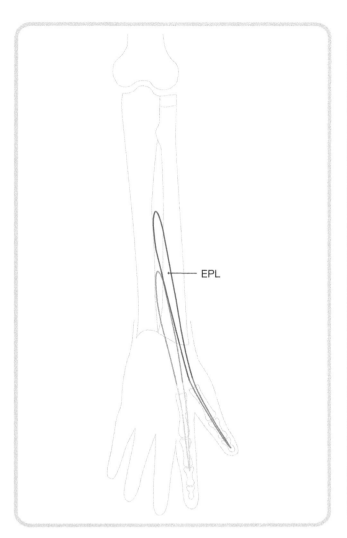

EPL

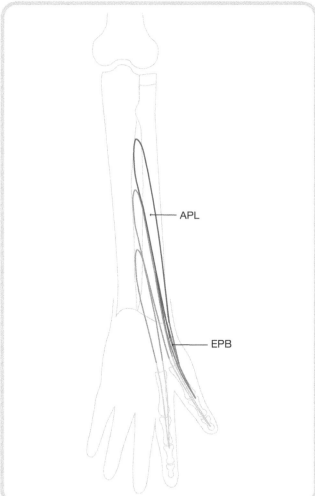

APL

EPB

STEP 5

- Draw in the **anconeus** (see Step 4 in *Section 7.7.1: Upper arm muscles*).
- Add the cut ends of 4 muscles that arise from the lateral epicondyle of the humerus: **extensor carpi radialis brevis**, **extensor digitorum**, **extensor digiti minimi** and **extensor carpi ulnaris**.
- Above these 4 muscles draw a diamond shape on the lateral side of the humerus to represent **extensor carpi radialis longus**. This originates from the lateral epicondyle of the humerus and inserts onto the posterior base of the 3rd metacarpal.
- Below the 4 muscles draw a triangle to represent **supinator** (see Step 1 in *Section 7.7.2: Muscles of the anterior compartment of the forearm*).

  How to draw

STEP 1

- Copy *Deep flexors of the forearm* Step 1 (see above): add distal phalanges for all digits, the metacarpals and proximal and middle phalanges of digits 2 and 5.
- Draw a flat-topped upright 'leaf' shape from the medial epicondyle and the olecranon process of the ulna down to insert on the base of the 5th metacarpal. This is the region of **flexor carpi ulnaris** that can be seen on posterior view (see *Superficial flexors of the forearm* Step 3).
- Draw a flat-topped leaf shape from the base of the radius to the end of the thumb to represent the deep extensor muscles shown in *Deep extensors of the forearm* Steps 2–4.

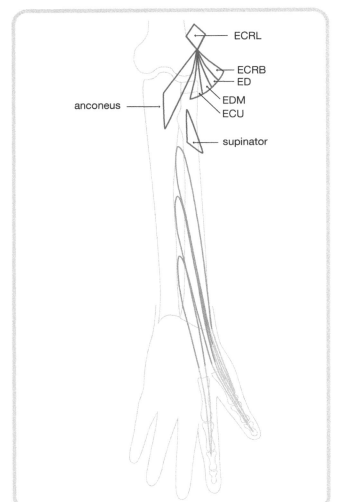

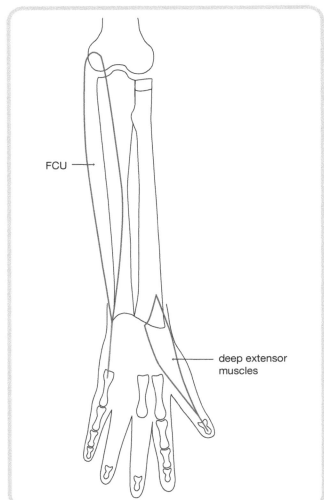

STEP 2

- Draw in **anconeus** as a triangular shape originating from the lateral epicondyle of the humerus and inserting into the olecranon process on the superior proximal part of the posterior ulna.
- Draw a curved triangular muscle shape from an origin on the humerus heading anteriorly around the forearm; this is the **brachioradialis**.

STEP 3

- Draw 3 muscles as narrow leaf shapes from the lateral epicondyle to the hand.
- Draw the tendon of **extensor carpi ulnaris** (ECU) inserting onto the base of the 5th metacarpal.
- Draw the tendon of **extensor digiti minimi** (EDM) inserting onto the base of the 5th proximal phalanx.
- For **extensor digitorum**, draw 4 tendons, each inserting onto the proximal phalanx (not shown), with a central part inserting onto the base of the middle phalanx and 2 collateral parts passing along the sides of the middle phalanx to insert onto the distal phalanx.
- Add 3 curved lines to represent juncturae tendinum, tendon-like connective tissue that aligns and stabilise the metacarpophalangeal joint during extension.
- Extensor indicis (see *Deep flexors of the forearm* Step 2) lies underneath the insertion of extensor digitorum on the ulnar side of the index finger.

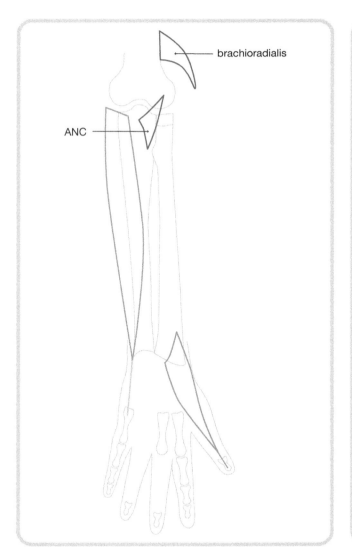

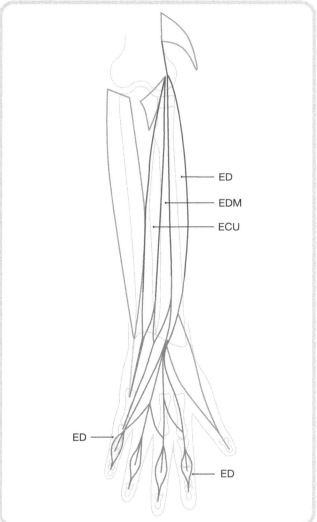

STEP **4**

Draw in 2 thin muscles just lateral to extensor digitorum, both originating from the common extensor tendon from the lateral epicondyle:

- Draw in the **extensor carpi radialis brevis** (ECRB) inserting onto the base of the 3rd metacarpal.
- Draw **extensor carpi radialis longus** (ECRL) inserting onto the base of the 2nd metacarpal.
- Both become tendons early on in the forearm, ECRL first and then ECRB.

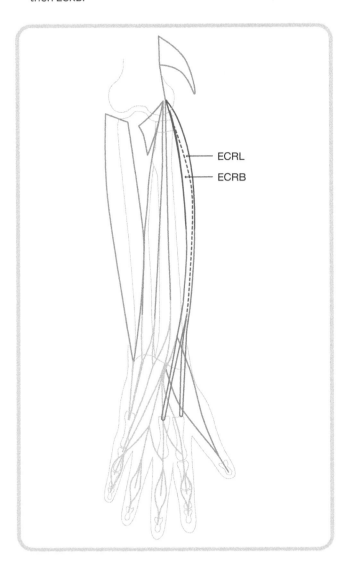

ECRL

ECRB

Intrinsic muscles of the hand

Intrinsic muscles are located entirely within the hand, as their name suggests. The origins of the intrinsic muscles are listed in Table 7.1; their insertions are shown in the images. Arteries and nerves supplying these muscles are listed in Table 7.2 and shown in *Section 7.1: Blood vessels* and *Section 7.5: Wrist*.

The intrinsic muscles produce finger and thumb movements. They are not the only muscles doing this; most forearm muscles do too, as extrinsic muscles of the hand (see Table 7.2 and *Sections 7.7.2* and *7.7.3*).

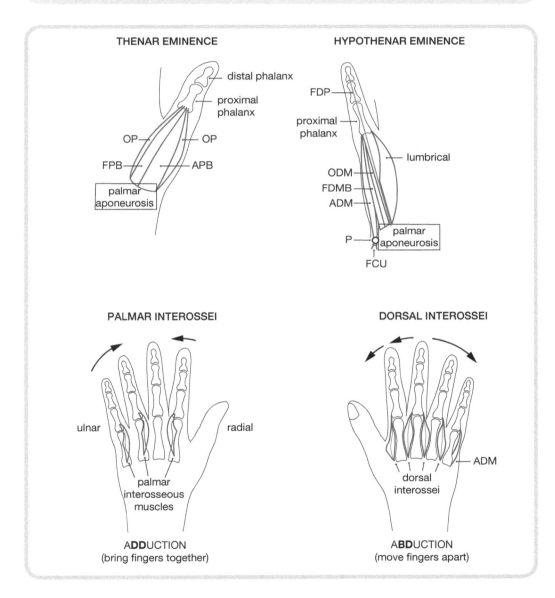

ADM	abductor digiti minimi	**FDMB**	flexor digiti minimi brevis	**ODM**	opponens digiti minimi
APB	abductor pollicis brevis	**FDP**	flexor digitorum profundus	**OP**	opponens pollicis
FCU	flexor carpi ulnaris	**FPB**	flexor pollicis brevis	**P**	pisiform bone

Table 7.1. Origins of intrinsic muscles of the hand

Muscle group	Muscle	Origins
Thenar	Opponens pollicis	Tubercle of trapezium, flexor retinaculum
	Abductor pollicis brevis	Scaphoid, flexor retinaculum, tubercle of trapezium
	Flexor pollicis brevis	Superficial head: flexor retinaculum, tubercle of trapezium bone Deep head: trapezoid and capitate bones
Hypothenar	Opponens digiti minimi	Hook of hamate, flexor retinaculum
	Flexor digiti minimi brevis	
	Abductor digiti minimi	Pisiform, pisohamate ligament, FCU tendon
Lumbricals	Lumbricals	FDP tendons
Interossei	Dorsal Palmar	Metacarpals (see steps for more details of origins)

THENAR EMINENCE

Thenar is a Greek word, meaning palmar.

The ulnar nerve innervates most intrinsic muscles of the hand, excluding opponens pollicis, abductor pollicis brevis and the 2 lateral lumbrical muscles. The median nerve innervates 4 muscles. You can remember this using the mnemonic LOAF or FOAL:

F: flexor pollicis brevis
O: opponens pollicis
A: abductor pollicis brevis
L: lateral 2 lumbricals.

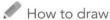 How to draw

 STEP **1**

- Draw the outline of the right thumb and palm.
- Draw the proximal and distal phalanx of the thumb.

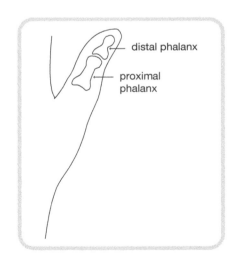

distal phalanx

proximal phalanx

STEP 2

- In brown, draw a 'flat-bottomed leaf' shape to insert on the base of the proximal phalanx of thumb.
- Divide this into 4. The outer 2 parts are 1 muscle, **opponens pollicis**. This lies deep to the **flexor pollicis brevis** and **abductor pollicis brevis**.

NOTE: FPB is innervated by the median nerve in 1/3 of people, ulnar nerve in 1/2 and both nerves in the rest of the population.

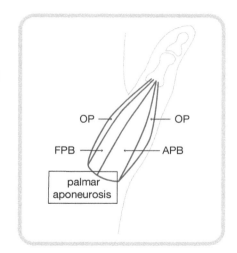

HYPOTHENAR EMINENCE

 How to draw

STEP 1

- Draw the outline of the little finger of the right hand and its 3 phalanges.
- Draw a small circle at the lower edge of the hand to represent the pisiform bone.
- Draw a small segment of a tendon attaching proximal to the circle; this is **flexor carpi ulnaris**.

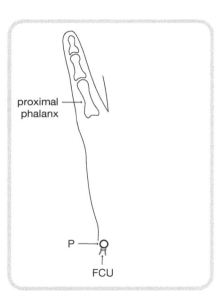

STEP 2

- Draw a grey line along the finger and inserting onto the base of the distal phalanx. This is the tendon of **flexor digitorum profundus** (FDP).

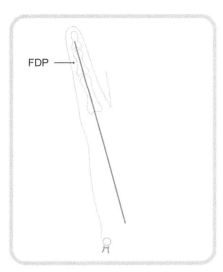

STEP 3

- Draw a curved triangle from an origin on the FDP tendon to insert on the medial side of the base of the proximal phalanx. This is a **lumbrical muscle**.

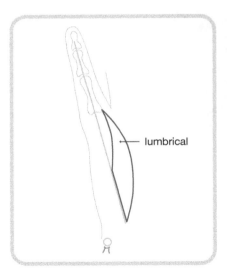

lumbrical

STEP 4

- Draw a rectangle across the palm of the hand to represent the palmar aponeurosis. Then draw a narrow triangle lateral to the FDP tendon and divide it into 2. The medial side is the **opponens digiti minimi** (ODM), the lateral side is the **flexor digiti minimi brevis** (FDMB).
- Draw a narrow 'leaf' shape from an origin on the pisiform to insert onto the lateral base of the proximal phalanx; this is the **abductor digiti minimi**.
- ODM and FDMB arise from the hamate as well as the flexor retinaculum.

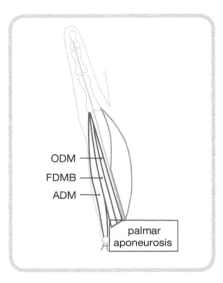

ODM

FDMB

ADM

palmar aponeurosis

PALMAR INTEROSSEOUS MUSCLES

The 3 **palmar interossei** help ADDuct the fingers, i.e. bring the fingers together.

How to draw

STEP 1

- Draw the outline of the palmar side of the right hand.
- Draw metacarpals (remember that these are numbered starting from the thumb) and phalanges for the 4 fingers.

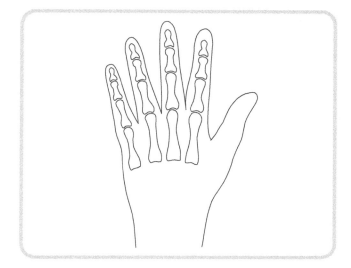

STEP 2

Draw 3 **palmar interosseous** muscles, each originating on a metacarpal (MC) and inserting onto the base of the corresponding proximal phalanx, as follows.

- The 1st from the ulnar side of the 2nd MC to the ulnar side of its proximal phalanx.
- The 2nd from the radial side of the 4th MC to the radial side of its proximal phalanx.
- The 3rd from the radial side of the 5th MC to the radial side of its proximal phalanx.

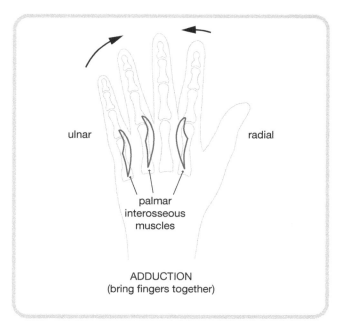

ulnar

radial

palmar
interosseous
muscles

ADDUCTION
(bring fingers together)

DORSAL INTEROSSEOUS MUSCLES

These muscles help ABDuct the fingers, i.e. separate them.

 How to draw

STEP 1

- Draw the outline of the back of the hand (dorsum).
- Draw the 4 metacarpals and phalanges for the 4 fingers.

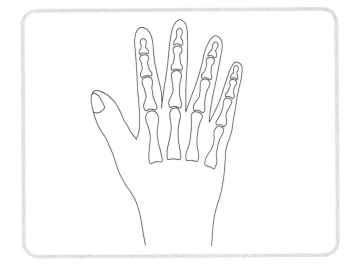

STEP 2

- Draw the **abductor digiti minimi** (ADM) on the lateral side of the little finger.
- Draw 4 **dorsal interosseous** muscles. They are bipennate (muscle fibres on each side of a central tendon). They originate from the adjacent MCs and insert into the base of the proximal phalanges, as shown, and extensor expansions. The middle finger has 2 dorsal interossei inserted on it, whereas the thumb and little finger have none.

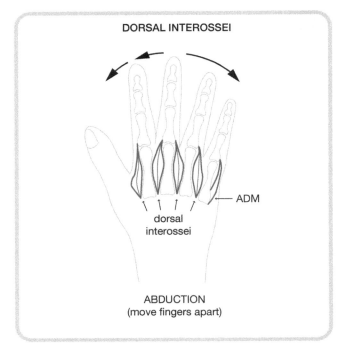

DORSAL INTEROSSEI

ADM

dorsal interossei

ABDUCTION
(move fingers apart)

7.7.5 Upper limb muscles (Table 7.2)

Table 7.2. Muscles of the upper limb

Area	Muscle group	Muscle	Nerve	Artery	Action
Shoulder		Deltoid	Axillary	Anterior and posterior circumflex, thoracoacromial	Abduction, flexion and extension of arm; medial and lateral rotation of arm
		Teres major	Lower subscapular	Subscapular and circumflex scapular	Adduction and internal rotation of arm
	Rotator cuff	Supraspinatus	Suprascapular	Suprascapular	Abduction of arm
		Infraspinatus	Suprascapular	Suprascapular and circumflex scapular	Lateral rotation of arm
		Teres minor	Axillary	Posterior circumflex humeral and circumflex scapular	Lateral rotation of arm
		Subscapularis	Upper and lower subscapular nerves	Subscapular	Adduction and medial rotation of arm
Arm	Anterior	Coracobrachialis	Musculocutaneous	Brachial	Flexion of shoulder, adduction of arm
		Biceps brachii	Musculocutaneous	Brachial	Flexion of forearm and shoulder; supination of forearm
		Brachialis	Musculocutaneous, radial	Brachial and radial recurrent	Flexion of forearm
	Posterior	Triceps brachii	Radial	Profunda brachii (and posterior humeral circumflex for long head)	Extension of forearm, adduction of shoulder
		Anconeus	Radial	Profunda brachii	Extension of forearm; stabilises elbow joint during pronation and supination
Forearm	Anterior	Pronator teres	Median	Ulnar and radial	Pronation and flexion of forearm
		Flexor carpi radialis	Median	Ulnar and radial	Abduction and flexion of hand
		Palmaris longus	Median	Ulnar	Flexion of hand and palmar aponeurosis

(continued)

Table 7.2. Muscles of the upper limb *(continued)*

Area	Muscle group	Muscle	Nerve	Artery	Action
Forearm *(continued)*		Flexor carpi ulnaris	Ulnar	Ulnar	Flexion and adduction of hand
		Flexor digitorum profundus	Digits 2 and 3: anterior interosseus (median) Digits 4 and 5: ulnar	Anterior interosseous	Flexion of hand
		Flexor digitorum superficialis	Median	Ulnar	Flexion of fingers at middle phalanx, flexion of proximal phalanges, flexes hand at wrist and flexes at MCP joints
		Flexor pollicis longus	Anterior interosseous (median)	Anterior interosseous	Flexion of distal phalanx of thumb
		Pronator quadratus	Anterior interosseus (median)	Anterior interosseous	Pronation of forearm
	Posterior	Extensor digitorum	Posterior interosseous (radial)	Posterior interosseus	Extension of hand and fingers, separation of fingers, extension of forearm
		Extensor digiti minimi	Posterior interosseous (radial)	Posterior interosseous	Extension and adduction of little finger
		Extensor carpi ulnaris	Posterior interosseous (radial)	Ulnar	Extension and adduction of hand
		Brachioradialis	Radial	Radial	Flexion of forearm; helps with pronation and supination of forearm
		Extensor carpi radialis longus	Radial	Radial	Extension of hand and abduction of hand at wrist
		Extensor carpi radialis brevis	Posterior interosseous (radial)	Radial	Extension of hand and abduction of hand at wrist
		Supinator	Posterior interosseous (radial)	Radial recurrent	Supination of forearm
		Extensor indicis	Posterior interosseous (radial)	Posterior interosseous	Extension of index finger and hand
		Abductor pollicis longus	Posterior interosseous (radial)	Posterior interosseous	Abduction and extension of thumb
		Extensor pollicis brevis	Posterior interosseous (radial)	Posterior interosseous	Extension and abduction of thumb
		Extensor pollicis longus	Posterior interosseous (radial)	Posterior interosseous	Extension of thumb

(continued)

Table 7.2. Muscles of the upper limb *(continued)*

Area	Muscle group	Muscle	Nerve	Artery	Action
Hand	Thenar eminence	Opponens pollicis	Recurrent branch of median	Superficial palmar arch	Opposition of thumb with fingers
		Flexor pollicis brevis	Superficial head: recurrent branch of median Deep head: ulnar	Superficial palmar arch	Flexion of thumb at first metacarpophalangeal joint
		Abductor pollicis brevis	Recurrent branch of median	Superficial palmar arch	Abduction of thumb
		Adductor pollicis	Ulnar	Deep palmar arch	Adduction of thumb
		Palmaris brevis	Ulnar	Palmar metacarpal	Wrinkles skin of palm!
	Hypothenar eminence	Abductor digiti minimi	Ulnar	Ulnar	Abduction of little finger
		Flexor digiti minimi brevis	Ulnar	Ulnar	Flexion of little finger
		Opponens digiti minimi	Ulnar	Ulnar	Opposition of little finger with thumb
	Other intrinsic muscles of the hand	Lumbricals	First and second: median Third and fourth: ulnar	Superficial palmar arch and deep palmar arch	flexion of metacarpophalangeal joints, extension of interphalangeal joints
		Dorsal interossei	Ulnar	Dorsal and palmar metacarpal	Abduction of fingers
		Palmar interossei	Ulnar	Palmar metacarpal artery of the deep palmar arch	Adduction of fingers

Chapter 8

Lower limb

This is more complicated than the arm. I have included the main branches of arteries and veins.

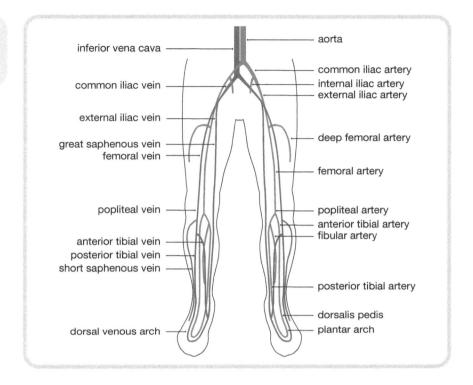

ARTERIES

You can learn the upper half of this diagram in *Section 5.6: Abdominal aorta.*

- The external iliac artery becomes the femoral artery behind the inguinal ligament.
- The femoral artery gives off a branch of the deep femoral artery and continues into the thigh as the femoral artery.
- The femoral artery then becomes the popliteal artery.
- It then divides into the anterior tibial artery (becomes the dorsalis pedis) and the posterior tibial artery; these join in the foot to form the plantar arch.
- The fibular artery is a branch of the posterior tibial artery.

VEINS

The veins are more complicated.

- The veins start in the foot as a dorsal venous arch; this drains into the posterior tibial vein, the anterior tibial vein, and the short and the great saphenous vein.
- The posterior and anterior tibial veins drain into the popliteal vein.
- The popliteal vein becomes the femoral vein; the great saphenous vein drains into the femoral vein.
- The femoral vein becomes the external iliac vein and then this becomes the common iliac vein.
- The common iliac veins join to form the inferior vena cava.

Lumbosacral plexus

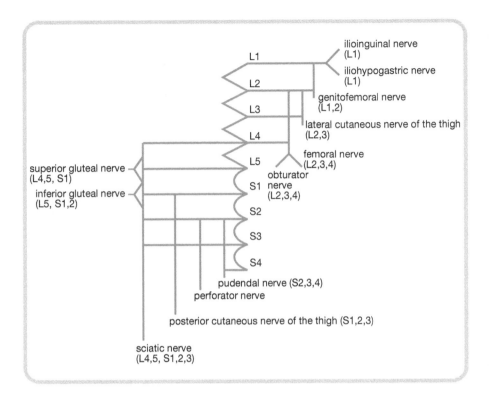

iliohypogastric nerve (L1)
ilioinguinal nerve (L1)
genitofemoral nerve (L1,2)
lateral cutaneous nerve of the thigh (L2,3)
femoral nerve (L2,3,4)
obturator nerve (L2,3,4)
L1
L2
L3
L4
L5
S1
S2
S3
S4
superior gluteal nerve (L4,5, S1)
inferior gluteal nerve (L5, S1,2)
pudendal nerve (S2,3,4)
perforator nerve
posterior cutaneous nerve of the thigh (S1,2,3)
sciatic nerve (L4,5, S1,2,3)

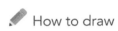 How to draw

STEP 1

- Draw 4 arrowheads pointing left and 4 semicircles pointing left below the arrowheads; label the nerve roots as shown.

STEP 2

- Add in the sciatic nerve.
- This has roots L4, 5 and S1, 2 and 3; join them together to form the sciatic nerve.
- Add in the superior gluteal nerve between roots L5, S1 and S2 and the inferior gluteal nerve between roots S2 and 3.

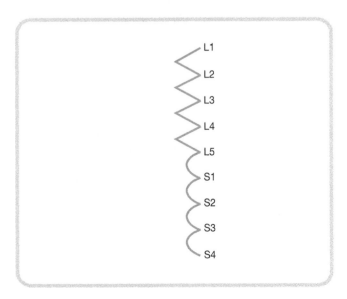

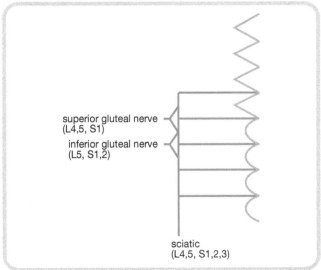

STEP 3

Add in 3 lines:

- One from S1, 2 and 3 – this is the posterior cutaneous nerve.
- One from roots S2 and 3 – this is the perforator nerve.
- One from S2, 3 and 4 should join to make the pudendal nerve.

 STEP 4

Add the lumbar part of the lumbosacral plexus.

- Add one line from L1 which splits into two: the ilioinguinal nerve and the iliohypogastric nerve.
- Add a second line from L2 and join it to L1, to form the genitofemoral nerve.
- Add another line from L3 and join this to L2, to form the lateral cutaneous nerve of the thigh.
- Draw another line from L4, join it to L2 and 3, split it in two and these will be the obturator nerve and femoral nerve.

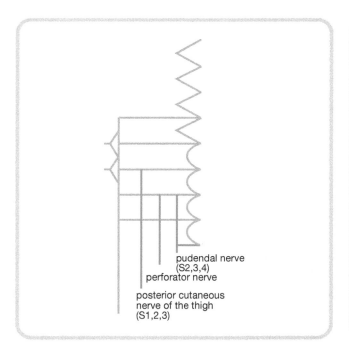

pudendal nerve
(S2,3,4)
perforator nerve

posterior cutaneous
nerve of the thigh
(S1,2,3)

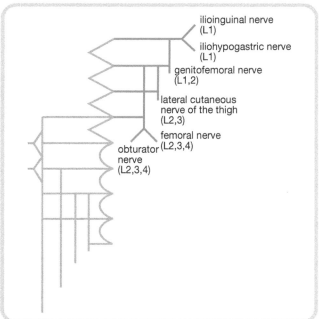

ilioinguinal nerve
(L1)

iliohypogastric nerve
(L1)

genitofemoral nerve
(L1,2)

lateral cutaneous
nerve of the thigh
(L2,3)

femoral nerve
(L2,3,4)

obturator
nerve
(L2,3,4)

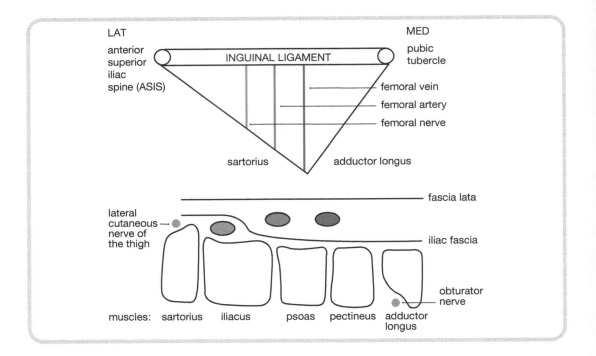

This image is to aid memory of the femoral canal. The femoral artery is actually palpated at the mid inguinal point not the middle of the inguinal ligament.

The two images look at the right femoral canal in a schematic way. The upper image is an anterior view and the lower image is a transverse view. Some people remember the order of the nerve, artery and vein using the word NAVY, where Y is for Y front! The Y is always medial, so if you consider the left side it is NAVY backwards.

How to draw the anterior view

STEP 1

- Draw a down-facing triangle under a horizontal rectangle with two circles at the ends to represent the inguinal ligament.
- The medial end is the pubic tubercle, the lateral end is the anterior superior iliac spine (ASIS).
- The borders below are, medially, the adductor longus muscle and, laterally, the sartorius muscle.

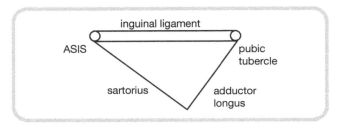

STEP 2

- Draw a blue line on the medial side from the inguinal ligament to the lower border. This represents the femoral vein.

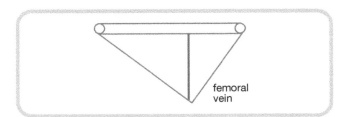

STEP 3

- Draw a red line down from the middle of the inguinal ligament. This represents the femoral artery.

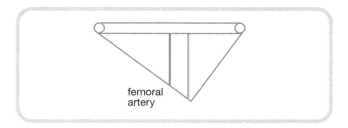

femoral artery

STEP 4

- Draw a green line on the lateral side from the inguinal ligament to the lower border. This represents the femoral nerve.

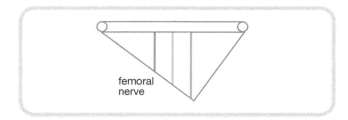

femoral nerve

 How to draw the transverse view

STEP 1

- Draw one horizontal line from left to right. Draw a second one below this, narrow at the lateral side and then wider at the medial side (as shown).
- The upper line is the fascia lata and the lower line is the iliac fascia.

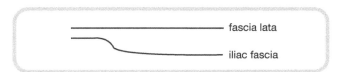

fascia lata

iliac fascia

STEP 2

- Draw 5 square (ish) shapes below these two lines, as shown. These represent the muscles that lie under/around the femoral triangle.
- The muscles can be remembered with the word 'SIPsPA'; not a real word, but it helped me! From lateral to medial: **s**artorius, **i**liacus, **ps**oas, **p**ectineus and **a**dductor longus.

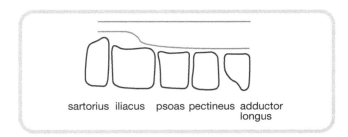

sartorius iliacus psoas pectineus adductor longus

STEP 3

- With a green pen add in the lateral cutaneous nerve of the thigh, lateral and superior to the sartorius muscle.
- Draw the femoral nerve superior to the iliacus.
- Draw the obturator nerve just below and lateral to the adductor longus muscle.

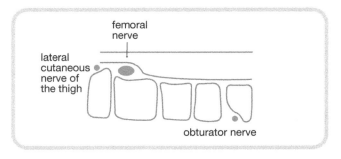

femoral nerve

lateral cutaneous nerve of the thigh

obturator nerve

STEP 4

- Draw in the femoral artery and the femoral vein (medially), between the fascia lata and iliac fascia.

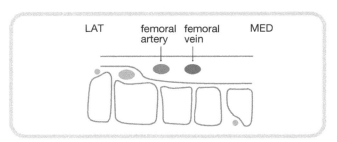

LAT   femoral   femoral   MED
         artery   vein

My memory prompt for the popliteal fossa is 'the diamond', due to the shape of the area.

Note: the order of structures from deep to superficial is: artery, vein then nerve

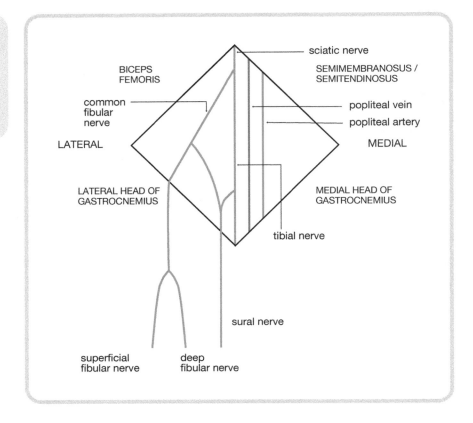

How to draw

STEP 1

- Draw a diamond shape as shown.
- Label the borders: superiolateral is biceps femoris, superiomedial is semimembranosus and semitendinosus, inferolateral is lateral head of gastrocnemius and inferomedial is the medial head of gastrocnemius.

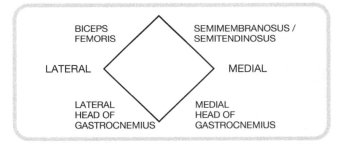

STEP 2

- Draw a straight red line down, off centre, to represent the popliteal artery (continuation of the femoral artery). The popliteal artery is the deepest structure in this image – an important aspect that may not necessarily be appreciated with a simple 2D drawing.

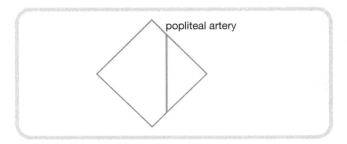

STEP 3

- Draw a straight blue line lateral to the popliteal artery to represent the popliteal vein. Although they are drawn next to each other, the vein is normally more superficial. The artery is deep to the vein and the nerves are often superficial to both.
- Draw a green line down from upper point to lower point. The top part is the sciatic nerve. This continues distally to become the tibial nerve medially and the common fibular nerve that runs laterally.

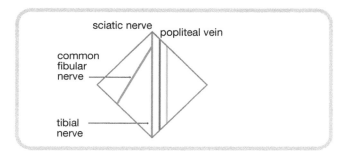

STEP 4

- Draw in the sural nerve. This can be formed from both the tibial nerve and the common fibular nerve.
- Add in the superficial and deep fibular nerves.

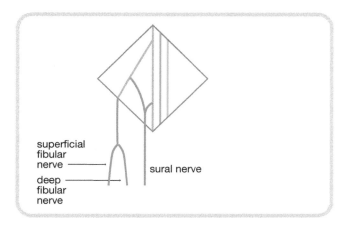

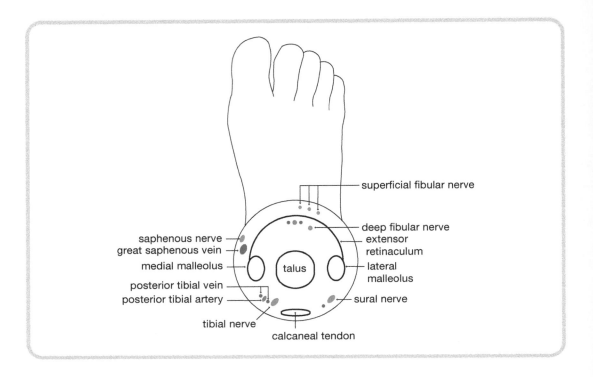

This diagram indicates where the 5 nerves to the ankle are located and shows a cross-section from the heel to the forefoot.

I always think it looks like a person wearing headphones.

✏️ How to draw

STEP 1

- Draw a large circle with a smaller circle in the middle – this central circle is the talus bone.
- Draw an oval on each side of the talus and join them with a semicircular line – these are the malleoli joined by the extensor retinaculum.
- Draw an oval at the base of the circle to represent the calcaneal tendon (or Achilles tendon).

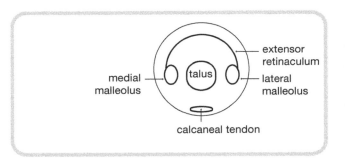

STEP 2

- Draw a blue dot and a green dot anterior to the medial malleolus – these represent the great saphenous vein (blue dot) and the saphenous nerve (green dot).

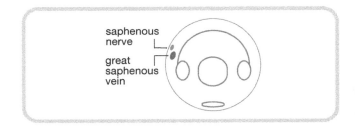

STEP 3

- Above the extensor retinaculum draw a few green dots to represent the superficial fibular nerves.
- Below the extensor retinaculum draw one red dot (dorsalis pedis artery), with 2 blue dots (dorsalis pedis veins) and a green dot (deep fibular nerve) laterally.

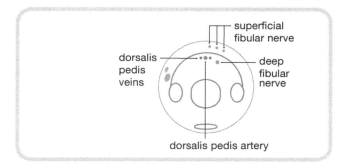

STEP 4

- Draw the sural nerve (green dot) and the small saphenous vein (blue dot) just posterior to the lateral malleolus and anterior to the calcaneal tendon.

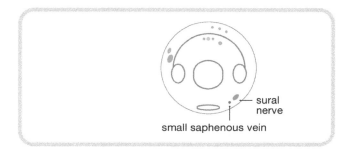

STEP 5

- Draw the posterior tibial artery (red dot), posterior tibial vein (blue dot) and tibial nerve (green dot), just posterior to the medial malleolus and anterior to the calcaneal tendon. Note that the tibial nerve is sometimes referred to as the posterior tibial nerve; however, this is not the correct name (possibly an error because the tibial vein and artery nearby have posterior as part of their names).

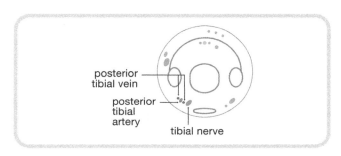

STEP 6

- Remember that the saphenous nerve is a branch of the femoral nerve, but the other 4 nerves are branches of the sciatic nerve (see *Section 8.4: Popliteal fossa*).

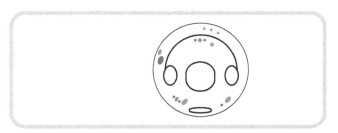

8.6 Bones of the lower limb

8.6.1 Femur

The femur is the longest and largest bone in the body. The head and neck of the femur are at an angle of 120–150°. The neck–shaft angle steadily decreases from 150° after birth to 125° in an adult and can reach values of below 120° in the elderly. The neck of the femur is 4–5 cm long. The length of the shaft is approximately 25% of a person's height.

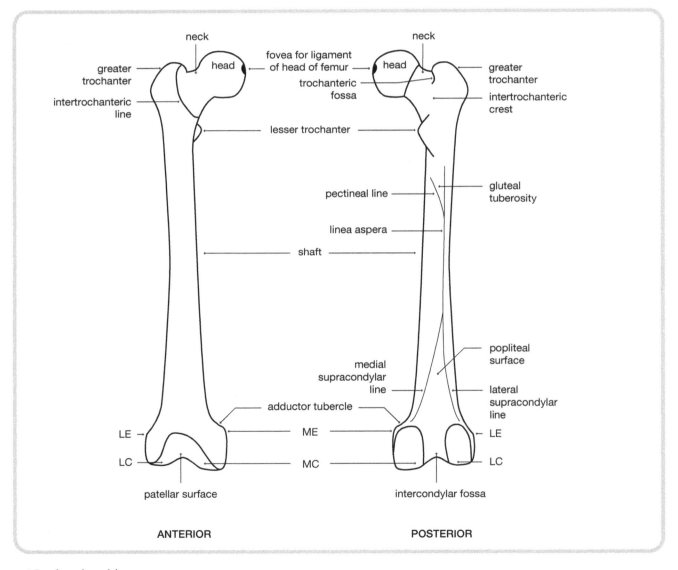

LC   lateral condyle
LE   lateral epicondyle
MC   medial condyle
ME   medial epicondyle

ANTERIOR VIEW

 How to draw

STEP 1

Start by drawing the outline of the femur.

- Draw a slightly curved line horizontally where the knee joint would be, then draw vertical lines upwards for a few centimetres. From here bring the 2 sides towards each other and draw directly upwards to represent the shaft of the bone.
- At the top, draw a protrusion on the lateral side and then a neck which joins to two-thirds of a circle representing the head of the femur. Join the lower side of the head to the medial side of the shaft.
- Label the greater trochanter as the protrusion on the lateral side, the neck medial to this and the head at the proximal end.
- Label the lateral and medial epicondyles distally.

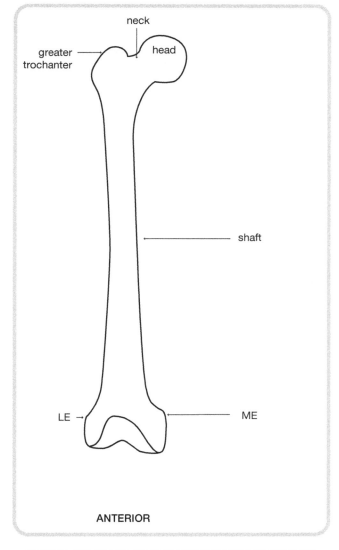

ANTERIOR

STEP 2

- Draw a black dot in the centre of the femoral head; this is the fovea for the ligament of the head of the femur.
- Draw a semicircle on the medial side just below the neck; this is the lesser trochanter.
- Draw an additional semicircle from the top of the lesser trochanter to the top of the greater trochanter.

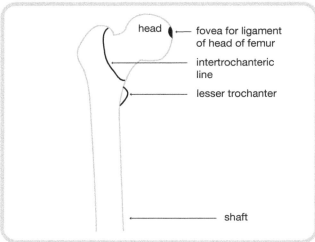

STEP 3

- Draw a semicircle between the medial and lateral epicondyle. The area within the line is the patellar surface, which articulates with the patella. At the sides, the areas under the line are continuations of the medial and lateral condyle (see *Posterior view* Step 3).
- The adductor tubercle is located superior to the medial epicondyle.

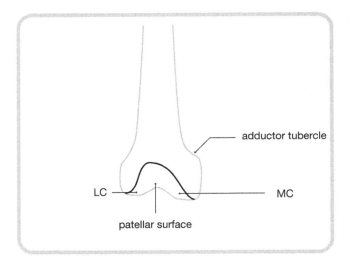

POSTERIOR VIEW

 How to draw

STEP 1

- Draw the mirror image of *Anterior view* Step 1 and label the head, neck, greater trochanter and shaft.
- Draw a slight 'lump' just inferior to the neck; this is the lesser trochanter.

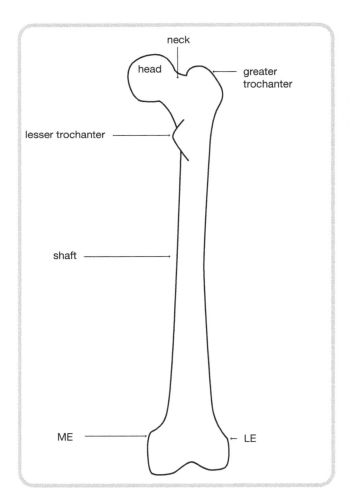

STEP 2

- Draw a line at the proximal end of the neck to delineate the head and neck. Draw a dot in the middle of the head for the fovea.
- Draw a line down from the protrusion of the greater trochanter and label the dip anterior to the greater trochanter as the trochanteric fossa.
- Draw a curved line below the trochanteric fossa to represent the lesser trochanter. The intertrochanteric crest lies between the greater and lesser trochanters.

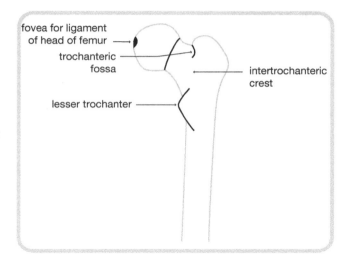

STEP 3

- Draw 2 inverted U shapes on the distal end of the femur; these are the medial and lateral condyles.
- Label the intercondylar fossa between them (attachment for several ligaments; helps stabilise the knee joint).

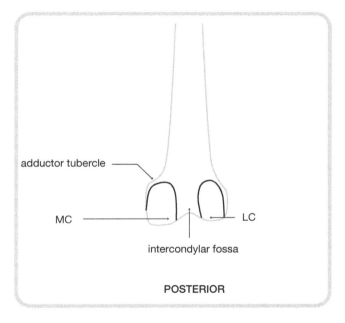

STEP 4

- Draw a line down the lateral edge of the shaft of the femur; this is the lateral supracondylar line (LSL). Draw a short line from just below the lesser trochanter laterally to join this line; this is the pectineal line, and the linea aspera continues distally.
- Draw a line from just lateral to the medial epicondyle to join the LSL; this is the medial supracondylar line (MSL).
- The gluteal tuberosity lies between the linea aspera and the LSL. The popliteal surface lies between the LSL and the MSL.

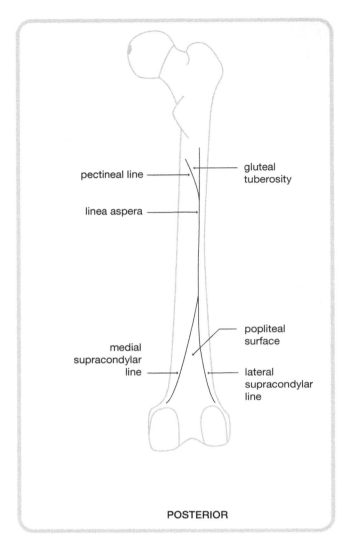

pectineal line

gluteal tuberosity

linea aspera

popliteal surface

medial supracondylar line

lateral supracondylar line

POSTERIOR

8.6.2   Tibia, fibula and patella

The tibia, femur and patella make up the knee joint. The fibula, tibia and talus bone form the hinged synovial ankle joint.

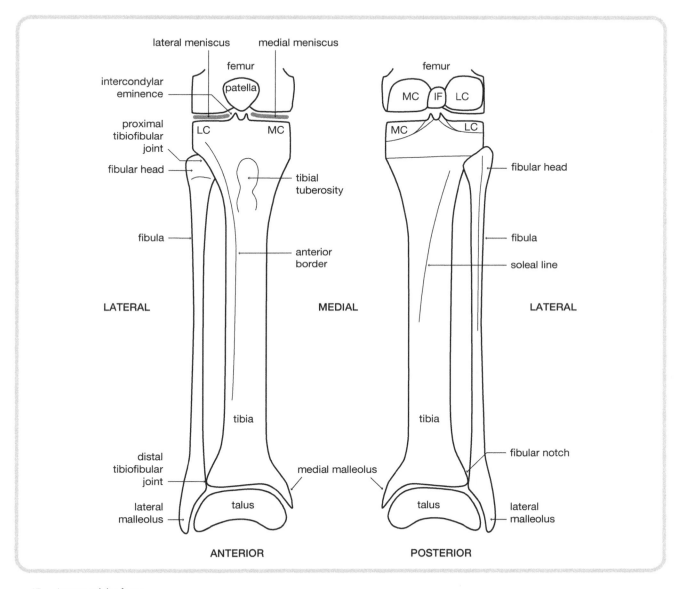

IF   intercondylar fossa
LC   lateral condyle
MC   medial condyle

ANTERIOR VIEW

 How to draw

STEP 1

- Draw a line across the top of the page with 2 little bumps in the middle. The 2 little bumps are the intercondylar tubercles of the intercondylar eminences.
- Draw a vertical line down at each end, gradually bringing them closer to form the shaft. Continue this down the page. At the bottom make the shape widen and draw a longer part on the medial side; this is the medial malleolus.
- Label the lateral and medial condyles.

STEP 2

- Draw a line down the lateral side of the shaft from the lateral condyle; this is the anterior border.
- Draw a 'monkey nut' without a bottom in the midline towards to the top of the tibia; this is the tibial tuberosity.

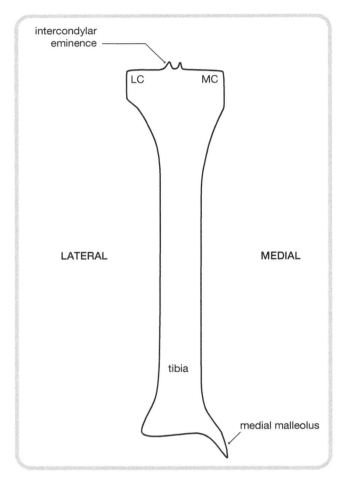

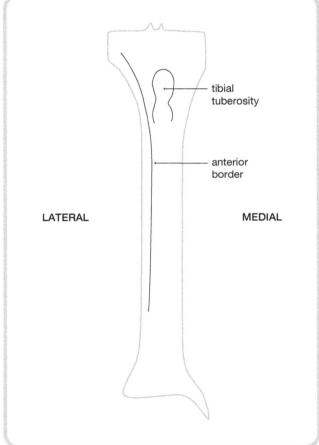

STEP 3

- Draw a narrow bone, the fibula, from just below the lateral condyle of the tibia to the lateral edge of the distal tibia. Make the medial side a similar length to the lateral side of the tibia. Then extend the lateral side further down as shown; this is the lateral malleolus.
- Label the distal tibiofibular joint, where the tibia and fibula touch.
- Label the proximal tibiofibular joint. Note that the fibula does not articulate with the femur or patella.
- Draw a line horizontally near the top of the fibula to show the fibular head.

STEP 4

- Draw the distal femur, with the patella in place above the 2 intercondylar tubercles.
- Draw the talus distally as shown.
- Draw the lateral and medial menisci in grey; these are fibrocartilaginous crescent-shaped structures that are located between the femur and tibia to provide stability and play a role in shock absorption.

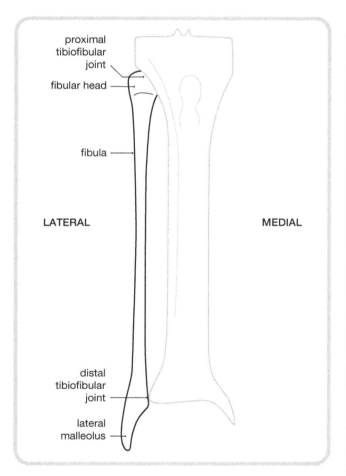

proximal tibiofibular joint

fibular head

fibula

LATERAL

MEDIAL

distal tibiofibular joint

lateral malleolus

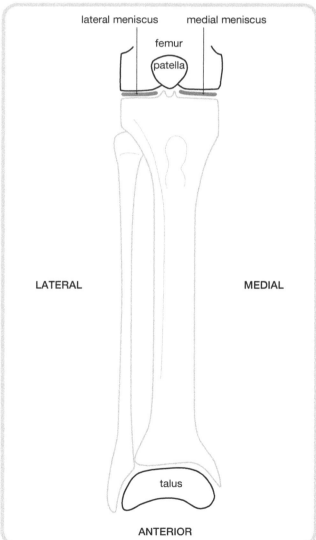

lateral meniscus

medial meniscus

femur

patella

LATERAL

MEDIAL

talus

ANTERIOR

POSTERIOR VIEW

 How to draw

STEP 1

- Draw a mirror image of the tibia from *Anterior view* Step 1 as shown, omitting a small area on the lateral condyle.

STEP 2

- Draw in the posterior view of the fibula (the mirror image of *Anterior view* Step 3).
- Draw a line from near the top along the lateral edge as shown; lateral to this is the lateral surface, medial to this is the posterior surface. The line represents a ridge along the posterior surface of the bone.
- Label the fibular notch on the lateral edge of the distal tibia.

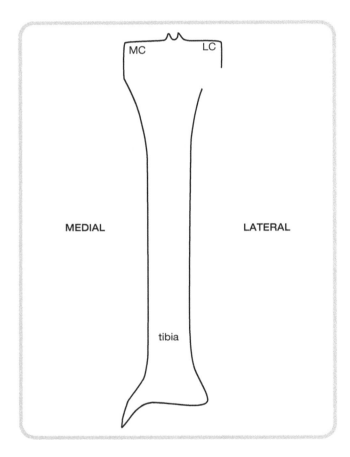

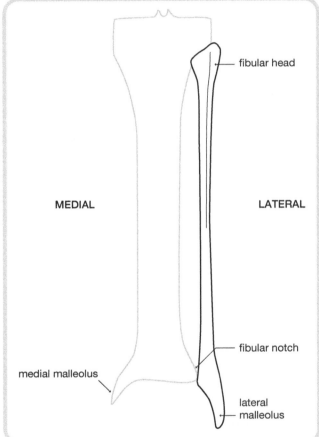

STEP 3

- Draw a line horizontally across the top of the tibia, just before the bone narrows. Draw a curved line on each side from the intertubercular tubercles to the edge of each side; the areas above these lines are the medial and lateral condyles.
- Draw a diagonal line from the upper lateral edge to the medial side, in the middle of the shaft. This is the soleal line.
- Draw the talus, one of the bones of the foot.

STEP 4

- Draw a copy of the posterior distal femur from *Section 8.6.1: Femur*.
- Label the medial and lateral condyles, the intercondylar fossa and the femur.

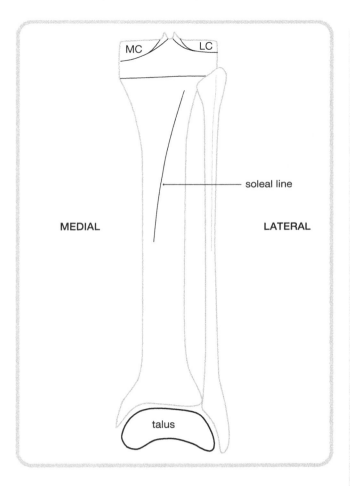

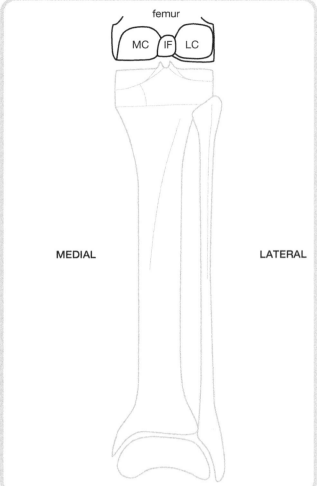

8.6.3 Bones of the foot

The ankle joint is formed where the distal ends of the tibia and fibula together form a deep socket (sometimes referred to as a mortise or malleolar mortise); they then articulate with the talus bone in the talocrural joint. It is a hinge-type joint that only permits flexion and extension.

The foot is described in 3 areas, hindfoot (calcaneus and talus), midfoot (navicular, cuboid and cuneiforms) and forefoot (metatarsals and phalanges). We will draw very simplified (schematic) dorsal, plantar, lateral and medial views.

C   cuneiform
      C1 medial (1st) cuneiform
      C2 intermediate (2nd) cuneiform
      C3 lateral (3rd) cuneiform
MT   metatarsal
MTP   metatarsophalangeal joint

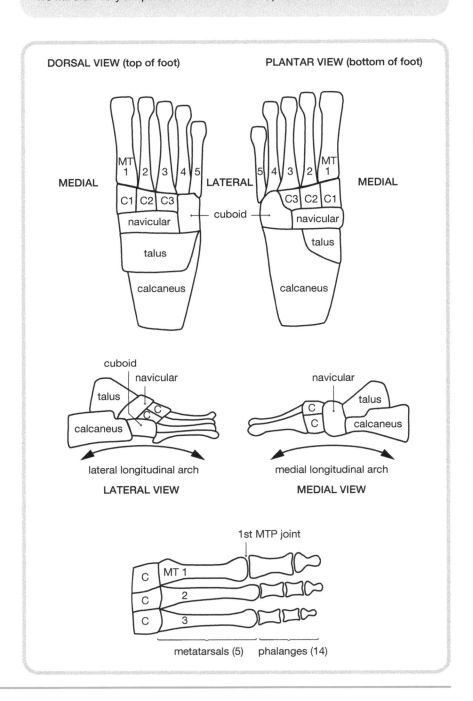

DORSAL VIEW (top of foot)

PLANTAR VIEW (bottom of foot)

MEDIAL

LATERAL

MEDIAL

LATERAL VIEW

MEDIAL VIEW

lateral longitudinal arch

medial longitudinal arch

metatarsals (5)   phalanges (14)

1st MTP joint

DORSAL VIEW

 How to draw

STEP 1

- Draw a 'bucket' shape on the page; this is the calcaneus.
- Anterior to the calcaneus draw an upside-down trapezoid shape. This is the talus.

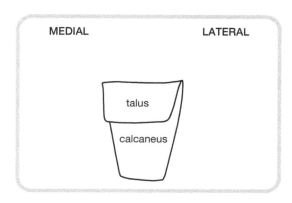

STEP 2

- Draw a rectangle from the medial side to two-thirds of the way across to the lateral side, in front of the talus. This is the navicular.
- Draw a 2nd rectangle at right angles to this on the lateral side. This is the cuboid.

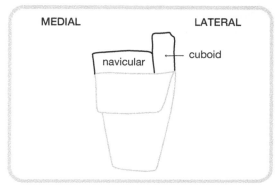

STEP 3

- Draw 3 squares above the navicular. These are the 3 cuneiform bones.

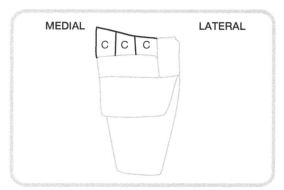

STEP 4

- Draw the 1st to 3rd metatarsals coming from each of the cuneiforms.
- Draw the 4th metatarsal anterior to the cuboid and draw the 5th metatarsal anterior and lateral to the cuboid.

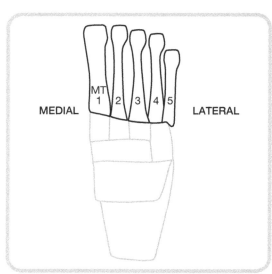

PLANTAR VIEW

✏️ How to draw

STEP 1

- Draw a long trapezoid shape to represent the calcaneus.
- On the medial anterior side draw a curved line cutting off the corner. The area anterior to this is the talus.

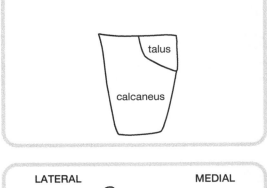

STEP 2

- Draw a rectangle anterior to the talus; this is the navicular.
- Medially and anterior to the calcaneus bone draw a slightly larger curved shape; this is the cuboid bone.

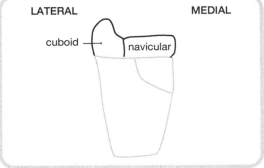

STEP 3

- Draw 3 squares anterior to the navicular; these are the cuneiform bones.

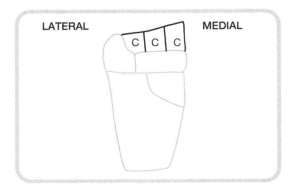

STEP 4

- Draw the 5 metatarsals as a mirror image of *Dorsal view* Step 4, i.e. 1 to 3 in front of the cuneiforms and 4 and 5 in front of the cuboid.

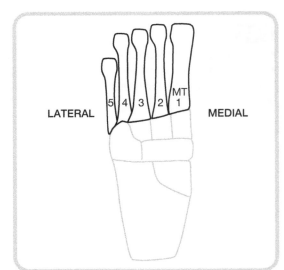

LATERAL VIEW

 How to draw

STEP 1

- Draw a horizontal rectangle with the anterior superior corner missing; this is the calcaneus.
- Superior to this draw a pentagon shape; this is the talus.

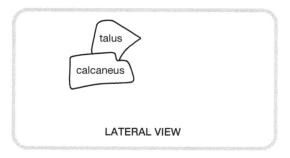

STEP 2

- Anterior to the talus draw a slanted rectangle; this is the navicular.
- Draw a square shape in front of the calcaneus; this is the cuboid.

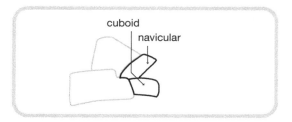

STEP 3

- Draw 2 of the cuneiforms above the cuboid; it is not possible to see the 3rd beyond the top of the foot in this view.

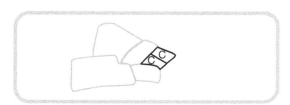

STEP 4

- Draw the 2nd to 5th metatarsals anterior to the cuneiform and cuboid bones. Because the metatarsals form the metatarsal arch proximally, these 4 are seen in this lateral view but the 1st metatarsal is out of sight, medial to them.
- Label the lateral longitudinal arch.
- Label the hindfoot, midfoot and forefoot.

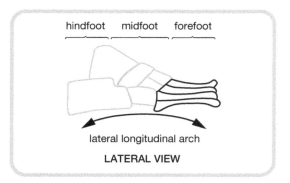

MEDIAL VIEW

 How to draw

STEP 1

- Draw the calcaneus and talus as a mirror image of *Lateral view* Step 1.

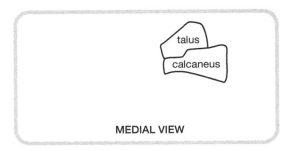

STEP 2

- Draw a vertical rectangle in front of the talus and calcaneus; this is the navicular.
- Draw 2 squares in front of the navicular; these are the 1st and 2nd cuneiforms.

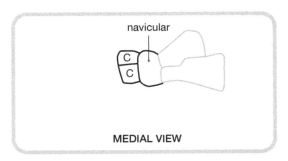

STEP 3

- Draw the 1st and 2nd metatarsals in front of the cuneiforms.
- Label the medial longitudinal arch.

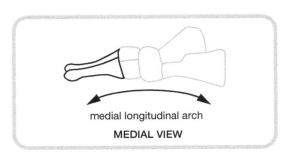

FOREFOOT (DORSAL VIEW, INCLUDING PART OF MIDFOOT)

 How to draw

- Draw the 3 cuneiform bones adjoining the 1st, 2nd and 3rd metatarsal bones.
- Draw the proximal and distal phalanx in front of the 1st metatarsal.
- Draw a proximal, middle and distal phalanx in front of the 2nd and 3rd metatarsals. The 4th and 5th toes have the same structure as the 2nd and 3rd.
- Label the 1st metatarsophalangeal joint.
- There are 5 metatarsals and 14 phalanges.

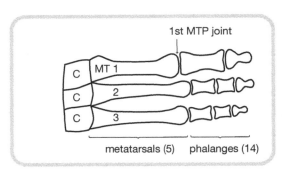

Muscles of the lower limb are summarised at the end of this section in Table 8.3; this gives their innervation, blood supply and actions. In the images, tendons are distinguished from their muscles by switching from the muscle brown colour to grey where a muscle belly ends and its long tendon starts.

Note the table lists muscles by anatomical group. However, each of the images you are going to draw shows the muscles seen in a specific view, which is not always exactly the same. For example, the gracilis is described and drawn in the anterior view of the thigh but belongs to the medial thigh anatomically speaking, as listed in Table 8.3.

8.7.1 Muscles of the gluteal region

We will first draw the muscles of the buttock. The arteries that supply them are listed in Table 8.1.

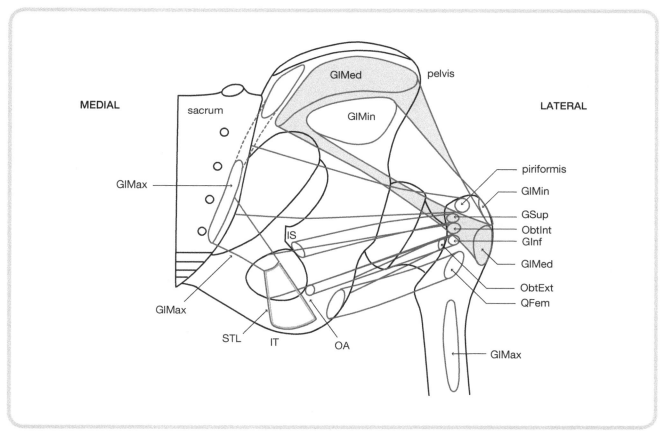

GInf	gemellus inferior	**GSup**	gemellus superior	**ObtExt**	obturator externus
GlMax	gluteus maximus	**IS**	ischial spine	**ObtInt**	obturator internus
GlMed	gluteus medius	**IT**	ischial tuberosity	**QFem**	quadratus femoris
GlMin	gluteus minimus	**OA**	obturator artery	**STL**	sacrotuberous ligament

✎ How to draw

STEP 1

- Draw the outline of half of the sacrum, coccyx, pelvis and upper portion of the femur, as shown.
- Label the ischial spine and ischial tuberosity.

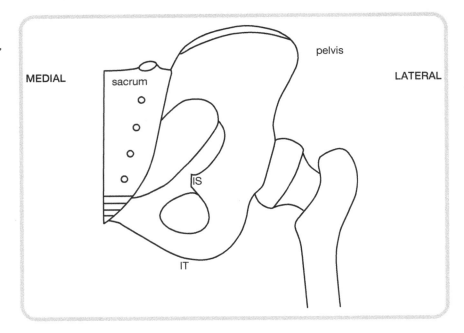

STEP 2

- Draw 2 ovals, one on the medial upper ilium and one on the lateral sacrum, lateral to the 2nd to 4th sacral foramina; these represent 2 of the origins of **gluteus maximus**. Draw dashed lines between the 2 ovals to indicate that the gluteus maximus muscle has origins from the sacrotuberous ligament and also the thoracolumbar fascia.
- Draw an almost 'bow-tie' shape from the sacrum to the ischial tuberosity, with a line in the middle over the obturator foramen. This is part of gluteus maximus; the part beneath the line represents the origin of the gluteus maximus from the lower part of the sacrotuberous ligament.
- Gluteus maximus has its origins on the ilium, thoracolumbar fascia (not shown), posterolateral aspect of the sacrum and coccyx and sacrotuberous ligament.
- Draw a thin oval in the lateral femur, below the neck; the gluteus maximus inserts onto the gluteal tuberosity here and (not shown) into the iliotibial tract. We will not draw the full body of the muscle because it covers most of the buttock area.

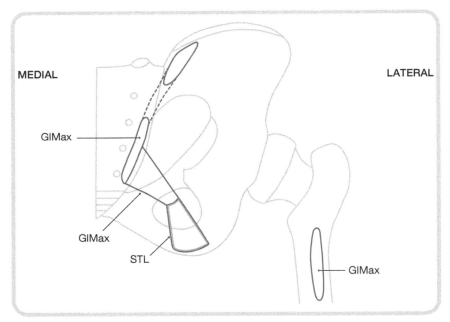

STEP ③

- Draw a triangular shape from just below the iliac crest to the lateral surface of the greater trochanter of the femur. This represents **gluteus medius**.
- Show its origin on the ilium and insertion onto the greater trochanter.
- Draw a smaller triangular shape under the gluteus medius, again drawing the origin on the ilium and insertion onto the anterior surface of the greater trochanter. This is the **gluteus minimus**.

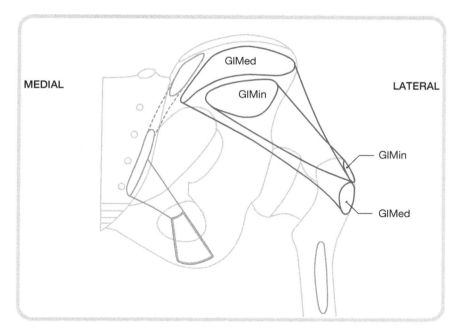

STEP ④

- Draw a triangular shape from the lateral sacrum to the medial edge of the greater trochanter of femur. This is the **piriformis**.
- Draw a circle to represent its insertion onto the superior border of the greater trochanter.

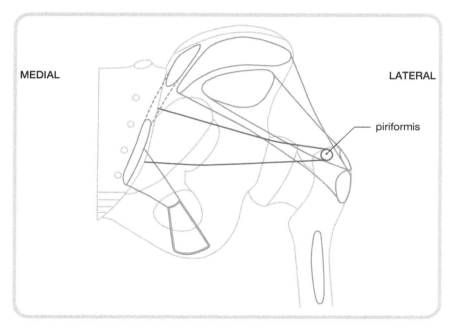

STEP 5

- Draw a slim rectangle from an origin on the ischial spine to insert just below the insertion of the piriformis muscle on the femur. This is the **gemellus superior**.
- The gemellus superior inserts into the medial surface of the greater trochanter.
- Draw a slim rectangle from an origin at the lower lateral edge of the obturator foramen, the ischial tuberosity, to insert below but in a similar femoral location as gemellus superior muscle. This is the **gemellus inferior**.
- The gemellus inferior inserts into the medial surface of the greater trochanter of the femur.
- The superior gemellus, obturator internus and inferior gemellus sometimes join before they insert onto the femur. This is known as the triceps coxae tendon (the 3 muscles together can be known as the triceps coxae muscle).

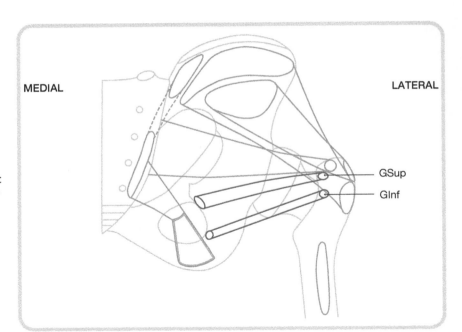

STEP 6

- Draw a line from the upper and lower edge of the obturator foramen to insert on the femur between the gemelli muscles. This is the **obturator internus**. It arises from the obturator membrane and the margins of the obturator foramen. It inserts onto the medial aspect of the greater trochanter as shown.
- Draw a slim rectangle from behind the ischium to the medial part of the femoral neck. This represents the **obturator externus**. It arises from the obturator membrane and foramen, and inserts onto the trochanteric fossa of the femur.

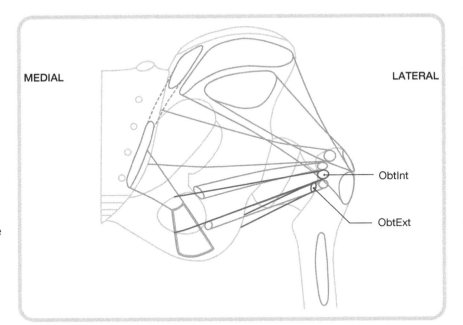

STEP 7

- Draw a slim rectangle from an origin on the lateral edge of the ischial tuberosity to insert onto the intertrochanteric crest of the femur. This is the **quadratus femoris**.

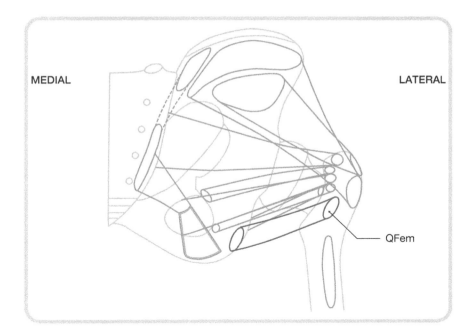

STEP 8

- Draw a green line from just above the ischial spine to lateral to the obturator foramen. This is the sciatic nerve (SN).
- Draw a red line to represent the superior gluteal artery (SGA) as shown. It comes from under gluteus medius and goes over gluteus minimus.
- Draw a red line from within the pelvis to the obturator foramen. This is the inferior gluteal artery (IGA). Add branches to the gluteus maximus, gemellus superior, gemellus inferior, obturator internus and quadratus femoris as shown. Add the obturator artery as a dashed line.
- Table 8.1 shows the arterial supply to the muscles of the buttock.

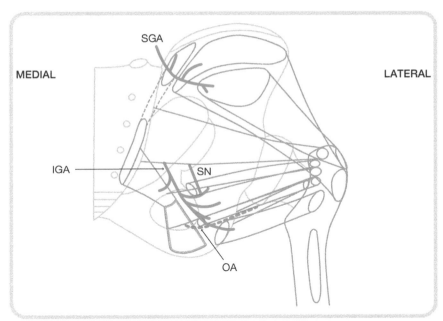

Table 8.1. Arteries supplying muscles of the buttock

Artery	Muscles supplied
Superior gluteal	Gluteus maximus, gluteus medius, gluteus minimus, tensor fasciae latae, piriformis
Inferior gluteal	Inferior and superior gemellus, quadratus femoris, obturator internus, piriformis
Obturator	Obturator externus

8.7.2 Muscles of the thigh

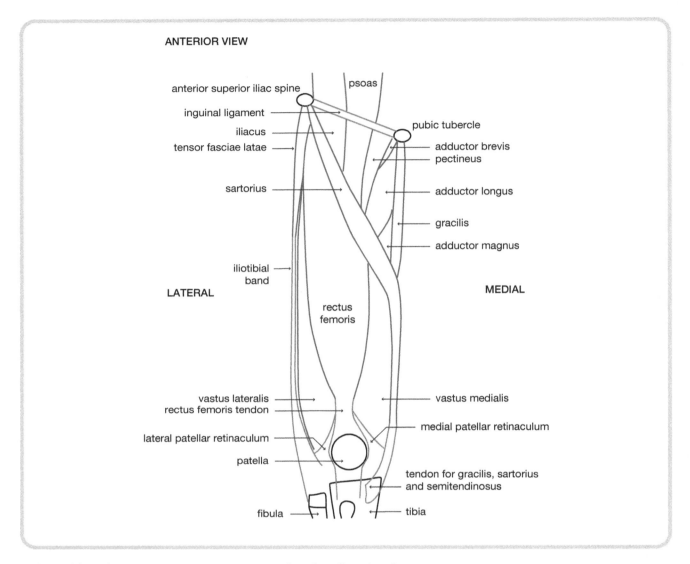

ANTERIOR VIEW

anterior superior iliac spine

psoas

inguinal ligament

iliacus

pubic tubercle

tensor fasciae latae

adductor brevis
pectineus

sartorius

adductor longus

gracilis

adductor magnus

iliotibial band

LATERAL

MEDIAL

rectus femoris

vastus lateralis
rectus femoris tendon

vastus medialis

lateral patellar retinaculum

medial patellar retinaculum

patella

tendon for gracilis, sartorius and semitendinosus

fibula

tibia

AdB	adductor brevis	LPR	lateral patellar retinaculum
AdL	adductor longus	MHG	medial head of gastrocnemius
AdM	adductor magnus	MPR	medial patellar retinaculum
ASIS	anterior superior iliac spine	Pc	pectineus
BFem	biceps femoris	Pl	plantaris
EI	external iliac	Ps	psoas
EO	external oblique	RFem	rectus femoris
G	gracilis	S	sartorius
GlMax	gluteus maximus	SM	semimembranosus
GlMed	gluteus medius	ST	semitendinosus
Il	iliacus	TFL	tensor fasciae latae
ITB	iliotibial band	VL	vastus lateralis
LHG	lateral head of gastrocnemius	VM	vastus medialis

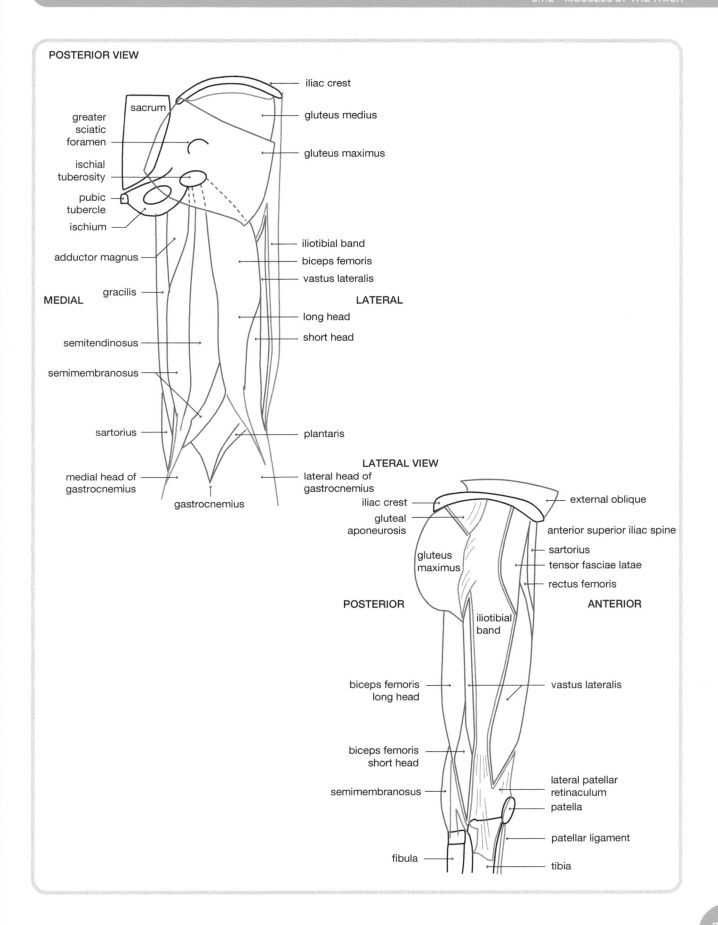

POSTERIOR VIEW

iliac crest

sacrum

greater sciatic foramen

gluteus medius

ischial tuberosity

gluteus maximus

pubic tubercle

ischium

adductor magnus

iliotibial band

biceps femoris

vastus lateralis

MEDIAL

gracilis

LATERAL

long head

short head

semitendinosus

semimembranosus

sartorius

plantaris

LATERAL VIEW

medial head of gastrocnemius

lateral head of gastrocnemius

gastrocnemius

iliac crest

external oblique

gluteal aponeurosis

anterior superior iliac spine

sartorius

gluteus maximus

tensor fasciae latae

rectus femoris

POSTERIOR

iliotibial band

ANTERIOR

biceps femoris long head

vastus lateralis

biceps femoris short head

semimembranosus

lateral patellar retinaculum

patella

fibula

patellar ligament

tibia

ANTERIOR VIEW

 How to draw

STEP 1

- At the top of the page draw a circle for the anterior superior iliac spine (ASIS), a circle for the pubic tubercle and a rectangle between them to represent the inguinal ligament.
- At the bottom of the page draw a circle in the middle to represent the patella.
- Below the patella, draw 3 sides of a square to represent the top of the tibia, and add a small semicircle near the top to represent the tibial tuberosity.
- Draw the fibular head lateral to the tibia, as shown.

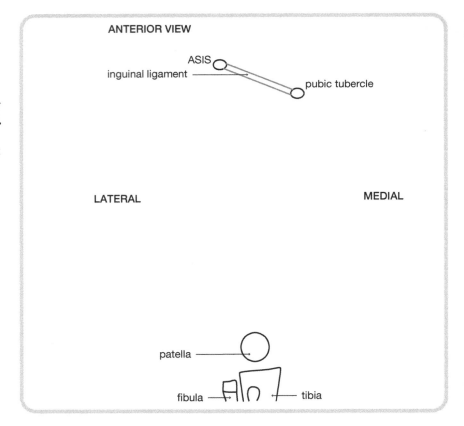

STEP 2

- Draw a long strap-like muscle from the ASIS crossing medially across to the middle of the thigh, then vertically downward to the medial part of the upper tibia. This represents the **sartorius**.
- The sartorius inserts on the pes anserinus. This is the common tendon for 3 muscles: the sartorius, gracilis and semitendinosus. Pes anserinus means 'goose foot', named due to the three-pronged look.

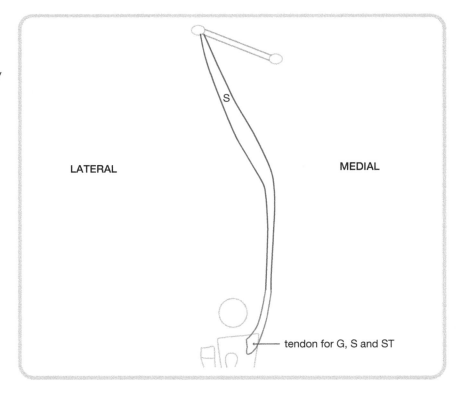

STEP 3

- Draw a thin rectangle from an origin at the pubic tubercle to run under sartorius. This is **gracilis**. It inserts on the pes anserinus.
- Draw 3 lines emerging from beneath the inguinal ligament, going down and behind the sartorius. Lateral to medial these delineate: **iliacus**, **psoas**, **pectineus** and **adductor longus**. See Table 8.2 for origins and insertions.

> NOTE: in the femoral canal we used SIPsPA to remember muscle order; you can use SIPsPAG for all of them!

- Draw a small triangle overlying the top of adductor longus; this is part of **adductor brevis**. This lies deep to pectineus and adductor longus.
- Draw a small triangle overlying the bottom of adductor longus; this is part of **adductor magnus**.

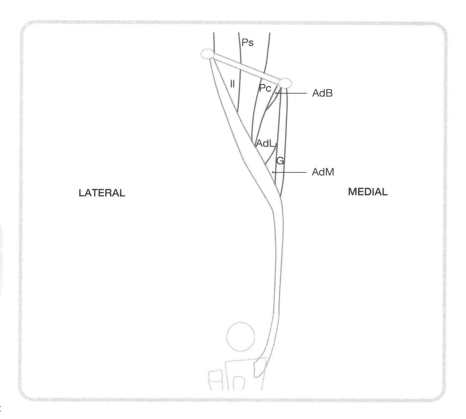

Table 8.2. Origins and insertions

Muscle	Origin	Insertion
Iliacus	Iliac fossa	Lesser trochanter
Psoas	Transverse process of T12 to L4	Lesser trochanter
Pectineus	Pectineal line on the superior pubic ramus of the pubic bone	Pectineal line of femur
Adductor longus	Pubic bone	Middle third of linea aspera
Adductor brevis	Anterior body of pubic bone and inferior pubic ramus	Proximal part of linea aspera and pectineal line
Adductor magnus	Adductor part: inferior pubic ramus and ischial ramus Ischial part: ischial tuberosity	Adductor part: gluteal tuberosity, medial part of linea aspera and medial supracondylar line Ischiocondylar part: adductor tubercle of femur

STEP 4

- Draw the **rectus femoris** emerging from beneath sartorius, forming the rectus femoris tendon just above the patella (also called patellar or quadriceps tendon). Continue the tendon over the patella to insert onto the tibial tuberosity. The rectus femoris arises from the anterior inferior iliac spine and the groove near the acetabulum on the ilium.
- Draw 2 grey lines curving away from the rectus femoris tendon. Label the areas below the lines as the medial and lateral patellar retinacula.
- Medial to rectus femoris label **vastus medialis**. This arises from the medial side of the femur; more specifically it arises from the intertrochanteric line, pectineal line, linea aspera and medial supracondylar line of the femur. It passes behind the medial patellar retinaculum to insert onto the rectus femoris tendon.

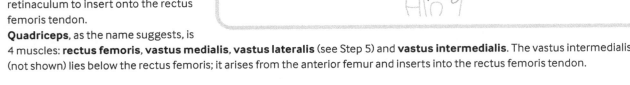

- **Quadriceps**, as the name suggests, is 4 muscles: **rectus femoris**, **vastus medialis**, **vastus lateralis** (see Step 5) and **vastus intermedialis**. The vastus intermedialis (not shown) lies below the rectus femoris; it arises from the anterior femur and inserts into the rectus femoris tendon.

STEP 5

- Draw a slim curved 'rectangle' shape from the ASIS down to the lateral condyle of the tibia. This is **tensor fasciae latae** (TFL) above and the iliotibial tract or band (ITB) further down. The TFL inserts onto the ITB.
- Medial to this, label the **vastus lateralis**, a quadriceps muscle which arises from the greater trochanter, intertrochanteric line and linea aspera. It inserts onto the base of the patella via the rectus femoris tendon and onto the tibial tuberosity (not shown).

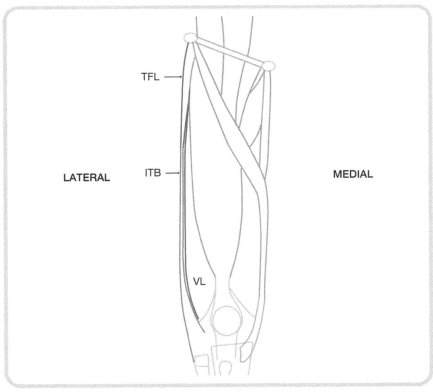

STEP 6

- Draw a nerve from above the inguinal ligament, crossing the tensor fascia latae laterally, with a descending branch that runs above vastus lateralis. This is the lateral cutaneous nerve of the thigh.
- Draw a nerve down the middle of the inguinal ligament to just above sartorius. Divide it into 2: the deep femoral and saphenous nerves. Add a branch from the saphenous nerve to the vastus medialis.
- Draw an artery medial to the femoral nerve and label it external iliac artery above and femoral artery below the inguinal ligament. Continue it down sartorius to vastus medialis. Here continue it as a broken line down and behind the patella; this is the popliteal artery.
- Draw a branch from the femoral artery, just above sartorius; this is the deep femoral artery. Add a branch laterally around the thigh, the lateral femoral circumflex artery; halfway along it, draw its descending branch.

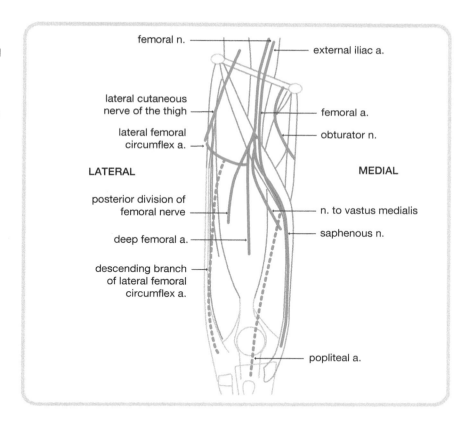

STEP 7

- Starting above the inguinal ligament, draw a vein medial to the femoral artery; this is the external iliac vein which drains the femoral vein. Draw and label the great saphenous vein, running up the medial side of the thigh to drain into the femoral vein.
- Add a blue line alongside the deep femoral artery upwards to join the femoral vein. This is the deep femoral vein.
- Draw a broken line alongside the popliteal artery; this represents the popliteal vein.

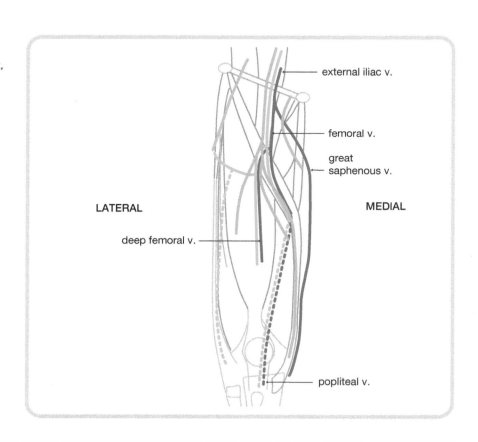

POSTERIOR VIEW

 How to draw

STEP ①

- Draw the outline of the iliac crest superiorly, the sacrum medially, and the pubic tubercle, ischium and ischial tuberosity inferiorly, as shown, occupying the top third of a page.

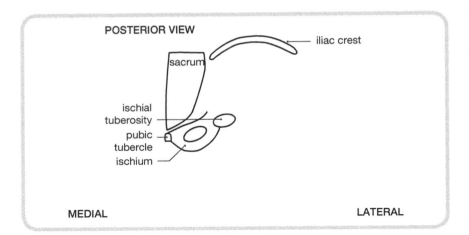

STEP ②

- Draw a large shape like a square flag over the buttock area as shown; this is the **gluteus maximus**.
- Above this add a vertical line to complete a shape that represents the **gluteus medius**.
- Draw a grey line at the top. This represents the gluteal aponeurosis, a fibrous membrane from fascia lata. It lies between the iliac crest and the superior border of the gluteus maximus. Part of the gluteus medius arises from here.
- The origins and insertions of the gluteal muscles are described in *Section 8.7.1 Muscles of the buttock.*

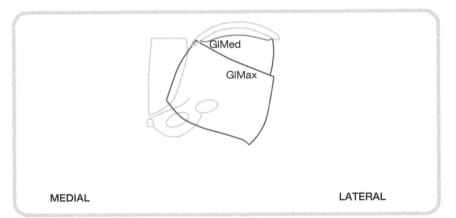

STEP 3

- From an origin on the ischial tuberosity draw a long curved shape laterally down to insert on the head of the fibula (not shown). This is the **biceps femoris**.
- Draw a line down from midway down the lateral side of biceps femoris to its distal tip. This divides the short head laterally and the long head medially. The 2 heads join to insert onto the head of the fibula. The short head arises from the linea aspera on the femur.

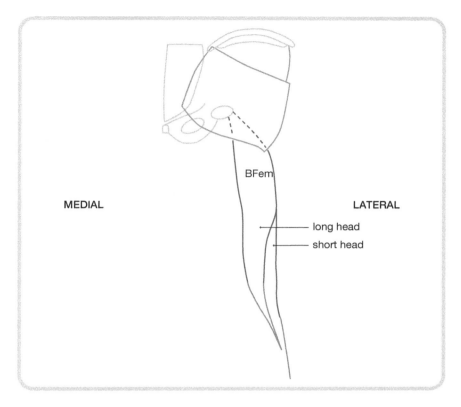

STEP 4

- Draw a thin muscle lateral to biceps femoris; this is the vastus lateralis.
- Lateral to this draw a long grey line; this is the iliotibial tract or band (ITB).

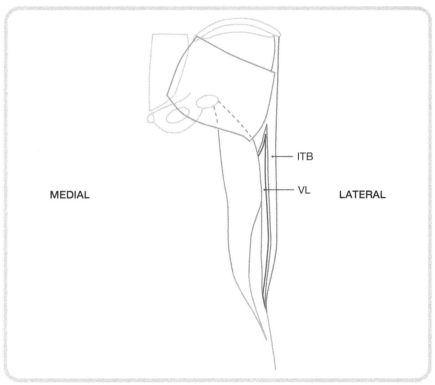

STEP 5

- From the ischial tuberosity, draw a leaf shape to insert medially where the medial condyle of the tibia would lie; this is the **semimembranosus**.

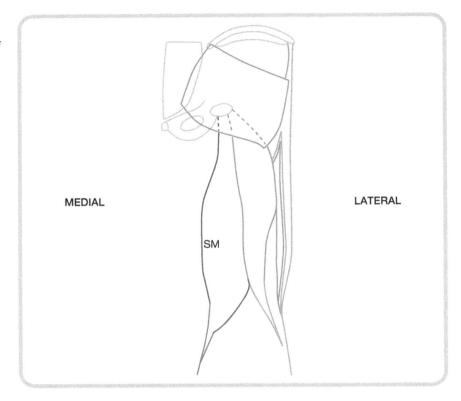

MEDIAL

LATERAL

SM

STEP 6

- Draw a slimmer leaf shape in the middle of semimembranosus; this is **semitendinosus**, which is superficial to semimembranosus. It has a long tendon of insertion, hence the name. Its origin is the ischial tuberosity, and it inserts onto the pes anserinus in the medial superior tibia.
- Draw a long rectangle from the ischium to the insertion point of semitendinosus; this is the **gracilis**. Just medial to this draw a slim triangle to represent the **sartorius** (see *Anterior view* Step 2).
- Between the gracilis and semimembranosus, label **adductor magnus** (see *Anterior view*).

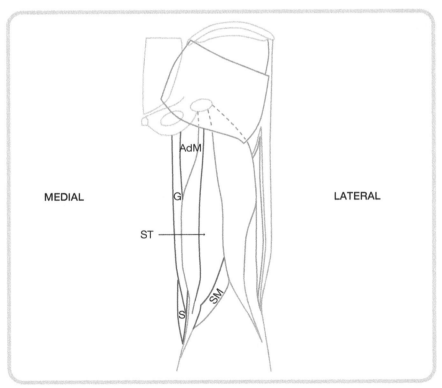

MEDIAL

LATERAL

AdM

G

ST

S

SM

STEP 7

- At the area of the posterior knee, we will draw a diamond shape that has semimembranosus superomedially and biceps femoris superolaterally.
- Draw a small triangle for the lower lateral edge of the diamond; this is **plantaris**, with the lateral head of **gastrocnemius** below (see *Section 8.7.4: Muscles of the posterior compartment of the lower leg* for origins and insertions).
- On the lower medial edge is the medial head of gastrocnemius. This outlines the popliteal fossa (see *Section 8.4: Popliteal fossa*).

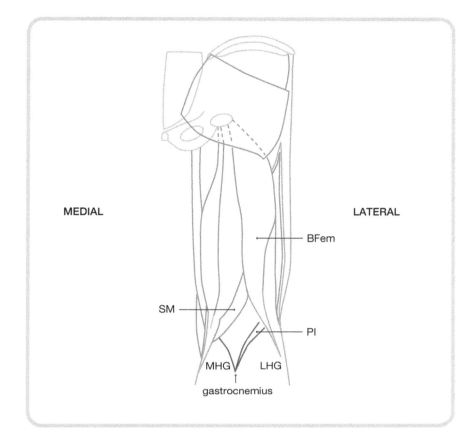

STEP 8

- Draw a semicircle posterior to the gluteus maximus; this represents the greater sciatic foramen.
- Draw a thick nerve from here, down into the popliteal fossa; this is the sciatic nerve. Draw branches to the biceps femoris, semitendinosus and plantaris.
- Proximally, draw a branch travelling upwards. This is the inferior gluteal nerve.
- Distally, show the sciatic nerve dividing into the tibial nerve and common fibular nerve. Add branches from each, joining to form the sural nerve, and draw an articular branch from the tibial nerve.
- Draw the popliteal artery and vein, next to the tibial nerve.
- Draw a second nerve exiting the sciatic foramen; this is the posterior femoral cutaneous nerve. Add its perineal branch medially, curving upwards.

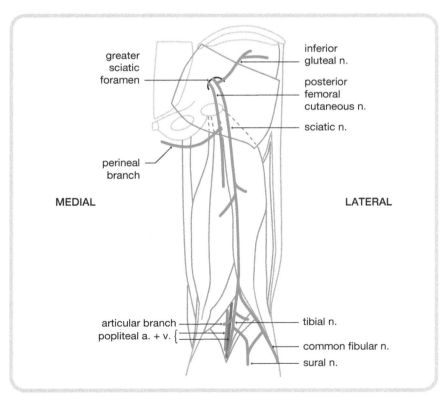

LATERAL VIEW

Origins and insertions of the muscles seen in the lateral view are described in the preceding sections.

✏️ How to draw

STEP 1

- Draw a curved shape at the top of the page. This is the iliac crest; anteriorly it is the anterior superior iliac spine (ASIS).
- At the bottom of the page draw the tibia, fibula and patella.

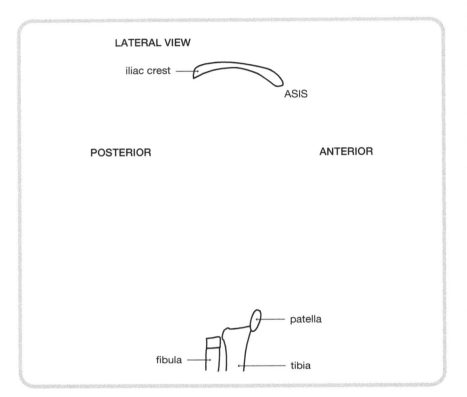

LATERAL VIEW

iliac crest
ASIS

POSTERIOR
ANTERIOR

patella
fibula
tibia

STEP 2

- From the posterior 2/3 of the iliac crest, draw grey lines representing the direction of fibres in the iliotibial tract, down the thigh to join the tibia and patella as shown.
- Label the gluteal aponeurosis superiorly.
- Label the iliotibial tract or band (ITB), which continues down to the knee and becomes the lateral patellar retinaculum and patellar ligament.

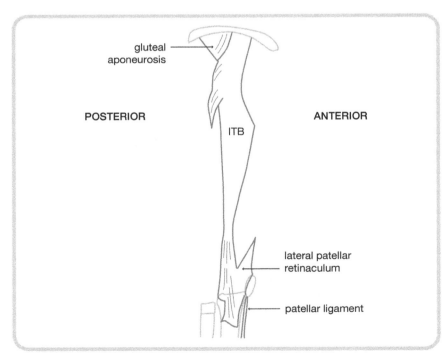

gluteal aponeurosis

POSTERIOR
ANTERIOR

ITB

lateral patellar retinaculum

patellar ligament

STEP 3

- Draw a curved rectangle above the iliac crest. This is the **external oblique** muscle.
- Draw a curve around the buttock to join the ITB. This is the **gluteus maximus**.
- Draw a line from the ASIS down, curving slightly to meet the lateral patellar retinaculum, as shown.
- Divide the area between this line and the ITB as shown: **tensor fasciae latae** (TFL) anterior to the ITB and **sartorius** anterior to this, then **rectus femoris** and **vastus lateralis** inferior to these.
- Draw a thin area posterior to the ITB; this is also the vastus lateralis. This is the largest quadricep muscle. It lies beneath the ITB, hence you see it in two areas on a lateral view.

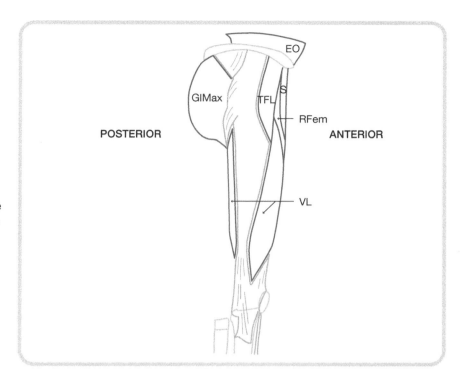

STEP 4

- Posterior to the vastus lateralis, draw the long and short heads of the **biceps femoris**.
- Inferior to this draw the **semimembranosus**.
- Draw the tendon of biceps femoris inserting into the head of the fibula and the posterior surface of the superior tibia.

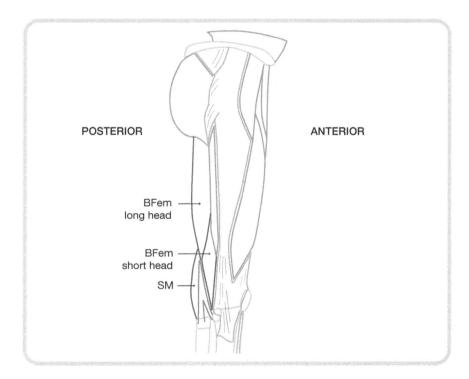

8.7.3 Muscles of the anterior compartment of the leg

The anterior compartment has 4 muscles:

- extensor digitorum longus
- tibialis anterior
- fibularis brevis
- extensor hallucis longus

NOTE: The terms fibularis and peroneus are both used and mean the same thing. Fibularis/fibular is current terminology.

EDL   extensor digitorum longus
EHL   extensor hallucis longus
FB   fibularis brevis
FL   fibularis longus
FT   fibularis tertius
GN   gastrocnemius
IER   inferior extensor retinaculum
MT   metatarsal
S   soleus
SER   superior extensor retinaculum
TA   tibialis anterior

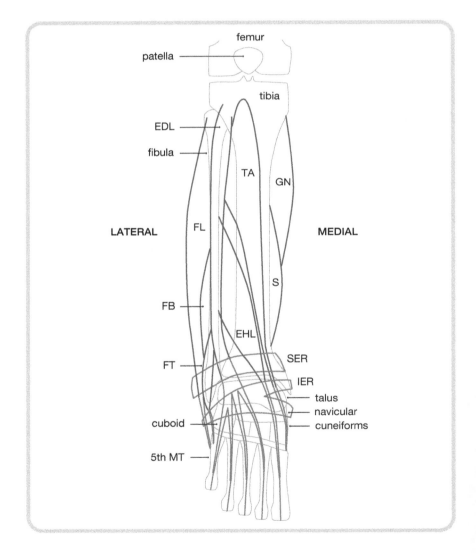

How to draw

STEP 1

- Draw the outline of the distal femur, patella, tibia and fibula, talus, navicular, cuboid, 3 x cuneiforms and 5 metatarsals.

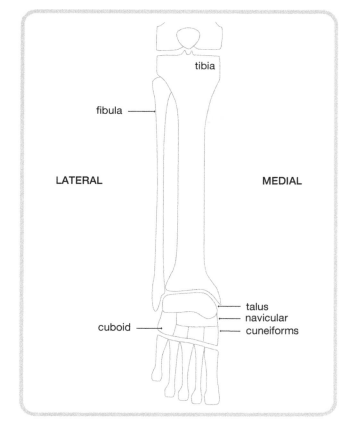

STEP 2

- Draw an open-ended leaf-shaped muscle from an origin on the lower one-third of the anterior fibula. Continue its tendon in grey down to inset onto the dorsal surface of the 5th metatarsal. This is the **fibularis tertius**.

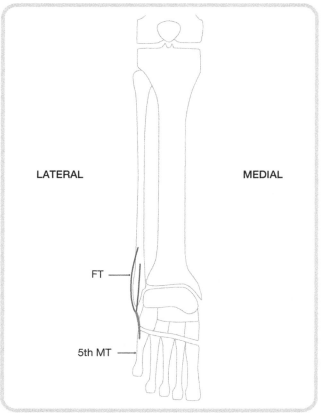

STEP 3

- Draw 2 lines from the middle of the anterior fibula towards the medial side of the ankle.
- From the distal end of these, draw a tendon passing downward. This is the **extensor hallucis longus** (EHL); it inserts onto the dorsal side of the distal phalanx of the great toe (see *Section 8.7.5 Muscles of the foot*).

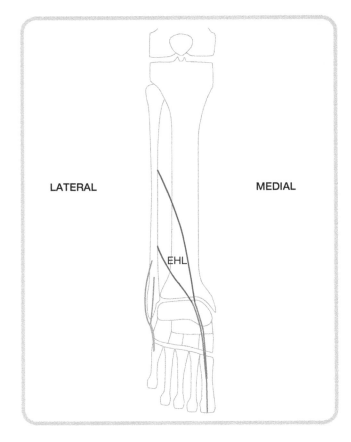

STEP 4

- Draw a curved muscle from an origin on the lateral tibial condyle down to the ankle. Continue it as 4 tendons down beyond the 2nd to 5th metatarsals; they insert onto the base of the middle and distal phalanges (see *Section 8.7.5 Muscles of the foot*). This is **extensor digitorum longus** (EDL), which lies superficial to EHL.
- Draw 2 lines from the lateral side of the tibia, from the upper tibia and from halfway down it, to almost join at the medial side of the ankle. This represents **tibialis anterior**, which lies superficial to EDL. It also originates from the interosseous membrane.
- From the proximal end draw the tendon, inserting into the medial cuneiform and the base of the 1st metatarsal. If you dorsiflex your foot you will feel the muscle just lateral to the anterior edge of the tibia.

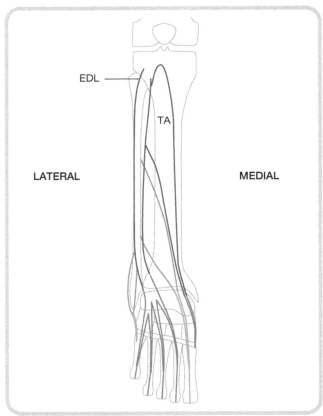

STEP 5

- Draw a triangle above the fibularis tertius; this is the **fibularis brevis**, which mainly lies under the fibularis longus. It arises from the lower 2/3 of the lateral side of the fibula and inserts onto the 5th metatarsal (not shown).
- From an origin at the top of the lateral fibula draw a line down the leg to the lateral side of the ankle, this is the **fibularis longus**. Continue its tendon down behind the lateral malleolus with fibularis brevis; it crosses the sole of the foot and inserts onto the lateral side of the base of the 1st metatarsal and the medial cuneiform bone (not shown).

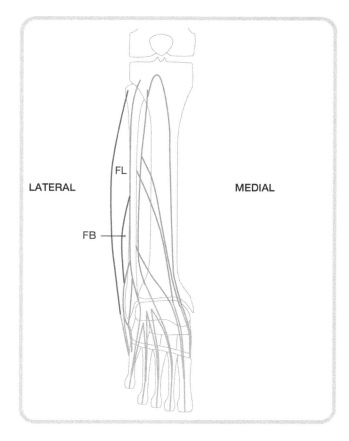

LATERAL   MEDIAL

FL

FB

STEP 6

- Draw an arc from behind the medial side of the middle of the tibia; this represents the **soleus**. This lies posteriorly but would be seen from an anterior view.
- Draw a convex line from below the medial condyle of the tibia to midway along the soleus muscle; this represents the **gastrocnemius**.
- For origins and insertions of these, see *Section 8.7.4: Muscles of the posterior compartment of the lower leg*.

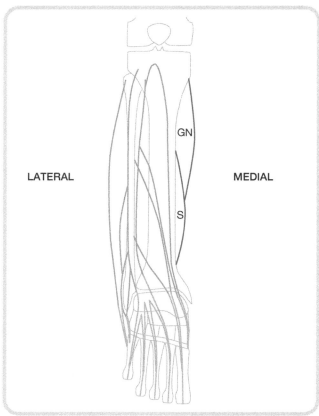

LATERAL   MEDIAL

GN

S

STEP 7

- Draw a grey rectangle across the distal end of the tibia and fibula. This is the **superior extensor retinaculum**. It binds down the tendons of fibularis tertius, EDL, EHL and tibialis anterior.
- Draw a horizontal Y shape below this, to represent the **inferior extensor retinaculum**. This has 2 layers: tendons for fibularis tertius and EDL pass between the 2 layers from lower leg to foot; medially it passes over EHL but encloses tibialis anterior.

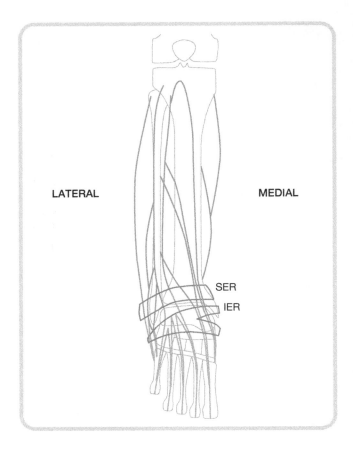

LATERAL

MEDIAL

SER

IER

8.7.4 Muscles of the posterior compartment of the leg

Muscles of the posterior compartment are flexors of the ankles and toes.

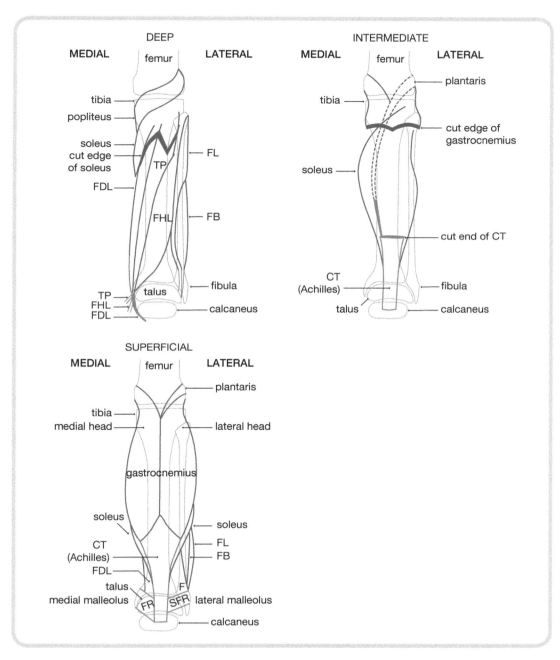

CT	calcaneal (Achilles) tendon	FL	fibularis longus
F	fibula	FR	flexor retinaculum
FB	fibularis brevis	SFR	superior fibular retinaculum
FDL	flexor digitorum longus	TP	tibialis posterior
FHL	flexor hallucis longus		

DEEP MUSCLES OF THE POSTERIOR COMPARTMENT

 How to draw

STEP 1

- Draw the posterior side of the distal femur, tibia and fibula, talus and calcaneus. Use black lines for the distal and proximal parts; use pencil in between these, where most of the muscle bellies will be drawn.

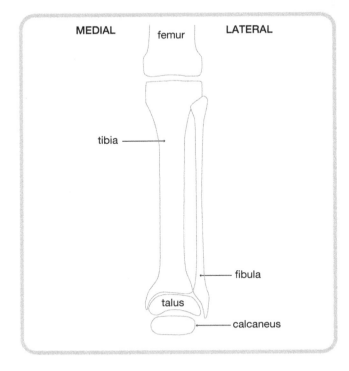

STEP 2

- Draw a flame shape from an origin at the lateral edge of the lateral epicondyle of the distal femur to insert on the posterior surface of the medial tibia above the soleal line (see *Section 8.6.2: Tibia, fibula and patella*). This is the **popliteus**.
- Along the lateral edge of the image draw the **fibularis longus** by starting with a straight line laterally and then curving to end in a grey tendon heading down under the foot (see *Deep plantar muscles* in *Section 8.7.5: Muscles of the foot*).
- Draw the **fibularis brevis** lateral to this as shown.

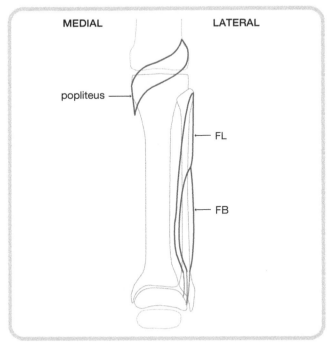

STEP 3

- Draw a leaf-shaped muscle that originates from the middle 1/3 of the posterior fibula heading medially downwards. This is the **flexor hallucis longus** (FHL).
- Show its tendon heading inferiorly; it inserts onto the base of the distal phalanx of the great toe.

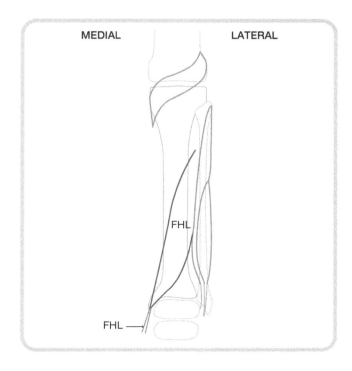

STEP 4

- Draw a line from the inner side of the fibula down to meet the end of the body of FHL, and continue its tendon downwards. This is the medial edge of **tibialis posterior**. Its origin is the inner edge of the tibia and fibula and the interosseous membrane between them. It runs medially and inserts into the tuberosity of the navicular bone, the cuboid bone, the cuneiform bones and metatarsals 2 to 4.

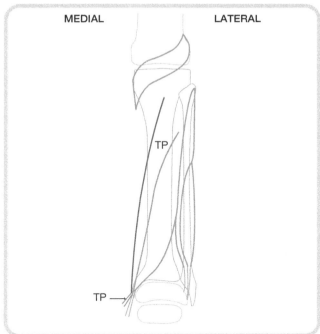

STEP 5

- Medial to TP, draw a line just inferior to the tibia's soleal line down the medial side of the lower leg; this is the medial edge of the **flexor digitorum longus** (FDL). The tendon runs behind the medial malleolus and passes along the sole of the foot. Behind the navicular it divides into 4 tendons which insert onto the distal phalanx of the 2nd to 5th toes.
- Draw a W shape above FDL, making the inner 2 lines thicker to represent the cut edge of the **soleus**. Its origin is the proximal one-third of the posterior surface of fibula and medial border of the tibia (soleal line); it inserts onto the posterior part of the calcaneus via the calcaneal tendon (tendo calcaneus) (see *Intermediate muscles of the posterior compartment*).

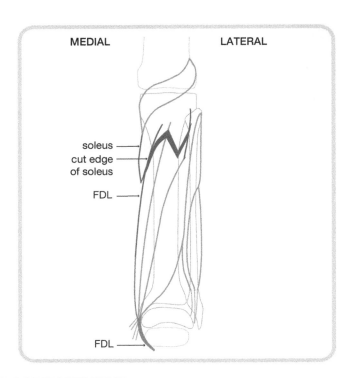

INTERMEDIATE MUSCLES OF THE POSTERIOR COMPARTMENT

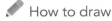 How to draw

STEP 1

- Draw the outline of the distal femur, the tibia and fibula, the talus and calcaneus.
- Draw the cut edge of the two heads of the **gastrocnemius**, arising from the lateral condyle and medial condyle of the femur.

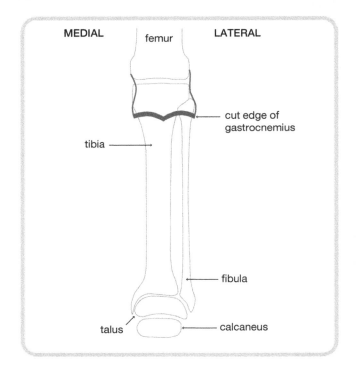

STEP 2

- At the middle of the calcaneus draw a trapezium upwards that is 'cut' at the end; this is the **calcaneal tendon (CT; Achilles tendon)**. It is the attachment for 3 muscles; gastrocnemius, plantaris and soleus.
- Draw a thin, long triangular muscle from just above the lateral head of gastrocnemius muscle on the lateral distal femur to behind the upper tibia bone; this represents the **plantaris**. Then continue it as a long grey line, the tendon that runs into the calcaneal tendon.

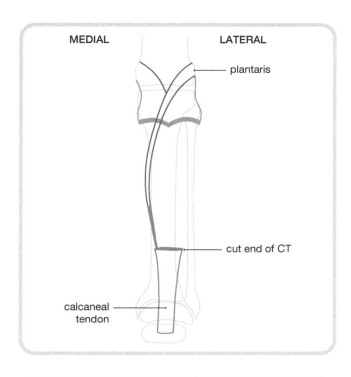

STEP 3

- Draw a large muscle originating from the upper part of the fibula, fibula head and soleal line of the medial upper tibia. This is the **soleus**. It runs down the posterior leg to join the calcaneal tendon with the gastrocnemius.

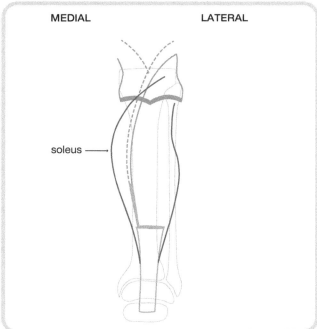

SUPERFICIAL MUSCLES OF THE POSTERIOR COMPARTMENT

 How to draw

STEP 1

- Copy the distal femur, the tibia and fibula, and the talus and calcaneus, as shown.

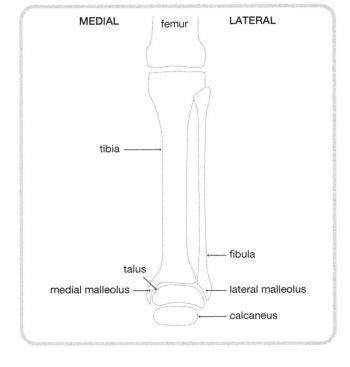

STEP 2

- Draw the **gastrocnemius** as 2 fish shapes starting with the 'tails' on the medial and lateral condyles of the femur and with the 'heads' about 3/4 of the way down the tibia.
- Draw a grey line from each 'fish head' to insert in a wide tendon on the calcaneus bone; this represents the calcaneal tendon.
- Label the medial and lateral heads of the gastrocnemius.
- Above the lateral head of the gastrocnemius draw a small triangle to represent the **plantaris** (as described previously).

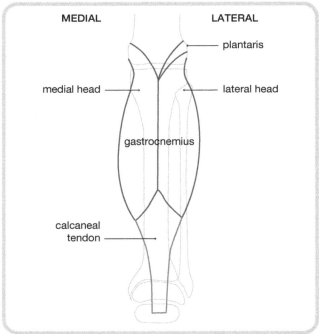

STEP 3

- On each side of the CT draw a sliver of muscle; this is the **soleus**, which is deep to the gastrocnemius (see earlier) and also inserts onto the CT.

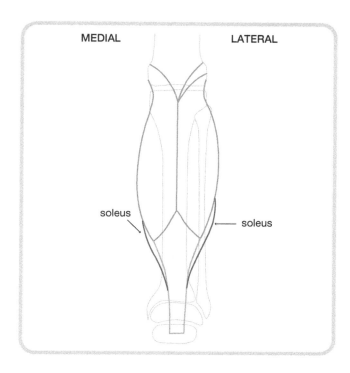

STEP 4

- Draw a line down from the middle of the lateral part of soleus to behind the lateral malleolus, and divide the area this creates with a vertical line to represent the **fibularis longus** and **brevis**.
- Draw a line down from the medial part of the soleus to the lower tibia. The area between this and soleus is the **flexor digitorum longus** (FDL).
- Draw a grey band from the medial malleolus to the CT over the calcaneus; this is the **flexor retinaculum**. The tibialis posterior and FDL run underneath it.
- On the lateral side draw a similar grey rectangle; this is the **superior fibular retinaculum** (the continuation of the lateral retinaculum in Step 7 of *Section 8.7.3: Muscles of the anterior compartment of the lower leg*).

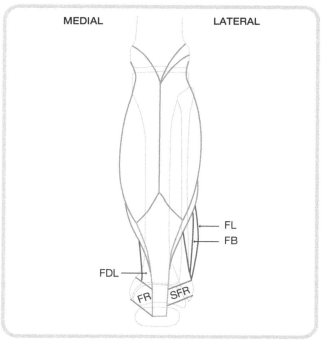

8.7.5 Muscles of the foot

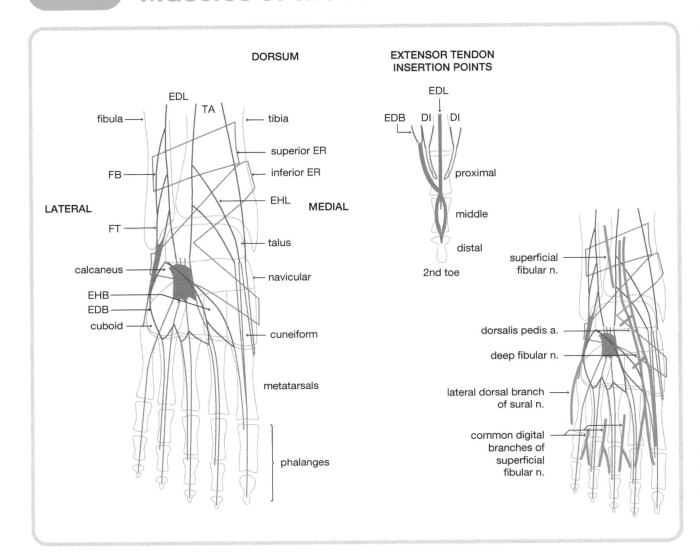

DORSUM

EXTENSOR TENDON
INSERTION POINTS

EDL

TA

fibula — tibia

— superior ER

FB — inferior ER

— EHL   MEDIAL

LATERAL

FT — talus

calcaneus — navicular

EHB

EDB

cuboid — cuneiform

metatarsals

phalanges

EDL

EDB   DI   DI

proximal

middle

distal

2nd toe

superficial
fibular n.

dorsalis pedis a.

deep fibular n.

lateral dorsal branch
of sural n.

common digital
branches of
superficial
fibular n.

AbDM	abductor digiti minimi	FDL	flexor digitorum longus
AbH	abductor hallucis	FDMB	flexor digiti minimi brevis
AdH	adductor hallucis	FHB	flexor hallucis brevis
CP	central part of plantar aponeurosis	FHL	flexor hallucis longus
		FL	fibularis longus
DI	dorsal interossei	FT	fibularis tertius
EDB	extensor digitorum brevis	L	lumbrical
EDL	extensor digitorum longus	LP	lateral part of plantar aponeurosis
EHB	extensor hallucis brevis		
EHL	extensor hallucis longus	P	plantar interossei
ER	extensor retinaculum	QP	quadratus plantae
FB	fibularis brevis	TA	tibialis anterior
FDB	flexor digitorum brevis	TP	tibialis posterior

DEEP MUSCLES OF THE SOLE OF THE FOOT

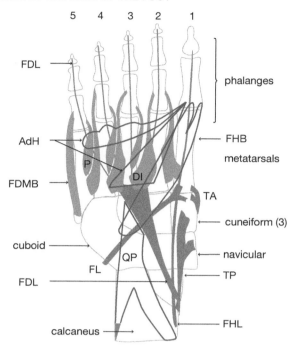

SUPERFICIAL MUSCLES OF THE SOLE OF THE FOOT

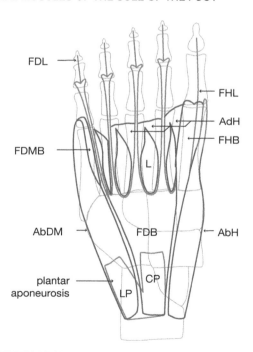

To understand tendons that insert onto the foot, first draw muscles of the lower leg (see *Sections 8.7.3* and *8.7.4*).

DORSAL MUSCLES

 How to draw

STEP 1

- Draw the outline of the distal tibia and fibula and the bones of the foot, as shown.

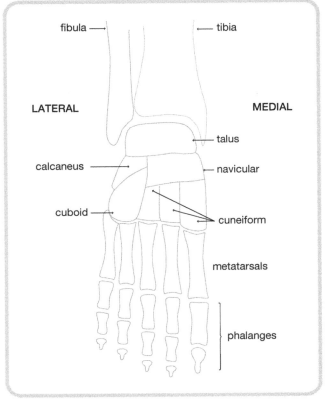

STEP 2

- Draw a small 'inverted tulip head' shape originating on the dorsum of the calcaneus and forming 3 tendons that insert onto the proximal part of the middle phalanx of the 2nd to 4th toes (see next step for insertion). This is the **extensor digitorum brevis** (EDB).
- Just medial to EDB draw a slim muscle from the calcaneus to insert onto the base of proximal phalanx of the great toe. This is the **extensor hallucis brevis** (EHB).

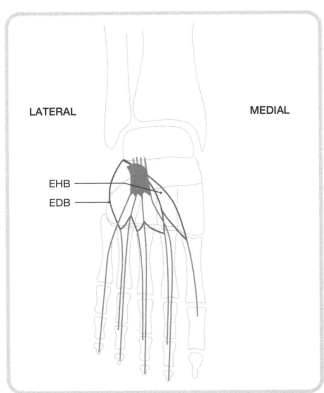

STEP 3

- From the top of the image, draw a long thin muscle, the distal end of **extensor digitorum longus** (EDL), as shown.
- Draw its 4 tendons inserting into the middle and distal phalanges of the 2nd to 5th toes.
- EDB tendons insert onto the lateral side of EDL tendons on the 2nd to 4th toes.

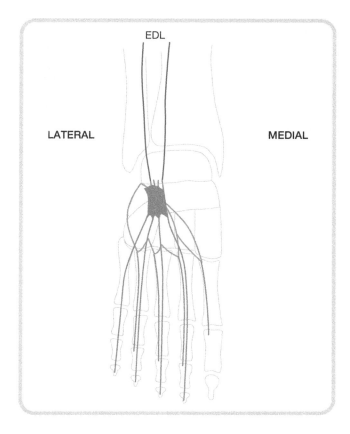

STEP 4

- Draw the distal end of the **fibularis tertius**, which has its origin (not shown) on the distal medial surface of the fibula, inserting into the base of the 5th metatarsal.
- Draw a small triangle to represent the **fibularis brevis** above fibularis tertius.

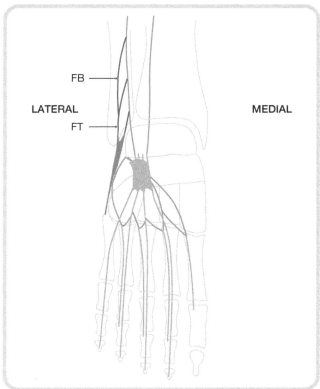

STEP 5

- Draw **extensor hallucis longus** (EHL) from the anterior surface of the middle part of the fibula (origin), passing medially to insert onto the distal phalanx of the great toe.
- Draw a triangle above EHL to represent **tibialis anterior**.
- Draw a grey line, the tendon, inserting into the medial cuneiform and the base of the 1st metatarsal.

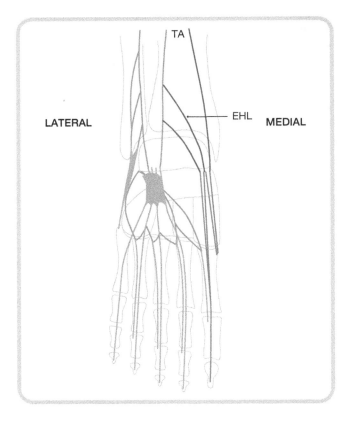

STEP 6

To make it clear how extensor tendons insert onto phalanges, we will draw a close-up.

- Draw the outline of the 3 phalanges of the 2nd toe.
- Down the middle, draw a thick grey line from the metatarsal to the base of the middle phalanx; this is the tendon of EDL.
- On each side of the metatarsal draw the **dorsal interossei** with tendons inserting into the proximal phalanx.
- Draw a leaf shape branching from the main tendon of EDL and inserting into the distal phalanx; this is the dorsal expansion of EDL.
- On the lateral side draw the EDB tendon coming in and inserting into the middle phalanx.

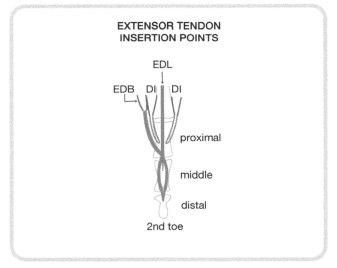

STEP 7

- Draw a green arrow over the middle of the ankle pointing down to represent the many branches of the superficial fibular nerves supplying the superficial area of the foot. These pass superficial to the retinacula (see next step).
- Draw the deep fibular nerve medial to this, passing deep to retinacula and tendon sheaths to branch into the great toe and 2nd toe.
- Draw the lateral dorsal branch of the sural nerve.
- Draw small Y-shaped branches between the 2nd to 5th toes. These are the common digital branches of the superficial fibular nerve.
- Draw an artery medial to the deep fibular nerve, passing towards the great toe. This is the dorsalis pedis artery.

NOTE: **D**orsalis **p**edis artery lies next to **deep** fibular nerve, DP–DP!

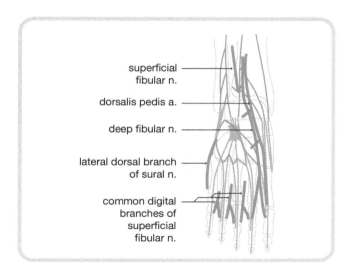

superficial fibular n.

dorsalis pedis a.

deep fibular n.

lateral dorsal branch of sural n.

common digital branches of superficial fibular n.

STEP 8

- Copy the **superior extensor retinaculum** and **inferior extensor retinaculum** from *Section 8.7.3: Muscles of the anterior compartment of the lower leg.*
- Of the structures shown in this image, only the superficial fibular nerve is superficial to these.

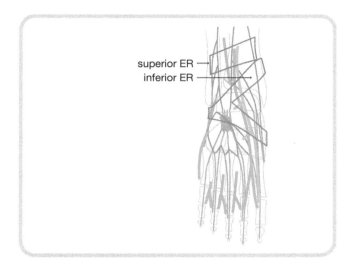

superior ER

inferior ER

DEEP PLANTAR MUSCLES

 How to draw

STEP 1

- Draw the bones of the foot as shown here.
- Draw the 3 **plantar interossei** originating midway along the medial side of the metatarsal and inserting on the medial base of the proximal phalanx of the 3rd, 4th and 5th toes.

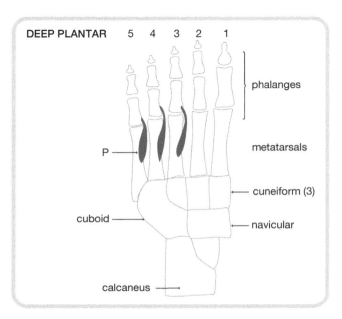

DEEP PLANTAR 5 4 3 2 1

phalanges

P

metatarsals

cuboid

cuneiform (3)

navicular

calcaneus

STEP 2

- Draw the 4 **dorsal interossei**. Each has 2 heads, 1 from the proximal half of each adjacent metatarsal bone. The 2 heads join and form a tendon which inserts onto the lateral side of the base of the 2nd, 3rd and 4th proximal phalanges; the most medial muscle inserts onto medial side of the 2nd toe.
- Draw the tendon of the **fibularis longus** emerging from above the cuboid bone and attaching to the medial cuneiform and the base of the 1st metatarsal.
- Draw the tendon of **tibialis posterior** emerging from the medial side of the calcaneus and attaching to the navicular and the medial cuneiform bone.

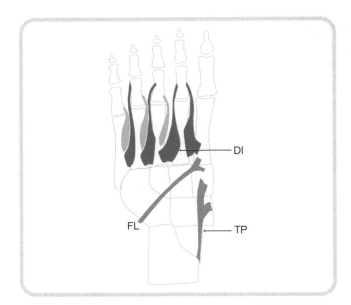

STEP 3

- **Adductor hallucis** has 2 heads that converge to insert on the lateral side of the base of the proximal phalanx of the great toe: oblique and transverse.
- Draw the oblique head from origins at the proximal ends of the 3 middle metatarsal bones to the insertion point.
- Draw the transverse head, looking cloud-like, from origins at the distal 3rd, 4th and 5th metatarsals (from the metatarsophalangeal ligaments) to the insertion point.

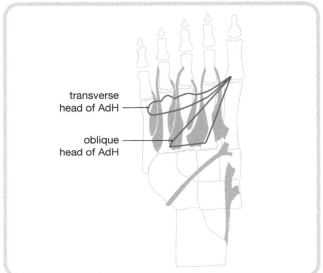

STEP 4

- Draw the **flexor hallucis brevis** muscle (FHB) as a 'lobster claw' shape.
- It originates on the medial part of the cuboid bone and part of the 3rd cuneiform bone. It divides into a lateral and medial head, which insert onto the sesamoid bones and the medial and lateral proximal phalanx of the great toe.

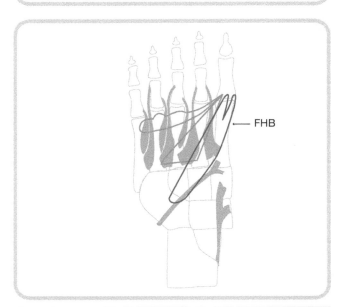

STEP 5

- Draw the tendon of the **flexor hallucis longus** (FHL) inserting onto the distal phalanx of the great toe. It originates on the posterior surface of the fibula.
- Draw the tendon of the **flexor digitorum longus** (FDL), inserting onto the distal phalanges of the 2nd to 5th toes. It originates on the posterior surface of the tibia.
- Draw the tendon of the **tibialis anterior** coming around the side of the 1st metatarsal and medial cuneiform and inserting on both.

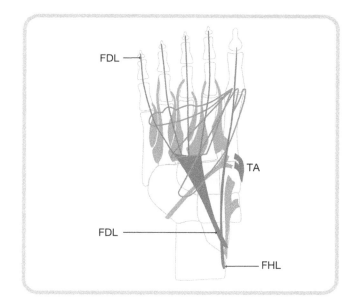

STEP 6

- Draw a thin muscle on the lateral side of the foot from an origin on the base of the 5th metatarsal to insert onto the base of the proximal phalanx of the 5th toe. This is the **flexor digiti minimi brevis**.
- Draw the **quadratus plantae** originating from the calcaneus to insert onto the tendon of the FDL. Quadratus plantae has 2 heads. The medial one is larger and more muscular; it arises from the medial side of the calcaneus. The lateral one is flat and more tendinous; it arises from the lateral border of the calcaneus and the long plantar ligament.

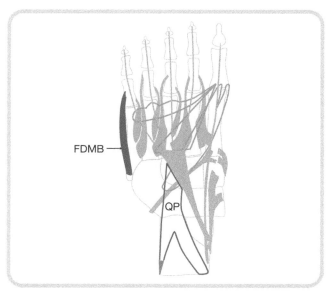

SUPERFICIAL PLANTAR MUSCLES

 How to draw

STEP 1

- Copy the bones of the foot from Step 1 of the section above on deep plantar muscles.
- Draw a long narrow muscle from an origin on the lateral process of the calcaneus to insert onto the lateral side of the base of the proximal phalanx of the 5th toe. This is the **abductor digiti minimi** (AbDM), which also has an origin at the plantar aponeurosis (not shown).
- Draw the **flexor digiti minimi brevis** (FDMB), inserting on the 5th toe with AbDM as shown. Its origin is the base of the 5th metatarsal and the fibularis longus tendon (not shown).

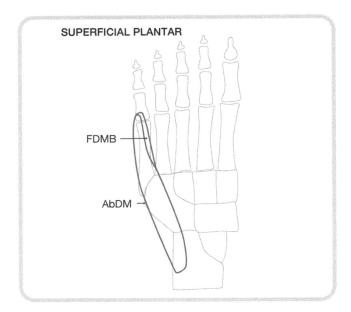

SUPERFICIAL PLANTAR

FDMB

AbDM

STEP 2

- Draw a long narrow muscle from the medial process of the calcaneus and the plantar aponeurosis (not shown), inserting onto the medial base of the proximal phalanx of the great toe. This is **abductor hallucis** (AbH).
- Draw the **flexor hallucis longus** (FHL) tendon emerging laterally to this and inserting into the distal phalanx of the great toe.

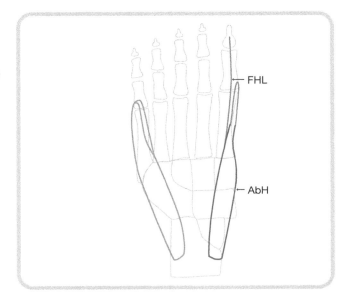

FHL

AbH

STEP ③

- Draw the **flexor digitorum brevis** (FDB) from its origin on the calcaneus to its insertion on the middle phalanx of the 2nd to 5th toes.
- Draw the tendon of the **flexor digitorum longus** (FDL) emerging from beneath the insertion of FDB to insert onto the end of the distal phalanx.
- Draw 4 **lumbrical** muscles emerging from beneath the FDB tendons. The lateral 3 have origins on both sides, and the medial 1 has its origin on the medial side of the FDL tendon of the 2nd toe. They insert onto the medial side of the 2nd to 5th proximal phalanges and the extensor tendons of the 4 lateral toes (not shown).

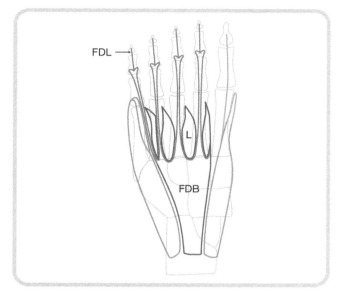

STEP ④

- Draw the parts of the transverse head of the **adductor hallucis** that are seen beneath the FDB and lumbricals and insert into the lateral part of the proximal phalanx of the great toe (for its origins, see Step 4 in the drawing of deep plantar muscles above).
- Draw the **flexor hallucis brevis**, which is seen lateral to and below AbH, inserting onto the medial part of the proximal phalanx of the great toe (for its origins, see Step 4 in the drawing of deep plantar muscles above).

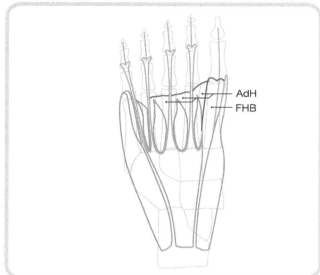

STEP ⑤

- Draw 2 grey rectangles over the calcaneus to represent the **plantar aponeurosis**, one in the middle (central part) and one on the lateral side (lateral part).

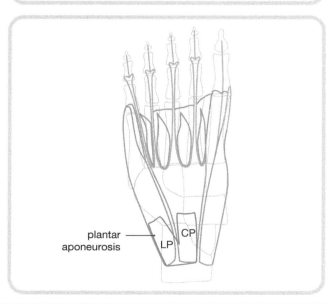

Muscles of the lower limb (Table 8.3)

Table 8.3. Muscles of the lower limb

Area	Muscle group	Muscle	Nerve	Artery	Action
Gluteal region		Gluteus maximus	Inferior gluteal	Superior gluteal and inferior gluteal	Extension and external rotation of hip
		Gluteus medius	Superior gluteal	Superior gluteal	Abduction and medial rotation of hip
		Gluteus minimus	Superior gluteal	Superior gluteal	Abduction and medial rotation of hip
		Tensor fasciae latae	Superior gluteal	Superior gluteal and lateral circumflex femoral artery	Hip joint flexion; trunk stabilisation
		Piriformis	Nerve to piriformis (S1,2)	Superior gluteal and Inferior gluteal	External rotation of hip
		Gemellus superior	Nerve to obturator muscle (L5, S1 and S2)	Inferior gluteal	Lateral rotation of hip joint
		Obturator internus	Nerve to obturator muscle (L5, S1 and S2)	Inferior gluteal	Abduction and lateral rotation of hip joint
		Gemellus inferior	Nerve to quadratus femoris (L4,5,S1)	Inferior gluteal	Lateral rotation of hip joint
		Quadratus femoris	Nerve to quadratus femoris (L4,5,S1)	Inferior gluteal	Lateral rotation and adduction of the hip joint
		Obturator externus	Obturator	Obturator	Adduction and lateral rotation of hip joint
Thigh	Anterior	Sartorius	Femoral	Femoral	Flexion, abduction and lateral rotation of hip joint; flexion and medial rotation of knee (when the knee is flexed)
		Quadriceps femoris (rectus femoris, vastus medialis, vastus intermedialis and vastus lateralis)	Femoral	Femoral	Extension of knee joint (RF also helps with hip flexion)
	Posterior	Biceps femoris	Sciatic: tibial part for long head and common peroneal part for short head	Deep femoral; also inferior gluteal and perforating arteries	Flexion of knee joint, lateral rotation of leg at knee (when the knee is flexed), extension of hip (by long head)
		Semitendinosus	Sciatic: tibial part	Inferior gluteal, perforating branches	Flexion of knee joint, extension of hip, medial rotation of leg at knee (when knee is flexed)
		Semimembranosus	Sciatic: tibial part	Inferior gluteal, profunda femoris, perforating arteries	Flexion of knee joint, extension of hip joint, medial rotation of leg at knee

(continued)

Table 8.3. Muscles of the lower limb *(continued)*

Area	Muscle group	Muscle	Nerve	Artery	Action
	Medial	Gracilis	Obturator	Obturator, femoral	Strong flexion and medial rotation of the knee joint when knee is semi-flexed; weak flexion and adduction of the hip joint
		Pectineus	Femoral, obturator	Obturator	Adduction and flexion of the hip joint
		Adductor longus	Obturator	Obturator, deep femoral	Adduction, flexion and medial rotation of hip joint
		Adductor brevis	Obturator	Obturator, deep femoral	Adduction of hip
		Adductor magnus	Obturator, sciatic (tibial part)	Obturator, deep femoral	Pelvis stabilisation: adductor part: flexion of the hip, external rotation and adduction of hip joint hamstring part: extension and internal rotation of the hip joint
		Iliacus	Femoral	Medial circumflex femoral	Flexion and external rotation of hip joint, anterior tilt of pelvis
Leg	Anterior	Tibialis anterior	Deep fibular	Anterior tibial	Dorsiflexion and inversion of foot
		Extensor hallucis longus	Deep fibular	Anterior tibial	Extension of great toe, dorsiflexion of foot
		Extensor digitorum longus	Deep fibular	Anterior tibial	Extension of toes, dorsiflexion of foot
		Fibularis tertius	Deep fibular	Anterior tibial	Dorsiflexion and eversion of foot
	Posterior	Popliteus	Tibial (sciatic)	Popliteal	Flexion and medial rotation of knee joint
		Tibialis posterior	Tibial (sciatic)	Posterior tibial	Inversion and plantar flexion of foot
		Flexor digitorum longus	Tibial (sciatic)	Posterior tibial	Flexion of toes and plantar flexion
		Flexor hallucis longus	Tibial (sciatic)	Fibular (branch of posterior tibial)	Flexion of great toe and plantar flexion of foot
		Fibularis longus	Superficial fibular	Fibular (branch of posterior tibial)	Plantar flexion and eversion of foot
		Fibularis brevis	Superficial fibular	Fibular (branch of posterior tibial)	Plantar flexion and eversion of foot
		Gastrocnemius	Tibial (sciatic)	Sural arteries	Plantar flexion and flexion of knee
		Soleus	Tibial (sciatic)	Popliteal, posterior tibial, fibular and sural	Plantar flexion
		Plantaris	Tibial (sciatic)	Sural	Plantar flexion and flexion of knee

(continued)

Table 8.3. Muscles of the lower limb *(continued)*

Area	Muscle group	Muscle	Nerve	Artery	Action
Foot	Plantar (sole of foot)	Abductor hallucis	Medial plantar	Medial plantar	Abducts and flexes great toe
		Flexor hallucis brevis	Medial plantar	Medial plantar	Flexion of great toe
		Flexor digitorum brevis	Medial plantar	Medial plantar and lateral plantar	Flexion of lateral 4 toes
		Abductor digiti minimi	Lateral plantar	Lateral plantar	Flexion and abduction of 5th toe
		Flexor digiti minimi brevis	Lateral plantar	Lateral plantar	Flexion and adduction of 5th toe
		Lumbrical muscles	Medial and lateral plantar	Medial and lateral plantar	Extends distal interphalangeal joints and flexes the proximal interphalangeal joints
		Adductor hallucis	Lateral plantar	Lateral plantar	Adduction of great toe
		Quadratus plantae	Lateral plantar	Posterior tibial	Flexion of distal interphalangeal joints and assists FDL in flexion
		Dorsal interossei	Lateral plantar	Deep plantar branch	Abduction of toes and flexion of the metatarsophalangeal joints
		Plantar interossei	Lateral plantar	Lateral plantar	Adduction of toes and flexion of the metatarsophalangeal joints
	Dorsum of foot	Extensor digitorum brevis	Deep fibular	Dorsalis pedis	Extension of toes 2–4
		Extensor hallucis brevis	Deep fibular	Dorsalis pedis	Extension of great toe

Chapter 9
Skin and immune system

9.1 Skin (integumentary system)

The skin is the body's first defence against pathogens and mechanical and chemical insults, providing a physical barrier, whereas the immune system is the body's internal defence against pathogens.

We will look at the layers of the skin in detail. Then in *Section 9.2* we will learn about lymphatic drainage, lymphatic circulation and anatomy of the thymus.

The skin is the largest organ in the body. It covers 1.5–2.0 square metres. It is a waterproof protective layer with several functions:

- helps regulate body temperature
- permits sensation of touch
- permits sensation of temperature
- provides a physical barrier
- protects against pathogens and chemical or mechanical injury.

Skin structure varies depending on whether it is hair-deficient or has hair follicles. In the image we will draw hair-deficient skin on the right and a hair follicle on the left.

The skin is more complicated than you first think, but it is easy to learn.

B	stratum basale
C	stratum corneum
G	stratum granulosum
L	stratum lucidum
M	melanocyte
P	papillary layer
PC	Pacinian corpuscle
R	reticular layer
S	stratum spinosum
SG	sebaceous gland

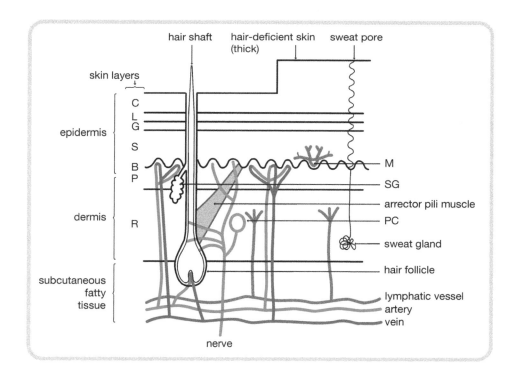

🖍 How to draw

On the left side of the page we will draw skin with a hair follicle and on the right side we will draw hair-deficient skin. Hair-deficient skin, for example the skin on the base of your foot, is normally thicker.

STEP ①

- First, we will draw the epidermis.
- Draw a line across the top of the page: start on the left, leaving a gap for a hair shaft, and then go a 'step' up for hair-deficient skin.
- Beneath this line, draw 3 more straight lines, all with a gap where the hair shaft will be.
- For a 5th line draw a wobbly line. This is the base layer or stratum basale.
- In order from top to bottom, label the 5 layers: stratum **c**orneum, stratum **l**ucidum, stratum **g**ranulosum, stratum **s**pinosum and stratum **b**asale. The stratum corneum is a dead layer of enucleated cells.

There are lots of ways to help remember the layers. An example is; '**C**ome **L**et's **G**et **S**un **B**urnt'. A good one, as you don't want to do this to your skin!

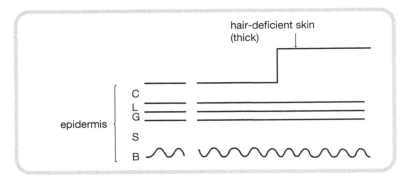

The innermost three layers of epidermis (stratum basale, stratum spinosum and stratum granulosum) are metabolically active compartments through which cells pass, changing their morphology as they undergo cellular differentiation. The two more superficial layers of cells undergo terminal keratinisation (or cornification, stratum corneum) which involves structural changes in keratinocytes, and also molecular and biochemical changes within the cells and their surroundings.

STEP ②

Next, we will draw the dermis, which has 2 layers, and the subcutaneous tissue.

- Underneath the stratum basale, draw 2 straight lines across the page, leaving a gap in each for the hair shaft and follicle. Leave a 2nd gap in the upper line as shown, for the arrector pili muscle (see Step 5). Ensure the layer above the upper line is shallower than the one below it.
- Label the upper layer as the papillary layer. This is loose connective tissue.
- Label the layer below this as the reticular layer. This is dense connective tissue. It is deeper than the papillary layer; show that in the drawing.
- Bracket the papillary and reticular layers with the label dermis.
- Label the layer below the dermis as subcutaneous fatty tissue (aka hypodermis). This is where the blood vessels, lymph vessels and nerves lie.

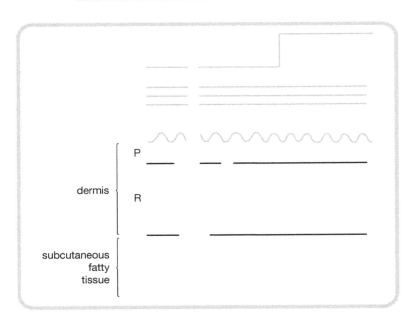

STEP 3

- From the edge of the gap in the stratum corneum on the left side, draw a hair follicle as a very long narrow triangle with a bulb at the bottom.
- Draw the hair with a thin outline, with an invagination at the bottom.
- Just below the stratum basale on the left side draw a little fluffy cloud on a hollow stalk between the papillary and reticular layer of the dermis; this is a sebaceous gland.

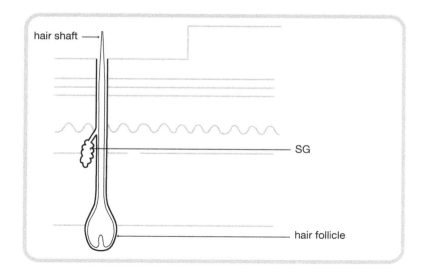

STEP 4

Sweat glands exist in both hair-deficient skin and skin that has hair. We will include the sweat gland only on the right side of the image for ease of drawing.

- Draw a squiggly ball deep in the reticular layer of the dermis; this is the sweat gland.
- From here draw a straight line to the stratum basale; this represents the sweat duct.
- Above the stratum basale, continue to draw up the page then draw a wiggly line to the top of the stratum corneum. This is the sweat pore.

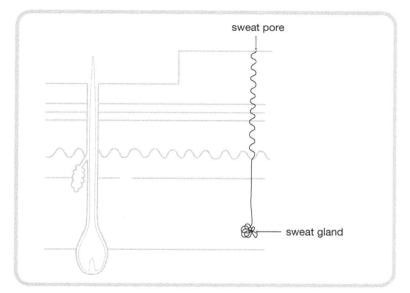

STEP 5

- Draw the arrector pili muscle as a triangular shape coming from the base of the hair follicle to the stratum basale.
- This tiny muscle contracts when you are cold, causing the hair to stand up on end. All the arrector pili muscles work at a similar time.

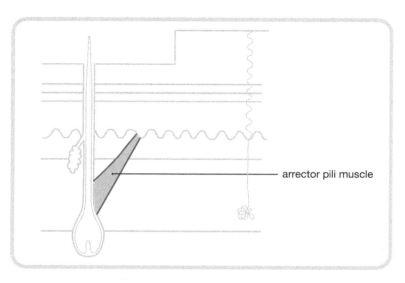

STEP 6

- Draw a melanocyte in the stratum basale layer, as shown.
- Melanocytes are cells that produce melanin, the brown pigment responsible for skin colouration. Sunlight increases melanin production to protect skin from harmful UV rays.

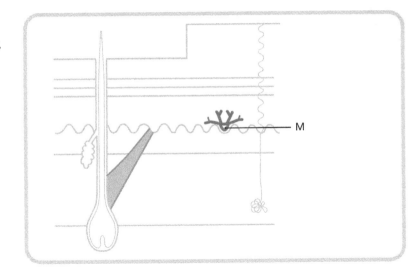

M

STEP 7

- Draw an artery along the base of the page.
- Draw 2 vertical branches up to the stratum basale to show how blood travels to the skin.
- Draw a small branch to the base of the hair follicle.
- Draw veins in a similar arrangement.
- Join the ends of the arteries and veins just under the epidermis to represent capillaries connecting the arteries and veins.

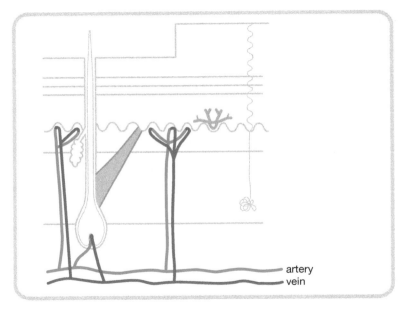

artery
vein

STEP 8

- Draw a nerve from the subcutaneous fatty tissue up to the top of the dermal layer.
- Add branches to the base of the hair follicle and the dermis.
- Draw a circle at the end of a branch in the dermis to represent a Pacinian corpuscle (PC). This is a pressure sensor. Pressure is detected by the PC and transmitted along the nerve. PCs transmit information about joint position to the brain; they have an important role in proprioception. Some areas, e.g. the fingertips, have more PCs than others.

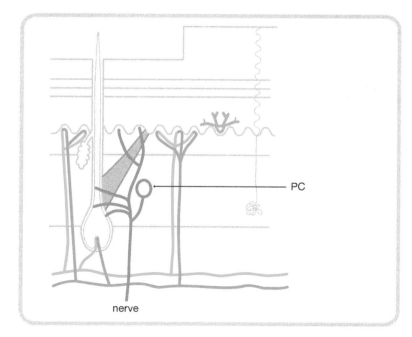

PC

nerve

STEP 9

- Draw in the lymph ducts in a similar way to the arteries and nerves.

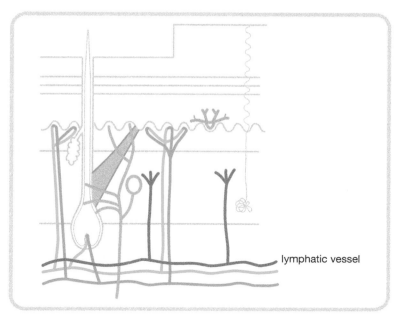

lymphatic vessel

9.2 Immune system

9.2.1 Lymphatic circulation

I am no expert in the lymphatic system or immunity, but I have tried to make it as simple as I can to explain the basics.

Lymphocytes are produced in the bone marrow. The 3 main types, which are found in the lymph fluid, are B cells, T cells and natural killer cells.

T stem cells originate in bone marrow and travel in the blood to the thymus. Here they differentiate into T helper cells or cytotoxic T cells. They continue to differentiate after leaving the thymus.

ADAPTIVE IMMUNITY

B cells (**B**one marrow cells) and T cells (**T**hymus cells) are the main components of the adaptive immune response. When B cells detect pathogens, they produce large amounts of antibodies which neutralise the pathogens.

T cells are involved in cell-mediated immunity. When a pathogen enters the body, T helper cells (Th) detect it and produce cytokines (proteins) that recruit other cells to mount an immune response. Cytotoxic T cells (Tc) produce toxic granules; these contain enzymes that kill human cells containing the pathogen.

T helper cells activate B cells to become plasma cells and memory cells.

After activation of B cells and T cells by a specific pathogen, memory cells are made. If the same pathogen is detected again the immune system will have a strong and rapid response.

INNATE IMMUNITY

Natural killer cells are part of the innate immune system. They find infected cells and tumours by detecting changes to the expression of major histocompatibility complexes (MHC) and other molecules present on the surface of infected or aberrant cells. When activated, natural killer cells release cytotoxic granules which destroy the cells.

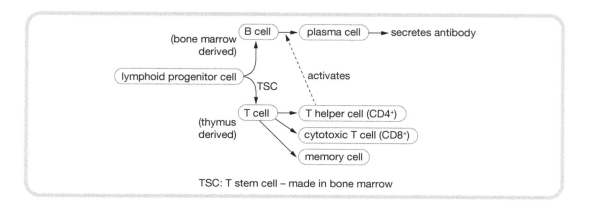

TSC: T stem cell – made in bone marrow

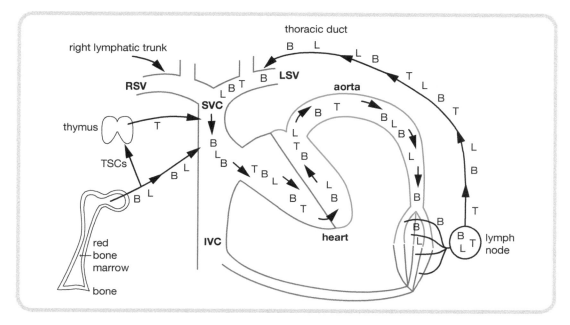

B	B cell
IVC	inferior vena cava
L	large lymphocyte (can be active B or T cells)
LSV	left subclavian vein
RSV	right subclavian vein
SVC	superior vena cava
T	T cell
TSC	T stem cell

The direction of cells is shown from the right side of the heart to the left side of the heart. This would be via the pulmonary circulation (not shown in the diagram to maintain simplicity).

✎ How to draw

STEP ①

- Draw the right side of the heart, the left and right subclavian veins, and the superior and the inferior vena cava in blue.
- Draw some capillaries on the right side of the page and a vein draining them into the IVC. Together, the blue vessels represent the venous system.
- In red draw the left side of the heart, and draw the aorta and a capillary network representing the arterial circulation.

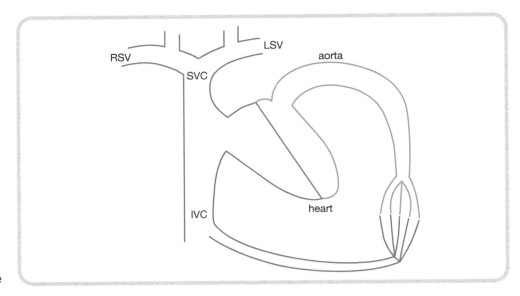

STEP ②

- On the left side of the page draw a bone with 2 layers. The inner area is red bone marrow.
- Above this draw a 'butterfly' shape. This represents the thymus.
- Draw an arrow from the bone marrow to the SVC. This represents B lymphocytes and other lymphocytes flowing from the bone marrow to the IVC.
- Draw a branch arrow to the thymus. This shows T stem cells made in bone marrow flowing to the thymus, where they mature into T helper cells and cytotoxic T cells.

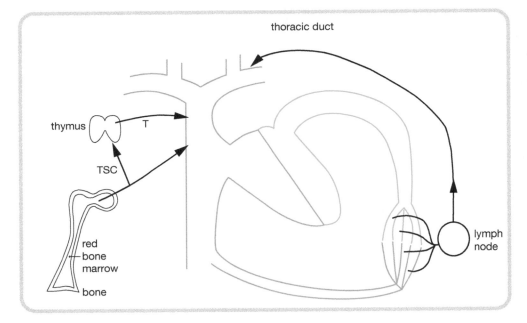

- Add an arrow from the thymus to the SVC to show T cells entering the circulation.
- Draw ducts perpendicular to the capillary network and joining together to connect to a circle; these represent lymphatic drainage from capillaries into a lymph node. From the node, draw an arrowed line to the left subclavian vein; this represents flow in the thoracic duct (see Step 7 in *Section 9.2.2 Lymphatic drainage*).

STEP 3

- Write Bs and Ls along the arrow from the bone marrow to the SVC. These represent B cells (B) and large lymphocytes (L) produced by the marrow; they enter the circulation, where large lymphocytes can function as natural killer cells.
- Add Bs and Ls through the right and left side of the heart and the arterial circulation to reach the capillary plexus. Continue them into the lymph node, along the thoracic duct into the venous circulation and back into the heart.

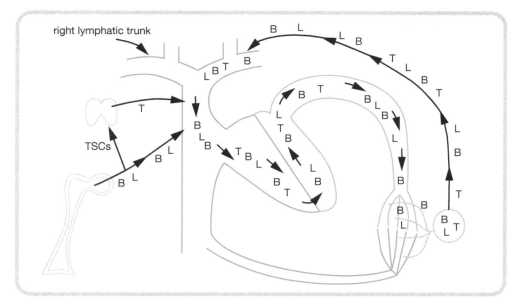

right lymphatic trunk

TSCs

- This forms a simplified version of the lymphatic circulation to help understand where cells are made and where they flow.
- On the arrow pointing to the thymus write 'T stem cells'. These are made in marrow and transported to the thymus where they mature into T cells – T helper cells (CD4+), cytotoxic T cells (CD8+) and memory cells.
- Add Ts from the thymus and throughout the circulation, alongside the Bs and Ls.
- Draw a short arrow into the right subclavian vein; this is the right lymphatic trunk.
- Add arrows to the circulation to confirm the direction of movement.

9.2.2   Lymphatic drainage

Lymphatic vessels carry lymphatic fluid from the lymph nodes. Ultimately, they all drain into the venous system near the junctions of the subclavian and internal jugular veins. However, there are differences in drainage routes on the left and right side of the body, as we will show in our drawings.

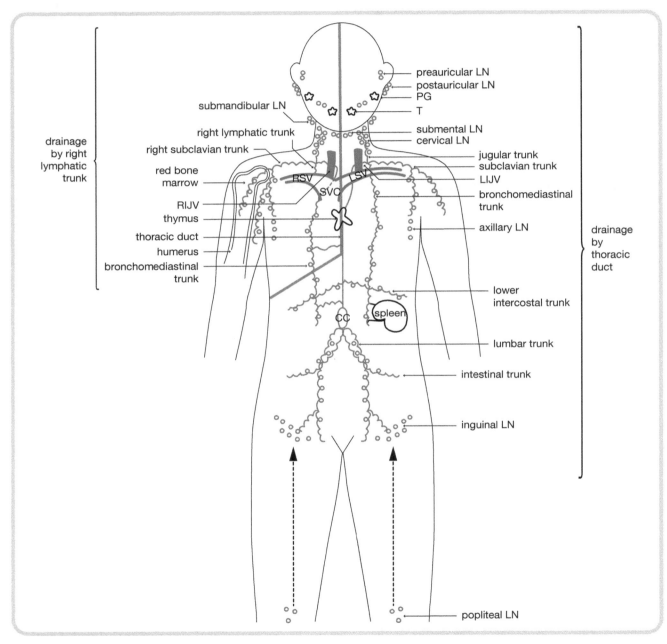

CC	cisterna chyli	**LSV**	left subclavian vein	**RSV**	right subclavian vein
LIJV	left internal jugular vein	**PG**	parotid gland	**SVC**	superior vena cava
LN	lymph nodes	**RIJV**	right internal jugular vein	**T**	tonsil (palatine)

How to draw

STEP 1

- Draw the outline of the body and head.
- Draw a grey line from the centre of the head down to the nipple line. From here draw a slanted line down towards the left side of the page to divide the body into a small and large segment.
- The right upper limb, chest and head – i.e. the upper left segment of the drawing – drain into the right lymphatic trunk. Label this as shown.
- The rest of the body drains into the thoracic duct. Label this as shown.

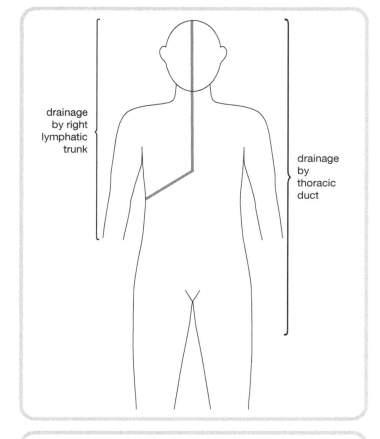

STEP 2

- Draw the superior vena cava and the right and left subclavian veins.
- Add the internal jugular vein on each side.

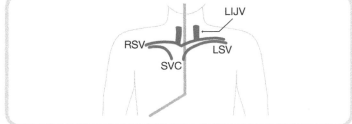

STEP 3

- Draw an 'X' shape midline below the left subclavian vein. This is the thymus.
- Draw a line from the top right side of the 'X' to loop behind the left IVC and drain into the left subclavian vein.
- Draw a line directly down from the lower middle of the 'X'. This is the thoracic duct. Draw an oval around the level of the umbilicus. This represents the cisterna chyli.
- Draw 2 bumpy lines with small circles fitted along them in an upside-down 'V' shape. These represent the lymphatic vessels and lymph nodes of the intestinal trunks.

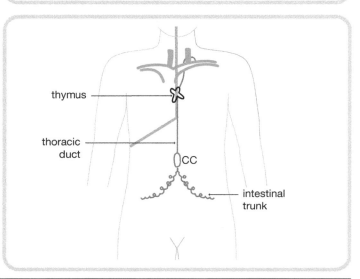

STEP 4

- From the cisterna chyli, draw a narrow upside-down U-shape as a bumpy line with small circles along it. This represents the vessels and lymph nodes of the lumbar trunks.
- At the bottom of each lumbar trunk, draw a second short branch in the same way. At the base of the lateral branch and along the groin line draw some small circles. These represent the inguinal lymph nodes.

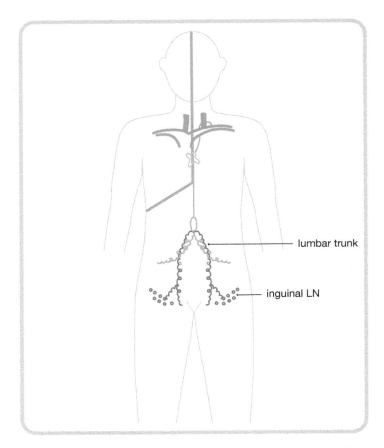

lumbar trunk

inguinal LN

STEP 5

- Draw a few nodes around the level of the knee; these are the popliteal lymph nodes.
- Draw a broken line up the leg to the inguinal lymph nodes. Lymphatic drainage of the leg is via these. There are superficial and deep inguinal lymph nodes. Lymph flows from here to the external iliac lymph nodes and then the para-aortic/lumbar lymph nodes (not shown) before entering cisterna chyli and the thoracic duct.

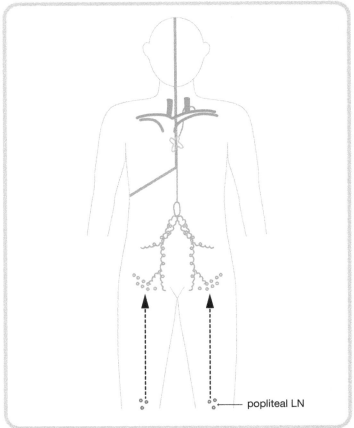

popliteal LN

STEP 6

- Draw a bumpy line from the upper left arm to join the thoracic duct entering the left subclavian vein. This is the subclavian trunk.
- Draw a further bumpy line going to the left subclavian trunk from the armpit. Draw axillary lymph nodes, which drain into the subclavian trunk.
- Draw a bumpy line just lateral to the left internal jugular vein, with associated small circles in the neck to represent the cervical lymph nodes. They drain into the jugular trunk on each side and then into the thoracic duct on the left and the right lymphatic trunk on the right (see Step 9).

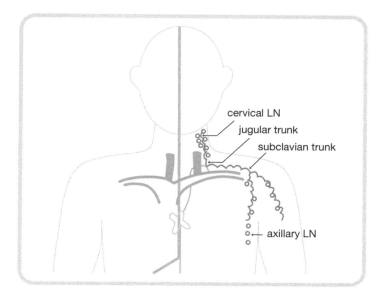

cervical LN
jugular trunk
subclavian trunk

axillary LN

STEP 7

- Draw a bumpy line from the waist line, up the middle of the left side of the body, to the upper end of the thoracic duct. This is the left bronchomediastinal trunk.
- Just below where the diaphragm would be, draw the spleen.
- Draw 2 black lines representing vessels joining the spleen to the lymphatic drainage system.
- Draw a bumpy line at approximately the level of the 12th rib. This is the lower intercostal trunk. It drains into the thoracic duct.

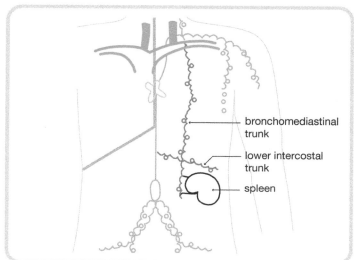

bronchomediastinal trunk

lower intercostal trunk

spleen

STEP 8

- On the head draw a few small nodes in front of the ear (preauricular lymph nodes), behind the ear (postauricular lymph nodes), below the middle of the jaw (submental lymph nodes), and below the back of the jaw (submandibular lymph nodes).
- Draw a little 'flower' anterior to the ear and another where the back of the mouth would be. These are the parotid gland and tonsils, respectively.

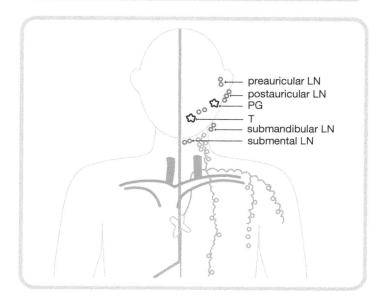

preauricular LN
postauricular LN
PG
T
submandibular LN
submental LN

STEP 9

Now we will draw the lymphatic drainage for the right side of the body.

- Referring to Step 8, draw mirror images of the parotid gland, tonsil, head and neck lymph nodes, and jugular trunk.
- Draw a line from the jugular trunk to the right subclavian vein. This is the right lymphatic trunk.
- On the right arm draw the humerus. Draw a second inner line in the same shape; this outlines the red bone marrow.
- Draw a bumpy line from here to the right lymphatic trunk. This is the right subclavian trunk. Add axillary lymph vessels and nodes as shown.
- Draw the upper part of the right bronchomediastinal trunk running up behind the SVC (broken line) to join the right lymphatic trunk. Add lymph nodes as shown.

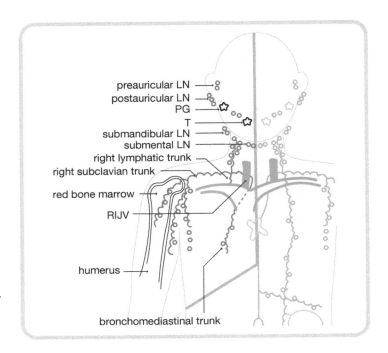

STEP 10

- Draw the lower part of the right bronchomediastinal trunk, starting at the same level as the left side. This trunk also has branches that drain into the thoracic duct: draw in 2 branches.
- Draw the lower intercostal trunk on the right side of the body, draining into the thoracic duct.

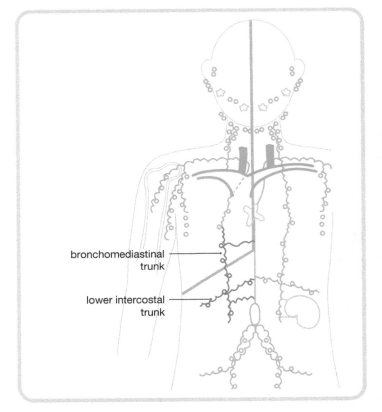

9.2.3 Thymus

The thymus is an important lymphoid organ that produces thymosin, a hormone that in turn stimulates T-cell maturation in the thymus. It is vital before birth and during childhood for protecting the body against autoimmunity.

As you get older, the thymus shrinks and lymphoid tissue gradually turns into fatty tissue (adipose tissue).

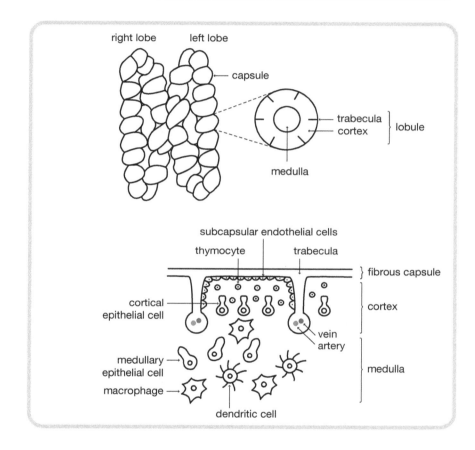

How to draw

STEP 1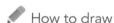

- In the top 1/2 of the page, draw 2 vertical cloud shapes joined in the middle; these represent the thymus.
- On both sides, fill the space with rough lumps joined together to show the capsules that make up the thymus.

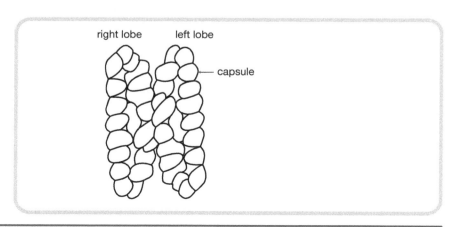

STEP 2

- Draw a cross section of one capsule by drawing a circle within a circle. The inner circle is the medulla. The outer circle is the cortex.
- Add a few short lines from the outer edge to the middle of the cortex; these are trabeculae. This shows a lobule.

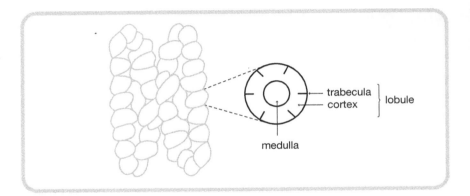

STEP 3

We will now draw a close-up image of part of a lobule.

- Draw a horizontal line along the page. Beneath this draw a second line with 2 gaps. The area between these 2 lines is the fibrous capsule.
- At each gap on the lower line, draw 2 vertical lines down and forming a circle at their lower end. These show 2 trabeculae. In the circle draw a red dot and a blue dot; these are the arteries and veins.
- Along the lower edge of the inner layer draw little bumps with dots in them. These represent the subcapsular endothelial cells.
- Label from just under the fibrous capsule to just below the trabecula as the cortex; label the medulla below this.

STEP 4

- Draw some 'dummy' shaped cells in the cortex and some in the medulla. These represent cortical and medullary epithelial cells.

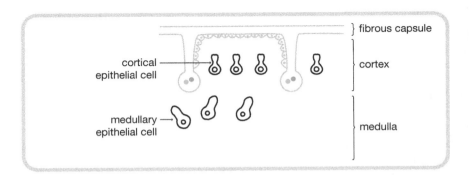

STEP 5

- In the cortex, draw some very small circles, each with a dot in its centre; these are thymocytes (lymphocytes in the thymus, e.g. immature T cells).
- In the medulla, draw 2 other types of cells as shown: dendritic cells and macrophages.

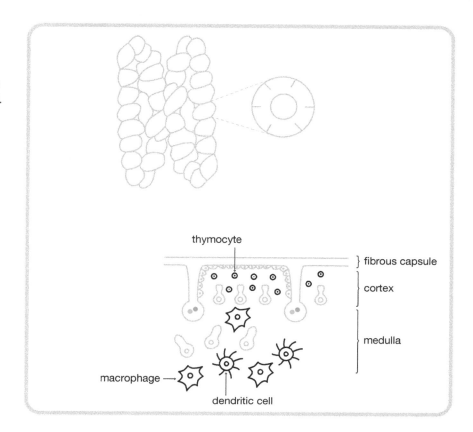